BLUEPRINTS IN
EMERGENCY MEDICINE

BLUEPRINTS in
EMERGENCY MEDICINE

Authors

Nathan W. Mick, MD
Clinical Fellow
Department of Emergency Medicine
Brigham and Women's Hospital
Boston, Massachusetts

Jessica Radin Peters, MD
Clinical Fellow
Department of Emergency Medicine
Brigham and Women's Hospital
Boston, Massachusetts

Scott M. Silvers, MD
Chief Resident of Emergency Medicine
Brigham and Women's Hospital
Boston, Massachusetts

Editor

Eric S. Nadel, MD
Residency Director
Department of Emergency Medicine
Brigham and Women's Hospital
Boston, Massachusetts

Faculty Advisor

Ron Walls, MD
Professor and Chairman
Department of Emergency Medicine
Brigham and Women's Hospital
Boston, Massachusetts

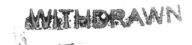

Blackwell
Publishing

© 2002 by Blackwell Science, Inc.
a Blackwell Publishing Company

Editorial Offices:
Commerce Place, 350 Main Street, Malden, Massachusetts 02148, USA
Osney Mead, Oxford OX2 0EL, England
25 John Street, London WC1N 2BS, England
23 Ainslie Place, Edinburgh EH3 6AJ, Scotland
54 University Street, Carlton, Victoria 3053, Australia

Other Editorial Offices:
Blackwell Wissenschafts-Verlag GmbH, Kurfürstendamm 57, 10707 Berlin, Germany
Blackwell Science KK, MG Kodenmacho Building, 7-10 Kodenmacho Nihombashi, Chuo-ku, Tokyo 104, Japan
Iowa State University Press, A Blackwell Science Company, 2121 S. State Avenue, Ames, Iowa 50014-8300, USA

Distributors:

The Americas
Blackwell Publishing
c/o AIDC
P.O. Box 20
50 Winter Sport Lane
Williston, VT 05495-0020
(Telephone orders: 800-216-2522;
fax orders: 802-864-7626)

Australia
Blackwell Science Pty, Ltd.
54 University Street
Carlton, Victoria 3053
(Telephone orders: 03-9347-0300;
fax orders: 03-9349-3016)

Outside The Americas and Australia
Blackwell Science, Ltd.
c/o Marston Book Services, Ltd.
P.O. Box 269
Abingdon
Oxon OX14 4YN
England
(Telephone orders: 44-01235-465500;
fax orders: 44-01235-465555)

Library of Congress Cataloging-in-Publication Data

Blueprints in emergency medicine / authors, Nathan W. Mick ... [et al.].
    p. ; cm. — (Blueprints USMLE steps 2 & 3 review series)
  ISBN 0-632-04626-0 (pbk.)
  1. Emergency medicine—Outlines, syllabi, etc. 2. Emergency medicine—Examinations, questions, etc. 3. Physicians—Licenses—United States—Examinations—Study guides.
  [DNLM: 1. Emergencies—Outlines. 2. Emergency Medicine—Outlines. WB 18.2 B6575 2002] I. Mick, Nathan W. II. Blueprints.
  RC86.92 .B58 2002
  616.02'5'076—dc21

2001007461

Acquisitions: Nancy Duffy
Development: Amy Nuttbrock
Production: Debra Lally
Manufacturing: Lisa Flanagan
Marketing Manager: Kathleen Mulcahy
Typeset by SNP Best-set Typesetter Ltd., Hong Kong
Printed and bound by Captial City Press

Printed in the United States of America
02 03 04 05 5 4 3 2 1
The Blackwell Science logo is a trade mark of Blackwell Science Ltd.,
registered at the United Kingdom Trade Marks Registry

Contents

Acknowledgements

Thanks to family and friends for their support through this effort and to future students of Emergency Medicine. May you find your study of the field as challenging and rewarding as we have.

Nathan Mick
Jessica Peters
Scott Silvers
August 2000

Notice: The indications and dosages of all drugs in this book have been recommended in the medical literature and conform to the practices of the general community. The medications described and treatment prescriptions suggested do not necessarily have specific approval by the Food and Drug Administration for use in the diseases and dosages for which they are recommended. The package insert for each drug should be consulted for use and dosage as approved by the FDA. Because standards for usage change, it is advisable to keep abreast of revised recommendations, particularly those concerning new drugs.

Preface

Medical Students, interns, and residents need high-yield, accurate, clinical, core content. The *Blueprints* series was developed to meet these needs and enable the reader to review the core material quickly and efficiently. We have since expanded our core content to include emergency medicine.

Although this series was designed for the medical student or resident reviewing for the USMLE, many students have stated that the books in the series have been helpful to them during their clerkship rotations and subinternships. Residents studying for the USMLE Step 3 often use the books for reviewing the areas that were their specialty. For instance, surgical residents will use the peds book for review since they have not has a peds rotation in over two years.

Blueprints in Emergency Medicine is not meant to be comprehensive, but rather it is composed of the high-yield topics that consistently appear on the boards. The topics in each book were chosen after analyzing over 2000 review questions, which we believed to be representative of the questions of the USMLE Step 2 & 3 exams. By concentrating on these high-yield topics the user will be reviewing the material most likely to be covered in each discipline on the boards.

Blueprints in Emergency Medicine includes USMLE style clinical questions to test your strengths in this unique area. These questions help prepare medical students and residents for questions likely encountered on the wards and as a review before the Step 2 & 3.

We hope you find *Blueprints in Emergency Medicine* informative and useful. We welcome feedback and suggestions you may have about this book or any in the Blueprints series. Send to blue@blackwellpub.com.

The Publisher
Blackwell Publishing, Inc.

Part I
ENT Emergencies

SIGNS AND SYMPTOMS

Ear Pain:

- Obstructed eustachian tube
- Foreign body
- Otitis media
- Otitis externa
- Mastoiditis
- Temporomandibular joint syndrome
- Perforated tympanic membrane
- Malignancy

Sore Throat:

- Mucosal trauma
- Pharyngitis
- Esophagitis
- Peritonsillitis
- Peritonsillar abscess
- Retropharyngeal abscess
- Epiglottitis
- Laryngitis (e.g., infectious or acid reflux)
- Ludwig's angina
- Allergic reaction
- Malignancy

Sinusitis

Sinus infection, or sinusitis, is an extremely common disease and is present in 5% of viral upper respiratory tract infections. The paranasal sinuses are air-filled structures named after the bone in which they are contained (e.g., frontal, maxillary, ethmoid, and sphenoid). Possible complications of sinusitis include orbital cellulitis, periorbital cellulitis, facial abscess, osteomyelitis, cavernous sinus thrombosis, meningitis, epidural abscess, subdural empyema, and brain abscess.

ANATOMY AND PATHOPHYSIOLOGY

Most paranasal sinuses drain into the nasopharynx. Knowledge of the sinus anatomy helps in understanding possible complications. For example, the blood supply to the ethmoid sinuses also connects with the ophthalmic vessels and cavernous sinus thereby predisposing these structures to extension of sinus infection (Fig. 1–1). Similarly, the optic nerve and carotid artery run along the lateral walls of the sphenoid sinus and are at risk for developing infection. Sinuses are normally sterile in healthy individuals. Sinusitis usually results from sinus drainage obstruction due to mucosal inflammation and thickened secretions. However, a dysfunctional mucus-clearing ciliary apparatus (resulting from viruses or tobacco smoke) and abnormal sinus anatomy may also predispose individuals to this condition. Viral upper respiratory tract infections and allergic rhinitis are the most common causes of sinus drainage obstruction leading to sinusitis. *Streptococcus pneumoniae*, *Haemophilus influenzae*, *Moraxella catarrhalis*, *Streptococcus pyogenes* (group A), *Staphylococcus aureus*, and viruses are the most common pathogens in acute sinusitis. Rarely, *Pseudomonas aeruginosa* and fungi cause infection. Chronic sinusitis refers to infection lasting longer than 3 months and typically involves anaerobic organisms.

HISTORY

Symptoms of acute sinusitis often include pressure or pain over the involved sinus, a mucopurulent nasal discharge, maxillary toothache, malaise, fever, and unresponsiveness to nasal decongestants. Discomfort from sinus obstruction tends to be localized in the region of the affected sinus.

PHYSICAL EXAMINATION

Physical findings that may be found with sinusitis include fever, mucopurulent nasal discharge, erythema, tissue warmth, tenderness over the involved sinus, and diminished direct light transillumination. Culture of nasal discharge is only warranted in cases of chronic sinusitis where less common or resistant organisms may be present. Although sinusitis is typically a clinical diagnosis, radiographic imaging is occasionally necessary

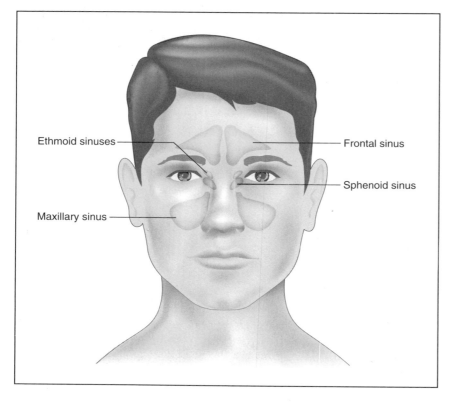

Ethmoid sinuses

Frontal sinus

Sphenoid sinus

Maxillary sinus

Figure 1–1   Paranasal sinuses.

for confirmation. Sinus plain films are unreliable for the detection of sinusitis. The imaging modality of choice for sinusitis is CT scan, but it requires clinical correlation.

TREATMENT

Most cases of acute sinusitis may be treated on an outpatient basis, and respond well to oral and nasal decongestants as well as antibiotics. The incidence of antibiotic-resistant organisms is increasing and varies among regions of the United States. For this reason, antibiotic choices ideally should be based upon the knowledge of local bacterial resistances. Antibiotics generally should be prescribed for a 10-day course. Treatment of nosocomial sinusitis following nasotracheal or nasogastric intubation should include coverage for *Pseudomonas* and methicillin-resistant *Staphylococcus aureus* (MRSA). Antihistamines may reduce sinus drainage and are not recommended in the treatment of acute bacterial sinusitis. Consultation with Otolaryngology and admission to the hospital should be consid-

ered in patients with severe disease, frontal or sphenoid air fluid levels, a compromised immune system, and for those at risk for medication noncompliance. Patients refractory to conventional medical treatments may require surgical drainage.

◆ KEY POINTS ◆

1. Viral upper respiratory tract infections and allergic rhinitis are the most common causes of sinus drainage obstruction leading to sinusitis.

2. *Streptococcus pneumoniae, Haemophilus influenzae, Moraxella catarrhalis, Streptococcus pyogenes* (group A), *Staphylococcus aureus*, and viruses are the most common pathogens in acute sinusitis.

3. Sinusitis is typically a clinical diagnosis.

4. The imaging modality of choice for sinusitis is CT scan.

2 Retropharyngeal Abscess

Retropharyngeal abscess refers to an abscess of the neck lying in the soft tissues between the cervical vertebrae and posterior oropharynx (Fig. 2–1). Retropharyngeal abscess is predominantly a disease of youth with 96% of cases occurring in children younger than 6 years of age. Infection readily travels in the retropharyngeal fascial planes. Complications of retropharyngeal infection include airway obstruction, sepsis, cervical osteomyelitis, mediastinitis, aspiration pneumonia, empyema, jugular vein thrombosis, and carotid artery erosion.

ANATOMY AND PATHOPHYSIOLOGY

Retropharyngeal lymph nodes are prominent in children less than 5 years of age but atrophy over subsequent years. Retropharyngeal abscess is believed to originate from an infected lymph node (i.e., lymphangitis) that progresses to cellulitis and ultimately abscess formation. In older patients, oropharyngeal trauma and the contiguous spread of mucosal cellulitis are more commonly the cause of retropharyngeal infection. Other risk factors include immunosuppression, oral procedures or instrumentation, dental infections, nasopharyngitis, and other oral, soft tissue infections such as peritonsillitis, lateral pharyngeal space infection, and Ludwig's angina. Retropharyngeal abscess is a polymicrobial infection most commonly caused by *Streptococci*, *Staphylococcus aureus*, *Prevotella*, *Bacteroides*, *Peptostreptococcus*, *Fusobacterium*, and rarely fungi. Tuber-culosis remains a significant pathogen in less developed regions of the world.

HISTORY

Individuals with retropharyngeal abscess are usually young children who may present with fever, sore throat, dysphagia (difficulty swallowing), odynophagia (painful swallowing), drooling, or muffled voice. They may also report neck or upper back pain with swallowing. Patients often prefer to keep their neck extended and lie supine to help reduce pharyngeal lumen obstruction.

PHYSICAL EXAMINATION

Typical physical findings of retropharyngeal abscess include fever, edema and erythema of the posterior oropharynx, tender cervical adenopathy, pain with tracheal movement, trismus, torticollis (contracted neck muscles), and stridor. Trismus and lower cervical infection may make direct visualization of swollen retropharyngeal tissues difficult. The diagnosis of retropharyngeal abscess is suspected by clinical presentation and confirmed by radiologic imaging. Plain films of the lateral neck may reveal prevertebral soft tissue swelling as well as forward displacement of the esophagus and trachea. The sensitivity of lateral neck plan films for retropharyngeal abscess is 88%. In cases of suspected retropharyngeal abscess, a chest x-ray should be

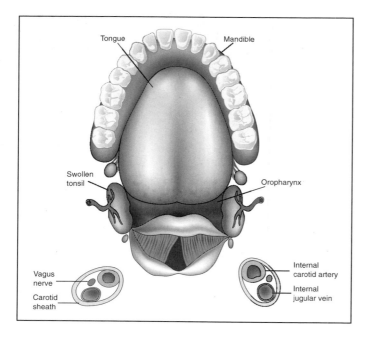

Figure 2–1 Horizontal section through the mouth and the oral pharynx.

obtained to help identify mediastinal extension. CT scan and MRI are more sensitive imaging modalities and better delineate the extent of disease. Laboratory blood evaluation usually adds little, if any, additional information and should not be necessary to make the diagnosis of retropharyngeal abscess.

TREATMENT

The initial management of all upper airway infections should focus on assuring a patent airway. Patients with retropharyngeal abscess should receive consultation by Otolaryngology, admission to the hospital, and intravenous antibiotics. Abscess incision and drainage by a surgeon in the operating room is indicated in most cases of retropharyngeal abscess.

◆ KEY POINTS ◆

1. Retropharyngeal abscess is predominantly a disease of youth with 96% of cases occurring in children younger than 6 years of age.
2. Trismus and lower cervical infection may make direct visualization of swollen retropharyngeal tissues difficult.
3. The diagnosis of retropharyngeal abscess is suspected by clinical presentation and confirmed by radiologic imaging.
4. Patients with retropharyngeal abscess should receive consultation by Otolaryngology, admission to the hospital, and intravenous antibiotics.
5. Retropharyngeal abscesses are drained by surgeons in the operating room.

3 Peritonsillitis

Peritonsillitis refers to the inflammation and infection of tissue surrounding the palatine tonsils. The disease ranges in severity from peritonsillar cellulitis to peritonsillar abscess. Peritonsillar cellulitis is an infection of the mucosa surrounding the pharyngeal tonsils. Peritonsillar abscess is often difficult to distinguish from cellulitis and is definitively diagnosed by the aspiration of pus from within the affected tissue. Complications of peritonsillitis include airway compromise, abscess rupture with aspiration of purulence, pneumonia, extension of infection to the mediastinum, necrotizing fasciitis, carotid artery erosion, jugular vein thrombophlebitis, cavernous sinus thrombosis, meningitis, and septic embolization.

ANATOMY AND PATHOPHYSIOLOGY

Peritonsillar cellulitis and abscess are believed to originate from an infection of the palatine tonsil that invades surrounding tissue. Peritonsillar abscesses tend to be polymicrobial, comprised of both aerobic and anaerobic pathogens.

HISTORY

Individuals with peritonsillar abscess frequently report symptoms of fever, sore throat, drooling, muffled "hot potato" voice, and trismus (i.e., inability to open the mouth completely due to pain). Other symptoms include dysphagia (difficulty swallowing), odynophagia (painful swallowing), otalgia (ear pain), pain with head rotation, and foul-smelling breath. If the tissue swelling is severe enough, stridor and airway compromise may be present.

PHYSICAL EXAMINATION

Common physical findings in peritonsillitis include fever, trismus, erythematous peritonsillar mucosa, and tender cervical adenopathy. Asymmetric swelling of peritonsillar soft tissue and deviation of the uvula to the opposite side is suggestive of a peritonsillar abscess.

DIAGNOSIS

If a peritonsillar abscess is suspected, large-needle aspiration may be performed to help identify purulence within the soft tissue. False-negative needle aspirations occur 10% of the time. The utility of aspirate gram stain and culture is controversial. Routine laboratory evaluation of blood does not aid in the diagnosis or treatment. Although radiologic imaging is seldom necessary in less severe cases, plain films, ultrasound, CT, and MRI may help to delineate the extent of more severe disease.

TREATMENT

The initial management of all upper airway infections should focus on assuring airway patency. Impending

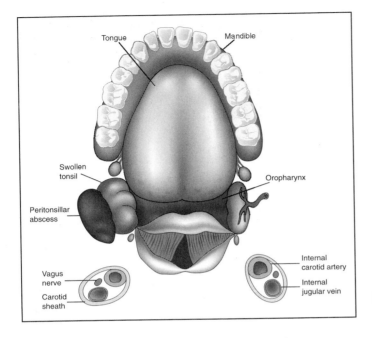

Tongue

Mandible

Swollen
tonsil

Oropharynx

Peritonsillar
abscess

Internal
carotid artery

Internal
jugular vein

Vagus
nerve

Carotid
sheath

Figure 3–1   Peritonsillar abscess.

airway compromise by an abscess may require emergent needle aspiration. Needle aspiration or incision and drainage may be performed. The needle or scalpel should be oriented medially to avoid penetration into the carotid sheath (Fig. 3–1). Less severe peritonsillitis may be treated on an outpatient basis with antibiotics, analgesics, and close follow-up. Otolaryngologic consultation, admission to the hospital, and IV antibiotics should be considered in cases of severe disease, a poorly visualized oropharynx, a nondiagnostic needle aspiration, immunocompromise (e.g., diabetes), severe pain, oral fluid intolerance, potential airway compromise, or when medication compliance and close follow-up are questionable.

◆ **KEY POINTS** ◆

1. Peritonsillar abscess with airway compromise may require emergent decompression.

2. Peritonsillar abscess is often difficult to distinguish from cellulitis and is definitively diagnosed by the aspiration of pus from the affected tissue.

3. During needle aspiration or incision and drainage, the needle should be medially oriented to avoid penetration into the carotid sheath.

4. Peritonsillar abscesses tend to be polymicrobial, comprised of both aerobic and anaerobic pathogens.

4 Otitis Media

Otitis media (OM) refers to inflammation of the middle ear due to an infectious etiology. OM is further classified as either acute otitis media (AOM), otitis media with effusion (OME), or chronic otitis media (COM). Risk factors for the disease include male sex, daycare attendance, parental smoking, a family history of middle ear disease, and anatomical abnormalities (e.g., cleft palate, Down's syndrome) that may affect drainage via the eustachian tubes. The term "recurrent otitis media" refers to three or more episodes over 6 months or four episodes within 1 year.

ANATOMY AND PATHOPHYSIOLOGY

The eustachian tube connects the middle ear to the nasopharynx and allows for pressure equalization, as well as drainage of secretions (Fig. 4–1). The greater incidence of OM among children is thought to result from the smaller diameter of the eustachian tube in children. Otitis media may be caused by viruses or bacteria. The most common bacterial pathogens in both children and adults are *Streptococcus pneumonia*, nontypable *Haemophilus influenzae*, and *Moraxella catarrhalis*, and less commonly *Streptococcus pyogenes*, *Staphylococcus aureus*, and *Pseudomonas aeruginosa*. Complications of OM include tympanic membrane perforation, cholesteoma, hearing deficit, mastoiditis, facial nerve injury, abscess, and meningitis.

HISTORY

Young children are sometimes unable to articulate focal ear complaints, making the diagnosis more difficult. Symptoms of OM include cough, poor appetite, diarrhea, vomiting, irritability, poor feeding, poor sleep, fever, ear pulling, and otalgia (ear pain). Otalgia often precedes any visible evidence of infection. Fever is often present, although up to one-quarter of patients may be afebrile.

PHYSICAL EXAMINATION

The external ear and canal should be inspected first for erythema, discharge, and tenderness. The diagnosis of OM requires direct visualization of the tympanic membrane (TM). The TM in a healthy individual without previous scarring appears clear or pearly white, and is mobile during air insufflation. Although many healthy individuals have a light reflex on the surface of the TM, this finding is unreliable. In OM, the TM first develops erythema, opacification, and less mobility, but later may develop an effusion evidenced by air-fluid levels or bubbles behind the membrane. In more severe or chronic cases, the TM may develop a perforation with purulent discharge. Erythema of the TM may also result from crying and local trauma. Examination of the opposite TM for symmetry may give additional information. Other diagnostic aides include tympanometry and

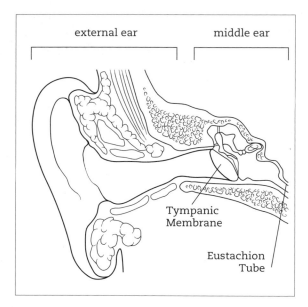

external ear   middle ear

Tympanic
Membrane

Eustachion
Tube

Figure 4–1   Cross section of the ear.

acoustic otoscopy, which are instruments that measure TM mobility by analyzing sound waves reflected off the TM. Laboratory blood analysis is not typically helpful in making the diagnosis of OM.

TREATMENT

Analgesics and antipyretics should be prescribed as necessary for symptom relief. Although 80% of cases of acute otitis media resolve spontaneously, identifying these patients at the time of presentation is not possible. Although controversial, many believe that antibiotics should be prescribed initially to patients with OM in order to prevent possible complications. The incidence of β-lactam (e.g., penicillins and cephalosporins)-resistant pathogens is increasing and varies among regions of the United States. Antibiotics should generally be prescribed for a 10-day course. Normal dose amoxicillin (40–45 mg/kg/day divided two or three times daily) is a reasonable first choice. High dose amoxicillin (80–90 mg/kg/day divided two or three times daily) or a non-β-lactam antibiotic may be more appropriate in areas of higher resistance. Currently, there is no evidence for the use of antihistamines, decongestants, or steroids in the treatment of AOM. Otolaryngology consultation should be considered for individuals who are not responding to oral antibiotics, and for those who have severe or recurrent disease.

♦ **KEY POINTS** ♦

1. Risk factors for OM: Male sex, daycare attendance, parental smoking, a family history of middle ear disease, and anatomical abnormalities.

2. 80% of cases of acute otitis media resolve spontaneously.

3. Antibiotics may be prescribed according to regional sensitivity data.

5 Otitis Externa

Otitis externa (OE) refers to inflammation of the external auditory canal. This disease has a spectrum that starts with dermatitis, and may progress to cellulitis, chondritis, and ultimately necrosis with osteomyelitis. Otitis externa is common among swimmers and referred to as "swimmer's ear" in this population. From 80 to 90% of necrotizing external otitis (i.e., NOE, also known as malignant external otitis) occurs in elderly diabetic patients. Complications of otitis externa include otitis media, mastoiditis, septic cerebral thromboembolism, meningitis, and brain abscess.

ANATOMY AND PATHOPHYSIOLOGY

The external auditory canal contains cerumen glands, within the layer of skin, that generate a protective lipid layer. When the lipid layer and skin are disrupted by heat, moisture, or local trauma, the area is exposed to bacteria and is at risk for infection. For this reason, the incidence of the disease appears to be highest in warm, humid environments. The most common organism in otitis externa is *Pseudomonas aeruginosa*; however, *Staphylococcus*, *Streptococcus*, *Proteus*, and fungi are other known pathogens.

HISTORY

Patients often present with a known auditory canal exposure to moisture or local trauma and otalgia (ear pain) that is worse with manipulation of the external ear. Individuals may also report a discharge from the ear canal or hearing loss due to canal swelling and obstruction.

PHYSICAL EXAMINATION

The auditory canal initially appears erythematous and, in more severe disease, may develop swelling and an exudative discharge. The presence of granulation tissue and erythema of the pinna or periaural soft tissue often signifies a necrotizing external otitis. In severe cases, cranial nerve palsies may occur that most commonly involve the ipsilateral seventh nerve (facial nerve). Since otitis externa can spread to the middle ear (otitis media), an attempt should be made to visualize the tympanic membrane. Conductive hearing loss may result from canal occlusion. Culture of canal exudates is rarely necessary. Serum glucose should be checked in patients with necrotizing infection since glucose regulation is important in treatment. Bone imaging with CT, MRI, or bone scan may be helpful in diagnosing osteomyelitis and delineating the extent of disease.

TREATMENT

Canal debris should be removed first with gentle irrigation and suctioning using tap water, sterile saline, Burrows solution, or 2% acetic acid. Mild to moderate disease limited to erythema and tenderness should be treated with a topical anti-inflammatory and antibiotics (usually a mixture containing polymyxin, neomycin, and hydrocortisone). Oral analgesics may be necessary also. If swelling obstructs the canal lumen, for 2 to 3 days a wick should be placed that absorbs the medicated drops and assists in the delivery of medicine to the inner canal. Patients should be instructed to avoid ear exposure to water and moisture for 2 to 3 weeks. If the tympanic membrane cannot be visualized, oral antibiotics should be considered for presumed concurrent otitis media. Patients with severe canal cellulitis may also benefit from oral or parenteral antibiotics that cover *Pseudomonas*. Patients without evidence of necrotizing infection are usually treated on an outpatient basis with close follow-up. Patients thought to have necrotizing external otitis should be evaluated by an otolaryngologist and admitted for intravenous antibiotics, possible tissue de-bridement, and tight control of diabetes if present. Hyperbaric oxygen therapy (HBO) may have a role in certain necrotizing infections.

◆ KEY POINTS ◆

1. The most common pathogen in otitis externa is *Pseudomonas*.

2. Topical steroid and antibiotic eardrops are the mainstay of treatment.

3. Consider oral antibiotics if the tympanic membrane is not visualized or with more severe cases of cellulitis.

4. Elderly diabetics are at risk for necrotizing external otitis.

6

Ludwig's Angina

The term *Ludwig's angina* is somewhat of a misnomer since the term does not refer to ischemic chest pain but rather a bilateral cellulitis of the floor of the mouth and neck originating in the submandibular space described by Ludwig in 1836. In most cases the infection begins at the site of dental trauma (e.g., extraction) or infection; however, foreign bodies, malignancies, isolated mucosal injury, fractured mandibles and other oral infections have also been implicated. Complications of Ludwig's angina include airway obstruction, osteomyelitis, mediastinitis, pericarditis, pneumonia, empyema, internal jugular vein thrombosis, carotid artery infection, necrotizing fasciitis, sepsis, and death. Asphyxiation is the most common cause of death.

ANATOMY AND PATHOPHYSIOLOGY

The dental molars are most often the origin of infection in Ludwig's angina since the molars extend deep into the mandible and only have a thin portion of mandibular cortex separating them from the soft tissues of the submandibular space. Ludwig's angina is usually a polymicrobial infection with *Streptococcus*, *Staphylococcus*, *Peptostreptococcus*, *Prevotella*, and *Bacteroides* most commonly isolated.

HISTORY

Individuals with Ludwig's angina may report dental disease, fever, painful swelling under the tongue, dys-phonia (i.e., muffled voice), dysphagia (i.e., difficulty swallowing), odynophagia (i.e., painful swallowing), and neck pain. Symptoms of dyspnea (i.e., difficulty breathing) should be taken seriously and may represent impending complete airway obstruction. Patients with a history of diabetes, end stage renal disease, alcoholism, and immunosuppression are at higher risk of developing infection.

PHYSICAL EXAMINATION

Physical examination may reveal fever, submandibular swelling with elevation of the tongue, tender induration of the submandibular soft tissues, trismus, drooling, dysarthria (difficulty articulating speech), and respiratory distress with stridor. Subcutaneous emphysema may also exist within affected tissue.

DIAGNOSIS

Laboratory blood evaluation seldom aids in diagnosis or treatment and is generally not useful. Drained fluid or purulence should be sent for gram stain and culture and sensitivity analysis. Blood cultures are not usually positive, but may reveal a causative organism. Plain films of neck soft tissues may aid in revealing soft-tissue swelling, gas collections, and airway narrowing. Chest radiography may reveal evidence of thoracic extension of infection. Although CT and MRI are the best imaging modalities for demonstrating and defining the extent of infection, they require that the patient lie flat on a table and may worsen airway obstruction. Patients with potential airway compromise should not leave the emergency department for imaging.

TREATMENT

Initial management of patients should focus on assuring a patent airway. Due to distorted anatomy, patients with Ludwig's angina represent a potentially difficult airway to manage. Further treatment consists of analgesia, intravenous antibiotics, otolaryngologic consultation, surgical drainage when appropriate, and admission to a closely monitored setting. Treatment with steroids has

thus far not been proven useful. Dental infections often require extraction of the affected tooth.

◆ KEY POINTS ◆

1. Ludwig's angina often originates at a site of dental infection.

2. Due to distorted anatomy, patients with Ludwig's angina represent a potentially difficult airway to manage.

3. Further treatment consists of analgesia, intravenous antibiotics, otolaryngologic consultation, surgical drainage when appropriate, and admission to a closely monitored hospital bed.

7 Epistaxis

Epistaxis (nosebleed) is more prevalent in drier climates. Causes of epistaxis include upper respiratory tract inflammation (i.e., infections, allergies), local trauma (i.e., nosepicking or blunt trauma), arterial-venous malformations, and coagulopathies. Although hypertension appears to worsen epistaxis, it has not yet been proven to cause it. Epistaxis is rarely a life-threatening condition.

ANATOMY

The nasal mucosa predominantly receives its blood supply via three major arteries that contain anastomosis between them: the sphenopalatine artery, the ethmoidal arteries (anterior and posterior), and the superior labial artery (branch of facial artery) (Fig. 7–1).

PATHOPHYSIOLOGY

Nearly all cases of epistaxis are arterial, and originate anteriorly within the mucosa of the nasal septum in a region known as "Kisselbach's plexus" or "Woodruff's plexus." Posterior epistaxis is less common and more difficult to manage since the application of direct pressure by pinching the nose does not compress the area.

HISTORY

Important historical considerations include the duration of hemorrhage, the amount of blood loss (often difficult to quantify), the precedence of trauma or recent surgery, preexisting medical conditions, the use of prescribed or illicit drugs (especially anticoagulants and cocaine), and a description of the frequency and severity of previous epistaxis.

PHYSICAL EXAMINATION

Epistaxis rarely is severe enough to compromise the airway. Vital signs should be checked to assess for evidence of volume depletion and shock. Hypertension is usually secondary to stress and anxiety. An attempt should be made to locate the site of hemorrhage. The posterior oropharynx should be examined for the presence of "streaming" blood, which may indicate the presence of active hemorrhage. A complete blood count (CBC), prothrombin or partial thromboplastin times (PT/PTT), and a blood type and screen are warranted in cases of significant hemorrhage or patients taking anticoagulants.

TREATMENT

Airway compromise and significant hemodynamic abnormalities should be treated first. Treatment of active hemorrhage begins with the patient blowing their nose to expel any retained clots. A gauze or cotton pledget (small rolled or molded cloth) may be moistened with a vasoconstrictive and anesthetic solution (e.g.,

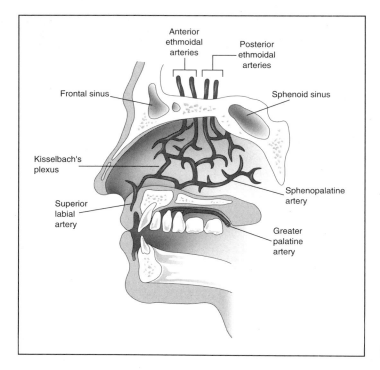

Figure 7–1 Nasal septum.

epinephrine with lidocaine), and inserted inside the nasopharynx with bayonet forceps. The patient is then instructed to hold direct pressure by pinching the soft part of his or her nose together and holding it for at least 10 minutes without releasing. Blood streaming in the posterior oropharynx during direct pressure usually indicates inadequate compression or hemorrhage in the posterior nasopharynx. If after pledget removal active bleeding is still present, chemical cautery with silver nitrate sticks may be attempted at sites of well-visualized, anterior hemorrhage where the bleeding has stopped or is extremely minimal. Chemical cautery should not be applied to directly opposite sides of the nasal septum due to the increased risk of cartilage necrosis. Electrical or thermal cautery has greater risk for septal perforation and is usually reserved for otolaryngologists. In cases of persistent hemorrhage, nasal packing should be placed using either "accordion layered" petrolatum-impregnated $1/4$-inch gauze or a commercially available device such as balloons, gelfoam, or the Merocel nasal sponge. Bilateral anterior packing may further help to tamponade active bleeding. Due to the fact that patients with posterior or bilateral anterior

packing are believed to be at increased risk for hypoventilation, cardiac dysrhythmias, and infection, such patients are usually admitted to the hospital for observation. Otolaryngology consultation should be sought in cases of continued epistaxis. Discharged patients should be prescribed topical, intranasal moisturizers, and receive instructions to follow up with their primary physician or otolaryngologist. Patients with nasal packing additionally should be prescribed prophylactic antibiotics for sinusitis, and receive instructions to return to the emergency department if they develop difficulty breathing, fevers, nausea, or vomiting.

◆ **KEY POINTS** ◆

1. Epistaxis is usually anterior and arterial in origin.

2. Patients receiving posterior or bilateral anterior nasal packing should be admitted.

3. Patients requiring nasal packing should be prescribed antibiotics to prevent sinusitis.

8

Epiglottitis

Although epiglottitis is typically considered a cellulitis of the epiglottic mucosa, a more accurate term would be supraglottitis (inflammation or infection above the vocal cords) since other supraglottic structures (e.g., tongue, vallecula, arytenoids, and tonsils) are often involved (Fig. 8–1). Epiglottitis is a life-threatening emergency usually occurring between 2 and 6 years of age. In adults, the disease is less common, and more likely to be missed. Epiglottitis may be confused with *Streptococcal pharyngitis*, croup (laryngotracheobronchitis), bacterial tracheitis, and foreign body obstruction. Complications of epiglottitis include complete airway obstruction, abscess formation, otitis media, cervical adenitis, pneumonia, pulmonary edema and meningitis.

ANATOMY AND PATHOPHYSIOLOGY

Since the introduction of the *Haemophilus influenzae* type B (HIB) vaccine, the incidence of epiglottitis has dropped dramatically. Currently, the most common pathogens of epiglottitis are *Streptococcus pyogenes* (group A), *Streptococcus pneumoniae*, and *Staphylococcus aureus*.

HISTORY

Children with epiglottitis usually present with the abrupt onset of high fever, sore throat, dysphagia (difficulty swallowing), muffled voice, drooling, and stridor. Unlike children, adults often present with a several day prodrome of upper respiratory tract infection, and a severe sore throat that is out of proportion to clinical findings.

PHYSICAL EXAMINATION

Children with epiglottitis are often febrile, toxic-appearing, drooling, prefer a position sitting upright and leaning forward, and may be in severe respiratory distress with stridor. Due to their smaller airways, children are less tolerant of supraglottic swelling and may progress to complete airway obstruction in hours. Phlebotomy is rarely helpful and may cause agitation with worsening airway obstruction. Noninvasive monitoring with pulse oximetry may be well tolerated and help to ensure adequate oxygenation. Plain film imaging of the lateral neck soft tissues during extension and inspiration typically reveals an enlarged, swollen epiglottis (i.e., thumb sign). Although direct visualization of the supraglottic structures with laryngoscopy allows for the definitive diagnosis of epiglottitis, the techniques should be performed with caution and with surgical backup if possible.

TREATMENT

The patient should be kept as calm as possible. Separation of a child from his or her parents may worsen agitation. Initial management should focus on assuring a

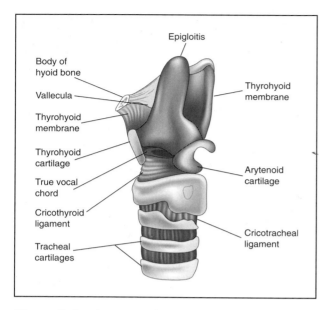

Epigloitis

Body of
hyoid bone

Vallecula

Thyrohyoid
membrane

Thyrohyoid
cartilage

True vocal
chord

Cricothyroid
ligament

Tracheal
cartilages

Thyrohyoid
membrane

Arytenoid
cartilage

Cricotracheal
ligament

Figure 8–1   Anatomy of the larynx.

patent airway. If necessary, bag valve mask ventilation and the needle insufflation of oxygen via the cricothyroid membrane are usually effective temporizing airway measures. Endotracheal intubation or tracheostomy is the definitive airway of choice. Cricothyroidotomy is usually contraindicated in children less than 10 years of age. Patients should be monitored in an intensive care unit and receive supportive therapy including humidified oxygen, intravenous fluid hydration, and intravenous antibiotics. Steroids may be useful. Heliox (mixture of helium and oxygen), which improves laminar airflow across an obstruction, is still under investigation.

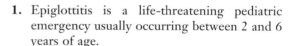

◆   **KEY POINTS**   ◆

1. Epiglottitis is a life-threatening pediatric emergency usually occurring between 2 and 6 years of age.
2. A previously common cause of epiglottitis, *Haemophilus influenzae* type B is now rare due to the available vaccine.
3. Lateral neck plain film x-rays may reveal a swollen epiglottis (i.e., thumb sign).
4. Initial management should focus on immediately establishing and protecting a patent airway.

Part II
Ophthalmologic Emergencies

SIGNS AND SYMPTOMS

Eye Pain:

- Foreign body
- Corneal abrasion or ulceration
- Keratitis (i.e., corneal inflammation)
- Entropion (i.e., ingrown lash)
- Dry eye
- Conjunctivitis
- Peri-orbital/orbital cellulites
- Episcleritis
- Scleritis
- Uveitis
- Iritis
- Chorioretinitis
- Endophthalmitis
- Vasculitis
- Glaucoma
- Sinusitis
- Migraine headache
- Chalazion
- Hordeolum
- Retrobulbar hemorrhage
- Malignancy

Eye Redness:

- Eye rubbing
- Foreign body
- Corneal abrasion
- Glaucoma
- Conjunctivitis
- Episcleritis
- Scleritis
- Iritis
- Chorioretinitis
- Subconjunctival hemorrhage

Acute Vision Abnormalities:

- Keratitis (i.e., corneal inflammation, corneal abrasion, or ulceration)
- Vitreal hemorrhage
- Retinal detachment
- Retinal hemorrhage
- Retinitis
- Dislocated lens
- Glaucoma
- Vitreitis
- Endophthalmitis
- Optic neuritis
- Ocular muscle entrapment

- Ocular muscle weakness (e.g., multiple sclerosis, myasthenia gravis, botulism)
- Central retinal artery occlusion
- Central retinal vein occlusion
- Stroke
- Arterial aneurysm
- Migraine
- Toxins (e.g., methanol, quinine)
- Malignancy

9 Traumatic Hyphema

The term *hyphema* refers to blood in the anterior chamber of the eye, between the iris and the cornea (Fig. 9–1). Hyphema has a spectrum of disease beginning with microhyphema (blood only visible under magnification), worsening to macrohyphema (blood grossly visible to the examiner's naked eye), and ultimately to an "8-ball eye" (blood that completely fills the anterior chamber, obstructing visualization of the iris.) As many as one-third of patients with hyphema will experience an episode of rebleeding over the subsequent 5 days, which is often worse than the initial event. Complications of traumatic hyphema include reduced vision, corneal bloodstaining, acute or chronic glaucoma, and synechiae formation (adhesions from the iris to the cornea or lens).

ANATOMY AND PATHOPHYSIOLOGY

Bleeding from traumatic hyphema results in torn blood vessels within the iris and ciliary body. Blood may obstruct the drainage of aqueous humor leading to elevated intraocular pressure (Fig. 9–2). Individuals with hemoglobinopathies (e.g., sickle-cell disease) are more prone to complications due to the increased susceptibility of their red cells to sickle in acidic and hypoxic environments.

HISTORY

Patients with hyphema usually report recent blunt trauma to the eye. Although patients with traumatic hyphema may present relatively asymptomatic, they may also complain of eye pain, decreased vision, or photophobia (light sensitivity).

PHYSICAL EXAMINATION

Evaluation of the eye should include the testing of visual acuity, visual fields, extraocular movements, pupillary light response, intraocular pressure, and the evaluation of the surface anatomy with fluorescein staining. Hyphema is typically diagnosed on slit lamp examination. In microhyphema, the slit lamp examination reveals floating red cells in the anterior chamber appearing similar to floating dust in a partially lit dark room. In macrohyphema, a meniscus of blood is visible in the dependent portion of the anterior chamber, between the cornea and the iris. In an "8-ball eye," the cornea appears darkish red, and it is difficult to see the iris due to the blood-filled anterior chamber.

The eye should also be evaluated carefully for evidence of corneal abrasions, globe rupture, and orbital hemorrhage. Globe rupture may present as an abnormally shaped eye, partial iris extrusion, or fluorescein stain "streaming." In the absence of globe rupture, individuals with traumatic hyphema should have their intraocular pressures measured.

TREATMENT

Management of traumatic hyphema often includes keeping the head elevated, limiting eye movements,

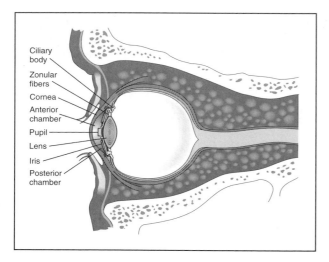

Figure 9–1 Eyeball and conjunctival sac.

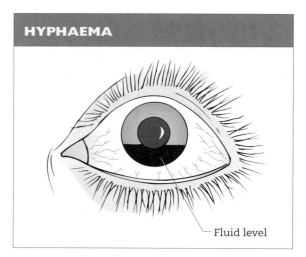

Figure 9–2 Macrohyphema.

analgesics, and the avoidance of anticoagulants. Other potentially helpful pharmacotherapies such as topical miotics, mydriatics, cycloplegics, steroids, and antifibrinolytics may be prescribed on a case-by-case basis after ophthalmologic consultation. Typically, patients receive a topical mydriatic (e.g., 1% atropine), a topical steroid (e.g., prednisolone), and an eye shield. Bed rest aimed at reducing the incidence of rebleed is controversial. The treatment of elevated intraocular pressure (>20 mmHg) with medications such as topical timolol, oral acetazolamide, or intravenous mannitol should be guided by an ophthalmologist. Smaller hyphemas are usually managed on an outpatient basis with close ophthalmologic follow-up. Severe cases should receive ophthalmologic consultation and may require hospital admission.

◆ **KEY POINTS** ◆

1. Hyphema refers to blood in the anterior chamber of the eye.
2. Individuals with traumatic hyphema are at risk for rebleed.
3. Complications include decreased visual acuity, corneal bloodstaining, glaucoma, and synechiae.

10 Periorbital and Orbital Cellulitis

Cellulitis is an infection of the skin and subcutaneous tissue. Periorbital (preseptal) cellulitis does not enter the orbit (eye socket), and remains anterior to the orbital septum. Orbital cellulitis refers to infection posterior to the orbital septum, within the orbit (Fig. 10–1). These infections are usually unilateral and tend to occur during youth. Periorbital and orbital cellulitis should be treated aggressively to avoid infectious extension into the brain via the cavernous sinus. The most common causes of periorbital and orbital cellulitis are sinus infections and local skin trauma.

ANATOMY AND PATHOPHYSIOLOGY

The orbital septum is a fascial plane that connects the rim of the orbit to the tarsal plate, forming a tissue barrier in front of the orbit. Venous drainage of the eye and surrounding tissues occurs via the cavernous sinus, which communicates with the brain. The most common pathogens responsible for orbital and periorbital cellulitis are *Staphylococcus aureus*, *Streptococcus pneumoniae*, *Streptococcus pyogenes* (i.e., group A), *Haemophilus influenzae*, and anaerobes.

HISTORY

Individuals with periorbital or orbital cellulitis may report sinusitis or recent local skin trauma. They often present with fever, redness, and tissue swelling. Reports of visual changes and ocular pain are more indicative of orbital cellulitis.

PHYSICAL EXAMINATION

Patients with periorbital or orbital cellulitis may be febrile, and typically present with warm, swollen, erythematous, periorbital soft tissue. Although conjunctival injection is more common with periorbital cellulitis, pain with extraocular movements, proptosis, increased intraocular pressure (>20 mmHg), and visual acuity deficits are more characteristic of orbital cellulitis. Orbital cellulitis may also affect the ophthalmic and maxillary branches of the trigeminal nerve resulting in sensory loss over these distributions. Gram stain and culture from blood, as well as soft-tissue aspirates, may reveal the offending pathogen; however, the yield from such tests tend to be minimal. Individuals suspected of having orbital cellulitis should undergo imaging with an orbital CT scan to look for evidence of orbital gas, abscess, and to better delineate the extent of infection. Plain films of the orbits are less sensitive and specific, and thus have limited value.

TREATMENT

Patients with orbital cellulitis or severe periorbital disease should have immediate ophthalmologic consultation, intravenous antibiotics, and be admitted to the

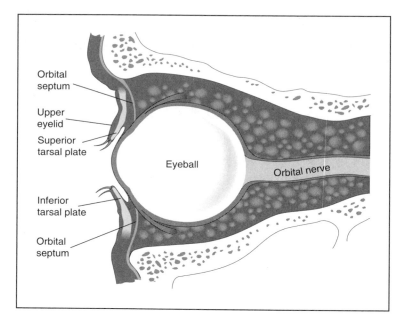

Orbital
septum

Upper
eyelid

Superior
tarsal plate

Eyeball

Orbital nerve

Inferior
tarsal plate

Orbital
septum

Figure 10–1   Sagittal section of the orbit.

hospital for observation. Orbital cellulitis often requires surgical drainage. Current antibiotic choices typically include a second or third generation cephalosporin, or penicillinase-resistant antibiotic. Early periorbital cellulitis may be managed on an outpatient basis with close observation and oral antibiotics.

◆ **KEY POINTS** ◆

1. Venous drainage of periorbital and orbital tissue occurs via the cavernous sinus, which may act as a conduit for intracerebral extension of infection.

2. Untreated orbital cellulitis can lead to loss of vision due to pressure on the optic nerve.

3. Ocular findings such as decreased visual acuity, ocular pain, increased intraocular pressure, and proptosis should raise the suspicion for orbital cellulitis.

4. Orbital CT scan is the imaging modality of choice for diagnosing orbital cellulitis and delineating the extent of infection.

5. Orbital cellulitis requires immediate ophthalmologic consultation, and possibly surgical drainage.

Orbital Hemorrhage

Orbital hemorrhage refers to bleeding that occurs within the orbit (eye socket), behind the globe (eyeball). Hemorrhage typically occurs when orbital vessels are damaged during trauma. Orbital hemorrhage is one of the true ophthalmologic emergencies that requires emergent treatment to salvage the eye.

ANATOMY AND PATHOPHYSIOLOGY

Orbital vessels may rupture during blunt orbital trauma causing hemorrhage that is contained behind the globe. Orbital pressure rises with hemorrhage and pushes on the posterior aspect of the eye. Increasing pressure transmitted to the globe may result in central retinal artery occlusion and optic nerve injury.

HISTORY

Individuals with an orbital hemorrhage may present with orbital pain, headache, blurry vision, and restricted or painful eye movement. Patients suffering significant facial trauma may present with an altered level of consciousness that interferes with their ability to perceive and report eye complaints. For this reason, the diagnosis of orbital hemorrhage should be considered in patients with evidence of significant orbital trauma and altered level of consciousness.

PHYSICAL EXAMINATION

Patients with orbital hemorrhage may exhibit periorbital ecchymosis, swelling, proptosis, decreased visual acuity, extraocular movement deficits, and increased intraocular pressure. Orbital CT scanning is the imaging modality of choice for diagnosing orbital hemorrhage.

TREATMENT

Orbital hemorrhage requires emergent ophthalmologic consultation and decompression. If the hemorrhage is believed to be compromising the retinal circulation, then it should be decompressed immediately in the emergency department by performing a lateral canthotomy. When the lateral canthus is incised, the globe is allowed to displace forward, thereby decompressing the orbit. Only health care providers familiar with the procedure should perform a lateral canthotomy. Anterior chamber paracentesis and intravenous mannitol are less effective therapies for decreasing orbital pressure related to orbital hemorrhage; however, they may provide some benefit if definitive decompression is not possible.

◆ KEY POINTS ◆

1. Orbital hemorrhage is a true ophthalmologic emergency that requires immediate decompression.

2. Increasing pressure transmitted to the globe may result in central retinal artery occlusion, and optic nerve injury.

3. Orbital hemorrhage should be considered in patients with evidence of significant orbital trauma.

4. If the hemorrhage is believed to be compromising the retinal circulation, then it should be decompressed immediately in the emergency department by performing a lateral canthotomy.

12 Corneal Abrasion

Corneal abrasion refers to a superficial disruption of the surface of the cornea that results from trauma. Similar to other soft-tissue injuries, corneal abrasions are prone to infection, including tetanus.

ANATOMY AND PATHOPHYSIOLOGY

The cornea is a round, avascular, sensate, clear structure positioned over the anterior aspect of the eye, which acts like a specialized window, refracting light and protecting the eye. It receives its nutrients from tears, aqueous humor, and adjacent vasculature along its perimeter at the limbus.

HISTORY

Individuals with corneal abrasion may report ocular pain, the sensation of a retained foreign body, blurred vision, and photophobia. The patient's tetanus status should be determined. A history of contact lens use should be elicited since contact lens wearers are more susceptible to ulceration with *Pseudomonas aeruginosa*.

PHYSICAL EXAMINATION

Patients with a corneal abrasion may present with a red eye due to conjunctival injection and visual acuity deficits resulting from refractive errors. A complete eye examination should be performed, which includes visual acuity testing, upper eyelid eversion, fluorescein staining, and a thorough slit-lamp examination. Fluorescein colors the tears and collects in the areas of the cornea where the epithelium has been disrupted, facilitating direct visualization of corneal abrasions. Although retained foreign bodies must always be considered among patients presenting with a red or painful eye, isolated corneal abrasions may feel like a retained foreign body. Ocular discomfort that migrates is more likely to result from a retained foreign body. Vertical corneal abrasions may indicate a foreign body trapped under the upper eyelid causing injury with blinking. Ocular pain relief following the application of a topical anesthetic may help differentiate a surface eye injury from other painful ocular diagnoses, and it also facilitates further examination of the eye.

TREATMENT

As previously stated, topical anesthetics such as tetracaine eyedrops afford immediate pain relief from corneal abrasions. Cycloplegic eyedrops (e.g., cyclopentolate and homatropine) may also help relieve pain by dilating the pupil and relaxing ciliary body spasm. Any dirt or foreign body should be removed with lactated Ringer's or normal saline irrigation. Patients without a retained foreign body or other eye injury may be safely discharged home on a 2- to 3-day course of a broad-spectrum topical eye antibiotic such as erythromycin or polysporin. A topical aminoglycoside or fluoroquinolone may be more appropriate for contact lens wearers due to their increased susceptibility to pseudomonal infection. During healing, patients should be advised not to wear a contact lens in their affected eye. Although eye patching was initially believed helpful, subsequent studies have failed to prove any benefit. Therefore, eye patching should not be routinely recommended for corneal abrasion. Patients should never be prescribed a topical eye anesthetic to take home, as its repetitive use impairs corneal healing, causes ulceration, and may lead to blindness. Oral analgesics such as acetaminophen and NSAIDs usually offer adequate pain relief. Patients should be referred to an ophthalmologist for follow-up within 24 hours. Patients not up-to-date on their tetanus should receive a booster vaccination in the emergency department.

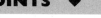

◆ KEY POINTS ◆

1. Isolated corneal abrasions may feel like a retained foreign body.

2. Vertical abrasions may represent a foreign body trapped under the upper eyelid causing injury with blinking.

3. Contact lens wearers are susceptible to infection with *Pseudomonas*.

4. Never prescribe topical eye anesthetics for home use.

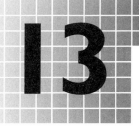

Central Retinal Artery Occlusion

Central retinal artery occlusion (CRAO) is an ophthalmologic emergency that occurs when the central retinal artery becomes occluded, causing retinal ischemia and painless vision loss. CRAO may lead to retinal infarction and irreparable damage if not corrected within approximately 90 minutes. The disease usually presents in patients between the ages of 50 and 70. Risk factors for CRAO include hypertension, cardiac disease (e.g., atrial fibrillation, or endocarditis), atherosclerosis, diabetes, collagen vascular disease, vasculitis, sickle cell disease, acute glaucoma, and orbital hemorrhage. Even with treatment, only 20 to 30% of patients with CRAO will recover useful vision in the affected eye.

ANATOMY AND PATHOPHYSIOLOGY

Blood supply to the retina occurs primarily via the internal carotid artery. Although CRAO may result from stenosis secondary to atherosclerosis, thromboembolic events are the most common etiology.

HISTORY

Individuals with CRAO typically present with acute, painless, monocular vision loss, in addition to risk factors for the disease.

PHYSICAL EXAMINATION

A rapid, complete eye examination should be performed that evaluates the visual acuity, visual fields, pupillary light response, retina, and intraocular pressure. Prognosis is directly related to visual acuity. Occlusions of smaller, more distal arterial branches within the retina usually manifest as partial visual field defects, whereas CRAO usually causes a complete visual field loss. Pupillary light responses may indicate an afferent pupillary defect (i.e., the loss of both direct and consensual pupillary constriction to light shone in the affected eye). Funduscopic examination typically reveals an edematous, gray-appearing retina in areas of infarction. The macula may develop a "cherry red spot" resulting from retinal thinning and better visualization of the underlying choroidal vasculature. Intraocular pressure may be elevated in cases of acute glaucoma and orbital hemorrhage. An electrocardiogram may identify thrombogenic dysrhythmias such as atrial fibrillation. Although echocardiography and carotid Doppler studies may add additional information, they are rarely indicated within the emergency department.

TREATMENT

Treatment of CRAO attempts to rapidly reestablish central retinal artery blood flow and retinal perfusion. Emergent ophthalmologic consultation should be obtained when considering CRAO as the possible diagnosis. Although treatment is generally futile in cases where complete obstruction has persisted for longer than 2 hours, some improvement may occur if partial retinal perfusion was present. Cases of compressive

CRAO (e.g., orbital hemorrhage) should be treated immediately with the appropriate decompressive maneuvers. Patients with noncompressive CRAO should initially be treated with global (i.e., eyeball) massage, which attempts to dislodge the clot by applying digital pressure over the closed eye for 5 second intervals. Carbogen (i.e., 5% carbon dioxide, 95% oxygen) breathing by the patient may help salvage ischemic retina by combining the vasodilatory effects of carbon dioxide with improved oxygenation. Anterior chamber paracentesis performed by an ophthalmologist may help to dislodge a clot to a more distal arterial branch by reducing the intraocular pressure and ultimately increasing the pressure gradient across the central retinal artery. Medications such as timolol eyedrops, intravenous acetazolamide, and intravenous mannitol may also help to reduce intraocular pressure. Selective intra-arterial thrombolysis of the retinal artery clot is another therapeutic option.

◆ **KEY POINTS** ◆

1. CRAO usually presents as painless monocular vision loss.

2. On funduscopy, the macula may develop a "cherry red spot" due to retinal thinning and better visualization of the underlying choroidal vasculature.

3. Delays in restoring retinal perfusion longer than 90 minutes may result in permanent vision loss.

4. CRAO usually signifies the presence of underlying cardiovascular or neurologic disease.

14

Acute Angle Closure Glaucoma

Glaucoma is an optic neuropathy caused by increased intraocular pressure that may result in permanent optic nerve damage. Acute angle closure glaucoma occurs when individuals with an anatomically small or narrow anterior chamber develop an obstruction in the outflow of aqueous humor leading to an increase in intraocular pressure and the potential for optic nerve injury. Untreated acute angle closure glaucoma may result in permanent deficits of visual acuity including blindness.

ANATOMY AND PATHOPHYSIOLOGY

A clear fluid-like substance, aqueous humor bathes the lens and cornea, providing nutrients and removing metabolic wastes. It is produced by the ciliary processes, and drains into the episcleral veins via the canal of Schlemm. Aqueous humor flows from the posterior chamber, through the pupillary aperture, into the anterior chamber, through the one-way trabecular meshwork lying at the junction of the iris and cornea, through the canal of Schlemm, and ultimately into the episcleral veins. Intraocular pressure is determined by the rate of production and clearance of aqueous humor. Pupillary dilation often causes iris retraction or folding, and may precipitate acute angle closure glaucoma in susceptible individuals.

HISTORY

Patients with acute angle closure glaucoma typically present with the sudden onset of eye pain, blurred vision, headache, nausea, and vomiting. They may also report a halo around lights.

PHYSICAL EXAMINATION

The physical examination of patients with acute angle closure glaucoma may reveal visual acuity deficits, conjunctival injection, a cloudy or steamy-appearing cornea, and a midway positioned or dilated pupil that is fixed or sluggish to react to light. By definition, the intraocular pressure should be elevated above 20 mmHg.

TREATMENT

Ophthalmology should be consulted immediately in cases of suspected acute angle closure glaucoma. Intraocular pressure reduction should be initiated as soon as possible. Three strategies for reducing intraocular pressure are: improving aqueous humor outflow, inhibiting aqueous humor production, and reducing aqueous or vitreous humor volume.

Improving Aqueous Humor Outflow

Pilocarpine 2% eyedrops, a miotic agent, should be applied—1 drop every 15 minutes—in the affected eye until pupillary constriction, and prophylactically—1 drop every 6 hours—in the unaffected eye. Cases refractory to multiple medical management may be definitively treated with peripheral or laser iridectomy performed by an ophthalmologist. This therapy effectively punches holes in the iris, allowing for the drainage of aqueous humor.

Inhibiting Aqueous Humor Production

Timolol 0.5% eyedrops, a β-blocker, reduces intraocular pressure within 1 hour and should be applied topically as 1 drop in the affected eye and repeated once after 30 minutes. Acetazolamide, a carbonic anhydrase inhibitor, helps to reduce intraocular pressure within 1 hour and is typically administered as an initial dose of 500 mg intramuscularly or intravenously, with repeated doses of 250 mg every 6 hours.

Reducing Aqueous or Vitreous Humor Volume

Intravenous mannitol administered at a dose of 1–1.5 mg/kg also helps to slowly and temporarily reduce the intraocular pressure by osmotically drawing water out of the aqueous or vitreous humor and into the circulation where excess fluid can be removed from the body in urine.

Anxious patients may benefit from relaxation with a sedative such as a benzodiazepine.

◆ KEY POINTS ◆

1. Acute angle closure glaucoma is an ocular emergency caused by increased intraocular pressure that may lead to irreversible damage.

2. Increased ocular pressure is due to the mechanical obstruction in aqueous humor drainage and made worse by pupillary dilation.

3. Cases refractory to conservative treatment may require peripheral or laser iridectomy.

Part III
Cardiovascular Emergencies

Chest Pain:
- Myocardial infarction
- Unstable angina
- Aortic dissection
- Pulmonary embolus
- Pneumothorax
- Esophageal rupture
- Angina
- Mitral valve prolapse
- Myocarditis
- Valvular disease
- Pericarditis
- Pneumonia
- Costochondritis
- Esophageal spasm
- Esophageal reflux
- Peptic ulcer disease
- Biliary colic
- Herpes zoster neuropathy

Cardiogenic Shock:
- Myocardial infarction
- Cardiomyopathy
- Myocarditis
- Papillary muscle dysfunction
- Cardiac tamponade
- Tension pneumothorax
- Cardiac valve failure
- Myocardial contusion
- Pulmonary embolus
- Dysrhythmia

Syncope:
- Autonomic dysregulation
- Vasovagal
- Benign positional vertigo
- Hypovolemia
- Arrhythmias
- Myocardial infarction
- Valvular lesions
- Subarachnoid hemorrhage
- Cerebral vascular accident
- Drug induced
- Seizure
- Psychogenic
- Pulmonary embolism

Syncope (cont.):

- Aortic dissection
- Leaking abdominal aortic aneurysm
- Hypoglycemia
- Hypoxemia
- Ruptured ectopic pregnancy
- Anaphylaxis
- Heat stroke
- Breath-holding spells

15 Dysrhythmias— Bradyarrhythmias

Dysrhythmias (also known as arrhythmias) are abnormalities of the cardiac electrical rhythm. They result from two basic mechanisms:

1. Disorders of impulse formation.
2. Disorders of impulse conduction.

Cardiac dysrhythmias may cause a decrease in cardiac output if the ventricular rate is too slow or too fast. Bradyarrhythmias are slow rhythms, with rates of less than 60 beats per minute (bpm). Tachyarrhythmias are fast rhythms, with rates of greater than 100 b.p.m. Tachyarrhythmias are covered in the following chapter.

ETIOLOGY

Bradyarrhythmias result from a specific cardiac or systemic disease process that leads to either a depression of SA node activity or delays in conduction.
    Causes include:

- Organic heart disease (myocardial ischemia or infarction, rheumatic heart disease, Lyme disease)
- Infiltrative heart disease (sarcoid, amyloid)
- Electrolyte abnormalities (hyperkalemia)
- Drugs (beta-blockers, digitalis, calcium channel blockers)
- Degenerative disease of the conduction system (aging)
- Hypothermia
- Hypothyroidism
- Exaggerated vagal tone

Bradyarrhythmias can be a normal physiologic finding (e.g., in trained athletes) and may not indicate a medical condition.

HISTORY

The need for emergent treatment is determined by the presence of symptoms associated with the bradyarrhythmia. Common symptoms include:

- Near syncope or lightheadedness
- Syncope or loss of consciousness
- Chest pain
- Shortness of breath

PHYSICAL EXAMINATION

Common signs of bradycardia requiring immediate treatment include:

- Hypotension (systolic blood pressure <90 mmHg)
- Pulmonary edema
- Shock (cyanosis, pallor, altered mental status, clammy or dusky skin)
- Congestive heart failure (elevated jugular venous pressure, pulmonary rales, dependent edema)

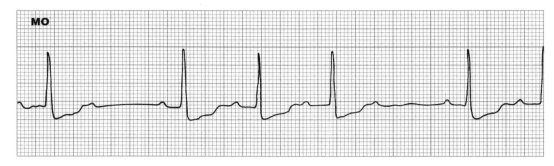

Figure 15–1   Type I second-degree block. The PR interval progressively lengthens until the fourth P wave is not conducted.

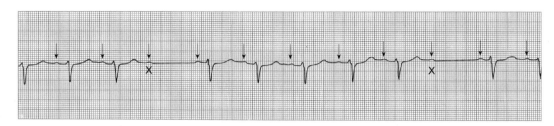

Figure 15–2   Note the constant PR interval. Type II second-degree block. The "X" indicates a P wave suddenly not conducted.

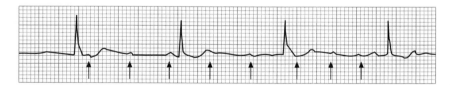

Figure 15–3   Complete AV block. Arrows indicate regular P waves with no relation to QRS.

DIFFERENTIAL DIAGNOSIS

Disorders of impulse formation (Table 15–1):

- Sinus bradycardia
- Sick sinus syndrome
- Atrioventricular nodal bradyarrhythmias
- Ventricular bradyarrhythmias

Disorders of Impulse Conduction (Table 15–2):

- Sinoatrial block
- Atrioventricular conduction

1. First-degree AV block
2. Second-degree AV block
   Mobitz Type I (Wenckebach)
   Mobitz Type II
3. Third-degree heart block

DIAGNOSTIC EVALUATION

The electrocardiogram (ECG) is the first diagnostic test to evaluate dysrhythmias.

Look for the presence or absence of P waves, and the relationship of the P waves to the QRS complex.

TABLE 15–1

Bradyarrhythmias—Disorders of Impulse Formation

Disorders of Impulse Formation	Atrial Rate	P wave	PR Interval	QRS	Causes	Treatment
Sinus bradycardia • Suppression of sinus node discharge rate	<60 bpm	Normal	Normal (0.12–0.20)	Narrow (0.04–0.10)	• Normal (athletes, during sleep, vagal stimulation) • Pharmacologic (beta-blockers, digoxin, Ca$^+$ channel blockers, narcotics) • Pathologic process (myocardial infarction/ischemia, hypothermia, hypothyroid, increased ICP)	If symptomatic and signs of hypoperfusion: • Atropine • Elective pacemaker • May need immediate external or internal pacing
Sick sinus syndrome (Sinus node dysfunction) • Group of disorders that manifests with both bradycardia and tachycardia in the same patient • Slow arrhythmias: Sinus bradycardia, sinus pause, sinoatrial block, atrial fibrillation, atrial flutter • Fast arrhythmias: Atrial fibrillation, atrial flutter, PSVT	Variable	Absent	Variable	Narrow (0.04–0.10) Wide (>0.10)	• Ischemic and rheumatic disorders • Myocarditis and pericarditis • Cardiomyopathies • Rheumatologic disease • Metastatic tumors • Surgical damage • Elderly patients with HTN • Beta-blocker, calcium channel blockers, and amiodarone may worsen the bradyarrhythmia	Most common indication for a permanent pacemaker
Atrioventricular nodal bradycardias • May be physiologic escape when SA node fails to generate impulse	Usually 45–60 bpm	Inverted (if conducted in a retrograde manner)—may appear before, during, or after QRS complex.	Variable	Identical to inherent QRS morphology	• The underlying disorder may be sinus bradycardia, sinus arrest, or AV block. • Beta-blockers and digitalis may also be responsible	Not indicated for asymptomatic patients with infrequent escape beats In symptomatic patients • Atropine • Artificial pacing
Ventricular bradycardia • A physiologic escape rhythm that arises in absence of stimuli from above pacemakers	30–45 bpm	Absent		Wide (>0.10)	• The underlying disorder may be sinus bradycardia, sinus arrest, or AV block • Beta-blockers and digitalis may also be responsible	Most patients are symptomatic • Atropine • Artificial pacing

TABLE 15–2

Bradyarrhythmias—Disorders of Impulse Conduction

Disorders of Impulse Conduction	Atrial Rate	P wave	PR Interval	QRS	Causes	Treatment
Sinoatrial block and escape rhythms • Absent atrial depolarization	If escape is AV node 45–60 bpm If escape is His-Purkinje 30–45 bpm	Absent		Narrow (0.04–0.10) Wide (>0.10)	• Cardiac ischemia or infarct • Hyperkalemia • Increased vagal tone • Pharmacologic (beta-blockers, digoxin, calcium channel blockers)	If symptomatic and signs of hypoperfusion: • Atropine • Elective pacemaker • May need immediate external or internal pacing
First-degree AV block • Usually due to slowing of conduction through the AV node	<60 bpm	Normal	Prolonged >0.20	Narrow	• Normal variant in healthy young adults • Electrolyte (hyperkalemia, hypermagnesemia) • Pharmacologic (beta-blockers, digoxin, Ca$^+$ channel blockers, narcotics) • Pathologic process (myocardial infarction/ischemia, hypothermia, hypothyroid, increased ICP, rheumatic fever, myocarditis)	Usually asymptomatic If symptomatic and signs of hypoperfusion: • Atropine • Elective pacemaker • May need immediate external or internal pacing
Second-degree AV block Type I (Wenckebach) • ECG shows grouped beating		Non-conducted P wave	Prolonging of PR interval until a P wave is completely blocked (Fig. 15–1)	Narrow	• Electrolyte (hyperkalemia, hypermagnesemia) • Pharmacologic (beta-blockers, digoxin, Ca$^+$ channel blockers, narcotics) • Pathologic process (myocardial infarction [inferior]/ischemia, hypothermia, hypothyroid, increased ICP)	Usually a benign finding and rarely progresses to complete heart block If symptomatic and signs of hypoperfusion: • Atropine • Elective pacemaker • May need immediate external or internal pacing
Second-degree AV block Type II • Conduction block in the His-Purkinje system		Non-conducted P wave	Normal (0.12–0.20) No prior lengthening of PR interval (Fig. 15–2)	Narrow or wide, depending on the site of block	• Cardiac ischemia (anterior wall) or infarct • Hyperkalemia • Increased vagal tone • Pharmacologic (beta-blockers, digoxin, calcium channel blockers)	This may progress to complete heart block; thus a permanent pacemaker is indicated. Emergent cardiology consultation should be obtained.
Third-degree heart block (Complete heart block) • AV dissociation with no relationship between P waves and QRS complexes • All atrial beats are blocked and the ventricles are driven by an escape focus distal to block	Atrial rate Unrelated to ventricular rate. Block at AV node rate: 40–60 Block occurs infranodal rate <40	Conducted P wave	(Fig. 15–3)	Narrow or wide, depending on the site of block	• Cardiac ischemia or infarct (inferior or posterior) • Pharmacologic (beta-blockers, digoxin, calcium channel blockers) • Lenegre's disease: fibrous degenerative changes in the conduction system that results from aging • Infectious and inflammatory processes: abscesses, tumors, infiltrative disease of myocardium, sarcoid nodules, myocarditis, and rheumatic fever	Treatment includes: • Atropine • Epi • Dopamine • Elective pacemaker May need immediate external or internal pacing

In order to differentiate between the types of brady-arrhythmias, determine the length of the PR interval and width of the QRS complex (Tables 15–1, 15–2).

Lab tests may help determine the underlying cause of the bradyarrhythmia, including electrolytes, CK and CK-MB, troponin I, and digoxin level.

TREATMENT

Consider treating the underlying cause such as correction of electrolyte abnormalities, management of acute coronary syndrome, or discontinuation of offending drugs like beta-blockers or digoxin.

Emergency treatment is required when:

- The heart rate is less than 50 bpm with clinical evidence of hypoperfusion (e.g., chest pain, shortness of breath, decreased level of consciousness).
- Bradyarrhythmias may progress to complete heart block.

Atropine is the first line agent, administered either by IV or through the endotracheal tube. Begin with 0.5 mg IV and repeat every 5 minutes until a dose of 2.0 mg is reached. For recurrent or persistent symptomatic bradycardia, transcutaneous or transvenous pacing is indicated. Dopamine 5–20 μg/kg/min or epinephrine 2–10 μg/min can be used when atropine is ineffective and transcutaneous pacing is unavailable (see Table 15–1).

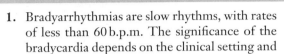

♦ KEY POINTS ♦

1. Bradyarrhythmias are slow rhythms, with rates of less than 60 b.p.m. The significance of the bradycardia depends on the clinical setting and can be a normal finding.

2. The need for emergent treatment is determined by the presence of symptoms associated with the bradycardia—for example, syncope, chest pain, shortness of breath, or decreased level of consciousness.

3. When treating bradyarrhythmias, consider underlying causes like myocardial infarction, drugs, and electrolytes.

4. Emergency cardiac pacing may be necessary if symptomatic bradycardia does not respond to medications.

16 Dysrhythmias— Tachyarrhythmias

Tachyarrhythmias are fast rhythms with rates greater than 100 bpm.

ETIOLOGY

Tachyarrhythmias result from mechanisms that cause an increase in the firing rate of conduction tissue. Common mechanisms include:

- Enhanced cellular automaticity in a normal or ectopic site.
- Reentry loops in a normal or accessory pathway.

Table 16–1 outlines the etiologies of specific tachyarrhythmias.

HISTORY

If stable, obtain a detailed history including:

- Current symptoms, for example, chest pain, dizziness, shortness of breath, syncope, diaphoresis, or palpitations
- Previous episodes
- Cardiac history
- Current medications

PHYSICAL EXAMINATION

Common signs of tachyarrhythmias requiring immediate treatment include:

- Hypotension (systolic blood pressure <90 mmHg)
- Pulmonary edema
- Shock (cyanosis, pallor, altered mental status, clammy or dusky skin)
- Congestive heart failure (elevated jugular venous pressure, pulmonary rales, dependent edema)

Auscultate the heart, listening for murmurs or irregular beats.

DIFFERENTIAL DIAGNOSIS

Narrow complex tachycardias (QRS <0.12) usually originate at or above the AV node. Examples of narrow complex tachycardias with regular rhythms include (Table 16–2):

- Sinus tachycardia
- Atrial tachycardia
- AV nodal re-entrant tachycardia
- Wolff-Parkinson-White (WPW) syndrome
- Atrial flutter
- Junctional tachycardia

TABLE 16–1

Etiologies of Tachyarrhythmias

Tachyarrhythmia	Definition	Etiology
Sinus tachycardia	• The sinus node pacing the heart at a rate >100 bpm with normal P waves and QRS complexes • Most often arises from sympathetic stimulation of the SA node	Conditions that drive the heart rate faster: • Pain • Fever • Anxiety • Drugs • Hyperthyroidism • Hypovolemia • Pulmonary embolism • Myocardial ischemia or infarction • Anemia
Paroxysmal supraventricular tachycardia (PSVT)	• Recurrent attacks of tachycardias usually with sudden onset and abrupt termination that originate from ectopic focus above the ventricles (atrial or junctional) • Generally caused by AV nodal re-entry or increased automaticity of an ectopic focus	• Premature atrial or ventricular contractions • Myocardial ischemia or infarction • WPW syndrome-congenital accessory tracts • Electrolyte disturbances • Drugs-digitalis toxicity
Junctional tachycardia	• Supraventricular tachycardias arising from the atrioventricular junction • Generally produces a rapid sequence of QRS-T cycles that may be slightly widened • Causes include AV nodal re-entry or increased automaticity of an ectopic focus	• Hyperthyroidism • Myocardial ischemia • Structural heart disease • Drugs • Alcohol
Atrial fibrillation	• A chaotic "irregularly irregular" rhythm caused by continuous, rapid firing of multiple atrial automaticity foci • Only an occasional atrial depolarization gets through the AV node to stimulate the ventricles, producing an irregular ventricular rhythm	• Hypertension • Myocardial ischemia or infarction • Mitral valve stenosis or insufficiency • Cardiomyopathies • Hyperthyroidism • Pulmonary embolus
Atrial flutter (Fig. 16–1)	• Originates from an atrial automaticity focus producing atrial depolarization that occurs in rapid succession • Characterized by a series of identical "flutter waves" in rapid back-to-back sequence • Most impulses are blocked at the AV node, so conduction to ventricles rate is a fraction of atrial rate (ex 2:1 block-atrial rate = 300 bpm, ventricular rate = 150 bpm)	• Myocardial ischemia or infarction • Valvular heart disease • COPD • Cardiomyopathies • Hyperthyroidism • Pulmonary embolus
Multifocal atrial tachycardia	• Multiple ectopic atrial foci that have achieved enhanced automaticity • The P wave morphology varies beat to beat • Generally seen in elderly patients with chronic lung disease and hypoxemia	• Chronic lung disease • Theophylline toxicity

TABLE 16–1 *Continued*

Etiologies of Tachyarrhythmias

Tachyarrhythmia	*Definition*	*Etiology*
Ventricular tachycardias (Fig. 16–2)	• Series of three or more premature ventricular complexes (PVCs) in a row produced by an automaticity focus in the ventricles • Produces wide QRS complexes with no P waves	• Myocardial ischemia or infarction • Cardiomyopathies • Drug toxicity • Hypoxia • Electrolyte abnormalities

Wolff-Parkinson-White (WPW) syndrome	• An abnormal connection between atria and ventricles through an accessory bypass tract—can be either a re-entry tachycardia or have normal sinus rhythm depending on direction impulse travels down accessory path
	• Reentry tachycardia appears similar to PSVT—impulse travels down AV node and up accessory pathway
	• Pre-excitation syndrome—impulse travels down accessory pathway and up AV node with the following characteristic ECG changes:
	  1. "Delta" wave-slurred initial deflection of QRS complex
	  2. Shortened PR interval
	• No "delta" wave present when tachycardia because ventricles depolarized by AV nodal reentry
	• "Delta" wave only present with NSR
		• Congenital cardiac defects
		• Cardiomyopathies

Torsades de pointes "twisting of the points"	• Rapid ventricular rhythm caused by a prolonged QT interval • Undulating rotations of the QRS complexes with constantly varying amplitudes gives a sinusoidal pattern	• Anti-arrhythmic drugs (Class IA & IC) • Tricyclic antidepressants • Myocardial ischemia or infarction • Electrolyte disorders-hypokalemia, hypomagnesemia • Congenital QT prolongation • CNS lesions—subarachnoid or intracerebral hemorrhage
Ventricular fibrillation (Fig. 16–3)	• Disorganized depolarization and contraction of small areas of ventricular myocardium producing an erratic, rapid twitching of the ventricles • Totally disorganized rhythm with no effective ventricular pumping activity	• Myocardial ischemia or infarction • Hypoxia • Hypothermia • Electrocution • Shock • Electrolyte abnormalities • Drugs—digoxin or quinidine

TABLE 16–2

Narrow Complex Tachycardias (QRS <0.12) with Regular Rhythms

Type	Atrial Rate	P Wave Morphology	Treatment
Sinus tachycardia	100–160 bpm	Normal	• No specific treatment is required but consider treating the underlying condition
Paroxysmal supraventricular tachycardia (PSVT)	150–250 bpm	Peaked or inverted	• Vagal maneuvers • Adenosine • Ca^{2+} channel or beta blockers • Synchronized cardioversion
AV nodal re-entry tachycardia (AVNRT)	150–250 bpm	Buried within QRS or inverted following QRS	• Unstable patients synchronized cardioversion • Stable patients—vagal maneuvers • Adenosine
WPW syndrome	150–250 bpm		• Unstable patients synchronized cardioversion • Stable patients—vagal maneuvers • Adenosine • Ablation of accessory tract
Atrial flutter (Figure 16–1)	250–350 bpm	"Sawtooth" shaped	• Unstable patients synchronized cardioversion • Stable patients—Ca^{2+} channel or beta blockers, or digoxin.
Junctional tachycardia	150–250 bpm	Inverted	• Treat underlying disorder • If cause is digoxin toxicity, discontinue drug • Amiodarone, beta blocker, or Ca^{2+} channel blocker

Narrow complex tachycardias with irregular rhythms include (Table 16–3):

- Multifocal atrial tachycardia
- Atrial fibrillation
- Atrial flutter with variable block

Wide complex tachycardias (QRS >0.12) can originate from any focus in the heart (supraventricular, AV nodal, or ventricular) and include (Table 16–4):

- Ventricular tachycardia
- Supraventricular tachycardia with aberrant conduction
- Torsades de pointes

DIAGNOSTIC EVALUATION

The electrocardiogram (ECG) is the first diagnostic test to evaluate tachyarrhythmias. Evaluate:

1. Ventricular rate—fast (>100 bpm), slow (<60 bpm), or normal (60–100 bpm)

2. Rhythm—regular or irregular

3. QRS width—narrow (<0.12 seconds) or wide (>0.12 seconds)

4. P wave—present or absent and its relationship to the QRS complexes.

Lab tests may help determine the underlying cause of the tachyarrhythmia, including complete blood count,

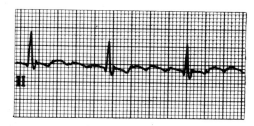

Figure 16–1 Atrial flutter with 4:1 block.

digoxin level, electrolytes, CK and CK-MB, troponin I, or thyroid function tests.

TREATMENT

If pulseless VT or VF, perform CPR until defibrillator is attached. Then follow the standard advanced cardiac life support (ACLS) protocol. If the patient is not in cardiac arrest, determine if the patient is hemodynamically stable or unstable. Treatment of tachyarrhythmias consists of intravenous drugs for clinically stable patients and synchronized cardioversion or defibrillation for unstable patients. Unstable patients in rhythms other than pulseless VT/VF require immediate synchronized cardioversion. For synchronized electrical cardioversion start with:

- 50 joules for PSVT and atrial flutter.
- 100 joules for atrial fibrillation and ventricular tachycardia.

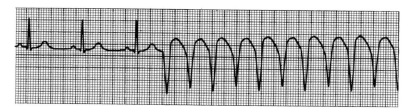

Figure 16–2 Sustained VT.

Isolated PVC's are common in the absence of organic heart disease. More complex forms, including paired PVC's and VT, may be the consequence of LV dysfunction or acute ischemia.

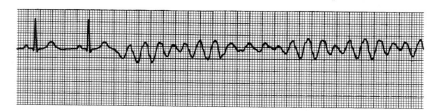

Figure 16–3 Ventricular fibrillation, the usual cause of sudden cardiac death.

TABLE 16–3

Narrow Complex Tachycardias (QRS <0.12) with Irregular Rhythms

Type	Atrial Rate	P Wave Morphology	Treatment
Multifocal atrial tachycardia	100–200 bpm	Varies from beat to beat (requires 3 or more differently shaped P waves with varying PR intervals)	• Treat underlying disorder • For decompensated lung disease, treat with oxygen and bronchodilators • Amiodarone, beta-blocker, or Ca^{2+} channel blocker
Atrial fibrillation	350–450 bpm	Fibrillatory waves— no distinct P wave	• Unstable patients need emergent synchronized cardioversion • Stable patients need rate control with Ca^{2+} channel blocker • Beta-blockers or digoxin • Because of risk of intra-atrial thrombi and arterial embolism, patients with Afib of >2 days should be anticoagulated (coumadin), first, for 3 weeks before attempts at electrical or chemical cardioversion
WPW syndrome with atrial fibrillation		Fibrillatory waves— no distinct P wave	• Unstable patients need emergent synchronized cardioversion • Stable patients need rate control with procainamide or amiodarone (Class I) • Do not use adenosine, digoxin, Ca^{2+} channel or beta-blockers as they may increase ventricular rate

If hemodynamically stable, various drugs can be used. Table 16–5 lists specific agents used in the treatment of tachyarrhythmias.

◆ KEY POINTS ◆

1. Tachyarrhythmias are fast rhythms, with rates greater than 100 beats per minute.

2. Symptomatic tachyarrhythmias are identified by chest pain, dizziness, shortness of breath, syncope, diaphoresis, or palpitations.

3. Tachyarrhythmias with evidence of hypoperfusion should be treated emergently with synchronized cardioversion.

TABLE 16–4

Wide Complex Tachycardias (QRS >0.12)

Type	Ventricular Rate	EKG	Treatment
Ventricular tachycardia (VT) (Figure 16–2)	150–250	• 3 or more consecutive PVCs • Wide QRS in a regular, rapid rhythm with a constant axis	• Unstable without pulse—defibrillate (unsynchronized cardioversion) • Unstable with pulse-synchronized cardioversion • Stable—amiodarone, lidocaine, procainamide, or sotalol
Torsades de pointes "twisting of the points"	250–350	• Undulating rotations of the QRS complexes • Constantly varying amplitudes give a sinusoidal pattern	• Treat underlying disorder—replete magnesium and potassium • Temporary cardiac pacing or isoproterenol to shorten the QT interval and overdrive the rhythm • TCA overdose, sodium bicarbonate
Ventricular fibrillation • Most life threatening (Figure 16–3)	350–450	• Fine course zigzag • No P waves or QRS complexes	• Immediate defibrillation (unsynchronized cardioversion) • If initial 3 attempts at defibrillation fail, CPR should be initiated and further defibrillations should occur after various intravenous drugs.

TABLE 16–5

Agents Used in the Treatment of Tachyarrhythmias

Drug	Indication
Adenosine	• First drug for narrow complex tachycardias PSVT • May be used diagnostically after lidocaine in wide complex tachycardias of uncertain type
Beta-blockers: metoprolol, atenolol, propranolol, esmolol, labetalol	• Second line agents after adenosine and digoxin for PSVT, Afib, Aflutter
Calcium channel blockers: verapamil or diltiazem	• To control ventricular rate in Afib or Aflutter • Used after adenosine to treat refractory PSVT with narrow QRS and stable BP
Digoxin	• To slow ventricular rate in Afib or Aflutter • Third line choice for PSVT after vagal maneuvers, adenosine, verapamil, and diltiazem
Lidocaine	• Stable VT, wide complex tachycardias of uncertain type, wide complex PSVT
Magnesium	• Torsades de pointes with pulse • Life threatening ventricular arrhythmias due to digoxin toxicity and tricyclic overdose
Amiodarone	• Used in a wide variety of atrial and ventricular tachyarrhythmias
Procainamide	• Recurrent VT not controlled with lidocaine • Refractory PSVT • Stable wide-complex tachycardia of unknown origin • Afib with rapid rate in WPW syndrome

17

Acute Coronary Syndromes

Coronary artery disease (CAD) is the leading cause of death among adults in the United States. It may be asymptomatic, but usually presents with symptoms like angina pectoris, acute myocardial infarction, or sudden death.

ETIOLOGY AND PATHOPHYSIOLOGY

Atherosclerosis produces narrowing of the coronary arteries and inadequate blood flow to the myocardium, leading to ischemia. Angina pectoris, the chest discomfort associated with myocardial ischemia, is caused by an imbalance between oxygen supply and oxygen demand. The lesion that causes angina is a smooth-surfaced atherosclerotic plaque that allows sufficient flow to the myocardium at rest but insufficient flow during times of increased exertion, causing symptoms. Symptoms subside at rest because oxygen demand has decreased, restoring the supply-demand balance. Unstable angina is thought to occur when a complex, irregular atherosclerotic plaque ruptures, causing thrombus formation, increased platelet activity, and increased coronary vasomotor tone (vasospasm). Unstable angina has a higher chance of progressing to an acute myocardial infarct. Acute myocardial infarction (AMI) is necrosis to a segment of heart muscle resulting from prolonged ischemia. It usually occurs when an acute thrombus or a ruptured atherosclerotic plaque suddenly occludes a coronary artery, resulting in myocardial ischemia and

ultimately tissue death caused by hypoxia. Myocardial infarcts are divided into two types, depending on the extent of necrosis within the myocardial wall (Fig. 17–1).

- Q wave infarctions: Typically result from full thickness (transmural) necrosis caused by total, prolonged occlusion of a transmural vessel.
- Non-Q wave infarctions: Usually result from incomplete coronary artery occlusion, causing ischemia of only the innermost layers of the myocardium (subendocardial).

Valvular heart disease, congenital heart disease, coronary artery vasculitis, and coronary dissection are nonatherosclerotic causes of ischemic heart disease.

HISTORY

A detailed history, including the onset and duration of symptoms, precipitating factors, and previous episodes, should be addressed. Risk factors for coronary artery disease should also be evaluated and include:

- Hypertension
- Hypercholesterolemia or hypertriglyceridemia
    High LDL cholesterol
    Low HDL cholesterol

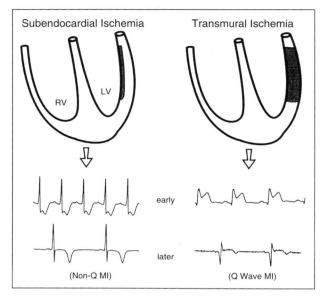

Subendocardial Ischemia   Transmural Ischemia

RV   LV

early

later

(Non-Q MI)   (Q Wave MI)

Figure 17–1 Patterns of myocardial ischemia. The coronary arteries rest upon the epicardial surface, and the subendocardial region is thus farthest from the source of nutrient supply. When there is tight stenosis of a coronary artery (but still some antegrade flow), a mismatch between oxygen supply and demand produces the pattern of subendocardial ischemia, ST segment depression. A good example of this is a positive stress test. Total occlusion of a coronary artery affects the full thickness of the myocardium, causing ST segment elevation, the pattern of transmural ischemia. This is usually the case with acute myocardial infarction. Note that *ischemia* does not equal *infarction*. If ischemia persists long enough to cause injury, the patterns of non-Q or Q wave infarction develop.

- Cigarette smoking
- Diabetes mellitus
- Family history of premature CAD <55
- Advanced age
- Males and post-menopausal women

Angina pectoris is a chronic, predictable pattern of substernal chest pain or uncomfortable sensation (pressure, squeezing, tightness, or burning) that occurs during physical exertion or emotional stress and is relieved by rest or nitrates within a few minutes. This discomfort can radiate to the neck, lower jaw, left shoulder, and left arm. It is often associated with diaphoresis, dyspnea, nausea, vomiting, or lightheadedness. Anginal symptoms typically last more than 15 seconds but less than 15 minutes.

Angina is considered unstable when it has one of the following three characteristics:

- New onset
- Has an increasing pattern: episodes are more frequent, last longer, or are not relieved by medications
- Produced by less exertion or while at rest

The symptoms of acute myocardial infarction may not be different from those of severe stable angina or unstable angina except the pain typically lasts longer.

PHYSICAL EXAMINATION

The physical exam can be normal. However, look for the following during your exam:

- Vital signs:
  - Tachycardia
  - Bradycardia
  - Hypertension
  - Hypotension (cardiogenic shock)
- Cardiac exam:
  - Systolic murmur (with papillary muscle or ventricular septal rupture)
  - S3 or S4 gallop (with decreased LV compliance)
  - Pericardial friction rub (with pericarditis)
- Pulmonary exam:
  - Bibasilar crackles or rales (with CHF)
- Neck exam: Jugular venous distention (with right ventricular MI)
- Extremities: pulse deficits, bruits, and lower extremity edema

DIFFERENTIAL

Life-threatening causes of chest pain:

- Acute myocardial infarct
- Aortic dissection

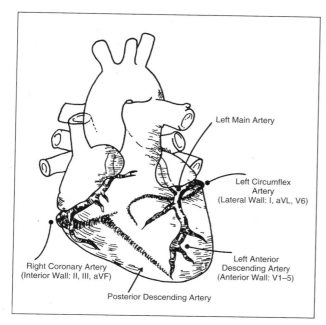

Figure 17–2 Coronary artery anatomy. The circumflex and right coronary arteries circle the heart in the atrioventricular groove; branches of the circumflex leave the groove to supply the lateral wall of the left ventricle. The major right coronary branch, the posterior descending artery, supplies the inferior wall. The anterior descending artery is located over the interventricular septum and sends branches into the septum and over the anterior wall of the left ventricle. The spatial orientation of the ECG leads allows groups of leads to be particularly sensitive to events in a given region of the heart (Table 17.1).

- Pulmonary embolus
- Pneumothorax
- Esophageal rupture

Other causes of chest pain include:

- Mitral valve prolapse
- Pericarditis
- Pneumonia
- Costochondritis
- Esophageal spasm

- Esophageal reflux
- Peptic ulcer disease
- Biliary colic
- Herpes zoster neuropathy

DIAGNOSTIC EVALUATION

In the emergency department, the ECG is the first test performed on patients having chest pain. Classic signs of myocardial ischemia include:

1. ST-segment depression
2. Symmetrically inverted T-waves

Classic signs of an acute MI are ST elevations of at least 1 mm in two continuous leads. Table 17–1 and Figure 17–2 help in determining localization of myocardial infarct. Figure 17–3 outlines the classic evolution of the typical Q-wave (transmural) MI. In the acute setting of a non-Q wave myocardial infarction, the ECG changes seen are more variable. There may be non-specific ST and T wave changes such as:

- Flat ST depressions
- T wave flattening or inversion.

Persistent T wave inversions can develop hours after a non-Q wave myocardial infarct. Repeat the ECG when the patient is pain free, looking for any transient changes. A chest x-ray is helpful in ruling out other causes of chest pain including pneumonia, pneumothorax, and widened mediastinum, suggesting aortic dissection. Lab studies include cardiac enzymes (CK, CK-MB fraction, and troponin I) coagulation profile (PT/aPTT), CBC, and electrolytes. Diagnosis of an AMI is based on a rise in cardiac enzymes and/or ECG changes with a clinical history suggestive of MI.

TREATMENT

Airway, breathing, and circulation should be addressed first. Patients should be placed on a monitor, pulse oximeter, blood pressure cuff, and have IV access. Treat life-threatening arrhythmias as well as hypotension and pulmonary edema. Immediate treatment of chest pain

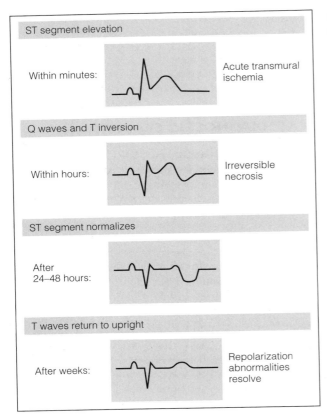

ST segment elevation

Within minutes: Acute transmural ischemia

Q waves and T inversion

Within hours: Irreversible necrosis

ST segment normalizes

After 24–48 hours:

T waves return to upright

After weeks: Repolarization abnormalities resolve

Figure 17–3   The changing pattern of the ECG in the affected leads during the evolution of myocardial infarction.

should begin with morphine, aspirin, nitroglycerin, and oxygen.

1. Oxygen by nasal canula at least at 2–4 L/min
2. Aspirin 160 mg–325 mg
3. Nitroglycerin (sublingual or spray)—dose is 0.4 mg every 5 minutes for continued pain unless systolic blood pressure <90
4. Morphine 2–4 mg IV if pain not relieved after 3 sublingual nitroglycerin tablets

Patients that have unstable angina or new-onset angina need to be admitted to a CCU or monitored bed and ruled out for myocardial infarction by serial enzymes. These patients should also receive:

- Beta blockers IV (propranolol, metoprolol)
- Heparin IV
- Nitroglycerin IV drip

Patients who have persistent symptoms, recurrent ischemia, depressed LV function or widespread ECG changes should go to cardiac catheterization if they are suitable for revascularization. Research is currently focusing on the glycoprotein IIb/IIIa inhibitors for the treatment of patients with unstable angina and myocardial infarction.

TABLE 17–1

Localization of Myocardial Infarction

EKG Changes (ST elevations, T wave inversions, or Q waves)	Area of Infarct	Artery Involved
II, III, aVF	Inferior	Right coronary artery
V1–V3	Anteroseptal	Left anterior descending
V2–V4	Anterior	Left anterior descending
I, aVL, V4, V5, V6	Lateral	Left circumflex artery
V1–V2	Posterior	Right posterior descending artery

- Tall R waves with ST depressions and tall upright T waves. This usually occurs in association with inferior MI.
- Obtain right-sided leads looking for ST elevations in V4R

TABLE 17–2

Contraindications to Thrombolytic Therapy

Absolute Contraindications	Relative Contraindications
• Active internal bleeding (excluding menses) • Hemorrhagic stroke at any time, or other CVA or TIA <1 year • Known intracranial tumor • Suspected aortic dissection • Diabetic retinopathy • Altered level of consciousness	• Severe uncontrolled hypertension (>180/110 mmHg) • Previous cerebrovascular accident (CVA) or other intracranial pathology • Non-compressible vascular punctures • Prolonged cardiopulmonary resuscitation (CPR) (>10 min) • Pregnancy • Active peptic ulcer disease • Recent trauma within 2 weeks • Major surgery within 3 weeks • Recent internal bleeding within 2–4 weeks • Current anticoagulation with INR 2–3 • Known bleeding diathesis • History of chronic severe hypertension • Prior streptokinase allergic reaction (should not give streptokinase)

The treatment of acute myocardial infarctions focuses on restoring blood flow and oxygen supply as rapidly as possible. Since most AMI are due to acute thrombosis within a coronary artery, the goal is to lyse the clot with thrombolytic agents such as t-PA and streptokinase. The goal is for patients to receive thrombolytics within 4 to 6 hours of symptom onset; however, benefit has been seen up to 12 hours. In the emergency department, treatment with thrombolytics should begin within 30 minutes of arrival. Any patient who is a candidate for thrombolytics but has a contraindication should be considered for immediate coronary angioplasty (Table 17–2). Emergent angioplasty is an alterna-

tive to thrombolytic therapy if treatment can occur within 60 minutes. Some patients require rescue angioplasty if thrombolytics fail to open the blocked vessel. Consider adjunctive treatments:

• Beta blockers—(metoprolol, atenolol) should be started on patients with AMI unless hypotension, bradycardia, or pulmonary edema is present
• Nitroglycerine IV
• Heparin IV

Thrombolytic agents are not part of the treatment of non-Q wave myocardial infarctions. However, these patients do benefit from nitrates and beta-blockers. In addition, they should also receive aspirin and heparin to help prevent further thrombus formation or extension. All patients with suspected myocardial infarction need to be admitted to either an intensive care unit or cardiac care unit.

Consider other causes of chest pain and acute myocardial infarctions, since ST elevation can also be seen with pericarditis, myocarditis, acute aortic dissection, acute cholecystitis, and pulmonary embolus. Table 17–3 outlines treatment options for acute coronary syndromes.

◆ KEY POINTS ◆

1. Risk factors for ischemic heart disease include hypertension, hyperlipidemia, smoking, diabetes mellitus, and a family history of premature CAD.

2. Unstable angina has one of the three following characteristics: new onset, increasing pattern (frequency/duration/severity), and angina at rest.

3. Acute thrombus or rupture of an atherosclerotic plaque is the most common cause of transmural MI.

4. Early administration of thrombolytic agents in the setting of AMI decreases mortality (door to drug <30 min).

5. Treat chest pain with morphine, aspirin, nitroglycerin, and oxygen.

6. Patients with unstable angina, new-onset angina, or potential AMI need to be admitted to a monitored bed.

TABLE 17–3

Treatments of Acute Coronary Syndromes

Treatment	Reason
Oxygen	• Increases the supply of oxygen to ischemic tissues
Aspirin	• Decreases platelet adhesiveness by blocking formation of thromboxane A2 • Studies show it decreases mortality and reinfarction after MI
Nitroglycerine	• Pain relief • Increases venous dilation, which lowers myocardial oxygen demand by diminishing venous return to the heart (preload) • Dilates coronary arteries and increases cardiac coronary flow
Morphine sulfate	• Pain relief • Reduces anxiety • Increases venous capacitance, which lowers myocardial oxygen demand by diminishing venous return to the heart (preload) • Decreases systemic vascular resistance, which lowers the force the myocardium contracts against in systole (afterload)
Beta-blockers (metoprolol, atenolol)	• Reduce myocardial work by decreasing the sympathetic drive to the myocardium (reduce HR and BP, thus reduce oxygen demand) • Decrease arrhythmias by decreasing catecholamine levels • Reduce myocardial contractility • Studies show they reduce the rate of reinfarction and recurrent ischemia • Do not give to patient with asthma, bronchospasm, or hypotension
Anticoagulants (heparin)	• Following thrombolytic therapy to maintain vessel patency • To prevent reinfarction if recurrent ischemia or unstable angina follows acute MI • To prevent thrombus formation when large regions of the LV have infarcted
Angiotensin converting enzyme (ACE) inhibitors	• Has been shown to limit infarct expansion if given in the first 24–48 hours
Thrombolytic therapy	• Dissolves the occluding thrombus and reopens the blocked artery
IIb/IIIa inhibitors (abciximab, eptifibatide, and tirofiban)	• Platelet glycoprotein IIb/IIIa receptor inhibitors block the final common pathway of platelet aggregation
Percutaneous transluminal coronary angioplasty (PTCA)	• Provides a method for mechanical reperfusion of the infarct-related artery (i.e., solves the true problem) • Provides an alternative method for patients who have contraindications to thrombolytic therapy • It provides the best outcome for patients with cardiogenic shock or pump failure • It provides the best outcome for patients with occluded vein grafts from coronary artery bypass

18 Congestive Heart Failure

Heart failure is the inability of the heart to pump blood adequately to meet the metabolic demands of the body. Since heart failure most commonly results from impaired left ventricular function, this chapter will only focus on left-sided heart failure. The hallmark of left heart failure is decreased effective cardiac output (CO). Left heart failure results in a backup of pressure and fluid behind the involved chamber causing abnormal fluid retention and pulmonary congestion, also known as congestive heart failure (CHF). Acute pulmonary edema is the most extreme form of left heart failure and is a life-threatening emergency.

ETIOLOGY

Heart failure may be the ultimate manifestation of almost every form of cardiac disease including:

- Coronary artery disease (myocardial ischemia or infarction)
- Hypertensive heart disease
- Cardiomyopathy (restrictive, dilated, and hypertrophic)
- Valvular heart disease
- Congenital heart disease
- Myocarditis
- Pericarditis

In addition, certain systemic diseases such as severe anemia, renal failure, and thyrotoxicosis can also cause CHF.

PATHOPHYSIOLOGY

There are two major mechanisms that cause heart failure.

1. Systolic dysfunction—due to impaired cardiac contractility (i.e., pump failure) with decreased ejection fraction.
2. Diastolic dysfunction—due to decreased compliance (i.e., relaxation) of the heart during ventricular filling with normal or supranormal ejection fractions.

There are three major compensatory mechanisms during heart failure.

1. Frank-Starling principle (as preload increases, the ventricle is stretched during diastole filling and the ejection fraction is increased)
2. Ventricular hypertrophy in response to LV dilation or high afterload
3. Neurohormonal activations in response to the fall in CO (adrenergic nervous system, renin-angiotensin system, and increased production of antidiuretic hormone [ADH])

These compensatory mechanisms are only temporarily effective and lead to increased myocardial work and worsening failure.

HISTORY

A detailed history, including any episodes of chest pain, previous episodes of heart failure, compliance or recent changes with medications, and dietary habits (i.e., excessive salt intake), should be addressed. The typical patient with CHF presents with:

- Dyspnea on exertion or at rest
- Decreased exercise tolerance
- Paroxysmal nocturnal dyspnea
- Orthopnea
- Ankle swelling and weight gain
- Nocturia
- Chest pain
- Nocturnal cough

PHYSICAL EXAMINATION

Common signs and symptoms include:

- Pulmonary rales
- Pleural effusion
- Pulmonary wheezes
- Tachypnea
- Tachycardia
- Hypotension
- Murmurs
- S3 or S4 gallop
- Cool extremities and cyanosis
- Lower extremity pitting edema
- Jugular venous distention

Differential diagnosis:

- Myocardial infarction
- Pulmonary embolism
- Cardiac tamponade
- COPD
- Constrictive pericarditis
- Pneumonia
- Pneumothorax
- Asthma
- Impacted foreign body
- Anaphylaxis

DIAGNOSIS

A chest x-ray may show cardiomegaly or pulmonary edema (plump vessels, interstitial or alveolar edema, and Kerley B lines). Obtain an ECG, looking for signs of ischemia, infarction, dysrhythmias, pericarditis, atrial or ventricular hypertrophy. Lab studies include CBC, electrolytes, CK, CK-MB, troponin, and digoxin level.

TREATMENT

For patients in respiratory distress, a trial of continuous positive airway pressure (CPAP) may help avoid intubation. Patients in severe respiratory distress who are hypoxic or unstable may need intubation and aggressive support until pulmonary edema is cleared. Keep patient sitting upright on stretcher if possible. Place Foley catheter to monitor urine output. The treatment goal is to reduce LV preload or filling pressure and ultimately increase myocardial contractility (i.e., CO) or decrease afterload. Medical treatment of CHF consists of:

1. Loop diuretics: Furosemide 20–40 mg IV q 30 minutes, may repeat several times, doubling dose each time if no response.
2. Morphine: 1–4 mg IV, repeat q 5–10 minutes for effect.
3. Oxygen: High-flow O_2 by mask, CPAP by mask and intubation.
4. Nitroglycerine: Sublingual NTG 0.4 mg × 3. May consider IV NTG if systolic BP >100.
5. Pressors: Dopamine IV if systolic blood pressure <100 or dobutamine if systolic BP >100 if in need of inotropic (pump) support.

Table 18–1 discusses the management of CHF and pulmonary edema.

Dialysis may be needed for patient with renal failure. When evaluating disposition, consider the following:

TABLE 18–1

Treatment of CHF and Pulmonary Edema

Treatment	Mechanism
Loop diuretics (furosemide)	• Decrease preload: — Decrease venous tone and increase venous capacitance — Cause diuresis
Morphine	• Decreases preload: — Dilates the capacitance vessels of peripheral venous bed reducing venous return to central circulation • Decreases afterload: — Mild arterial vasodilation
Nitroglycerine	• Decreases preload: — Dilates venous capacitance vessels inhibiting venous return to the heart. • Decreases afterload: — Decreases systemic vascular resistance and facilitates cardiac emptying
Oxygen	• Increases arterial PO_2 and causes pulmonary vasodilation • Nonrebreather masks with reservoirs can provide 100% O_2 • Continuous positive airway pressure (CPAP) can be applied during • spontaneous respirations with a tight-fitting mask to help prevent alveolar collapse and improve gas exchange • Intubation if patient cannot maintain adequate oxygenation despite 100% O_2 delivery or if signs of cerebral hypoxia (lethargy or obtundation) • Positive end-expiratory pressure (PEEP) can be used to prevent alveolar collapse and improve gas exchange
Position: place patient in sitting position with legs dependent	• Increases lung volume and vital capacity • Decreases work of respirations and venous return to the heart
Pressors (dopamine, dobutamine)	• Dopamine (pressure too low): If acute pulmonary edema with signs and symptoms of shock and initial SBP <100. • Dobutamine (normotensive pump failure): If acute pulmonary edema with SBP >100
Dialysis	• Decreases intravascular volume • Useful in renal patients when diuretics are ineffective
Digoxin: for patient with CHF and atrial fibrillation	• Slows the conduction through the AV node (controls rate) • Increases both the force and velocity of myocardial contraction (increases pump function)
Nitroprusside: for patients with hypertension as cause of pulmonary edema	• Vasodilates both arteriolar and venous beds

- Patients with new-onset CHF or pulmonary edema need to be admitted to the hospital either to ICU or a monitored bed.

- Patients with chronic CHF and mild worsening of symptoms that respond well to IV diuretics in the ED may be discharged home after consultation with a primary care physician. These patients often need adjustments in their chronic drug regimen, and close follow-up within 24 to 48 hours.

- Chronic CHF patients with more severe symptoms or other complicating factors (e.g., new dysrhythmias or suspected ischemia) should be admitted for observation, evaluation, and adjustments in drug regimen.

◆ KEY POINTS ◆

1. Heart failure is the inability of the heart to pump blood forward to meet metabolic demands either from pump failure or impaired LV filling.

2. Congestive heart failure is caused by an elevation of end-diastolic volume and pressure that is transmitted to the left atrium, pulmonary veins, and capillaries resulting in pulmonary congestion and edema.

3. The most common presenting symptom of CHF is shortness of breath.

4. Treatment of CHF and pulmonary edema involves loop diuretics, morphine, nitroglycerine, oxygen, and pressors.

5. Successful treatment of heart failure requires identifying and treating the underlying cause and eliminating precipitating factors.

19

Infective Endocarditis

Infective endocarditis (IE) is a condition characterized by infection of the endocardium and heart valves. The spectrum of disease varies from a smoldering infection to one of acute onset frank sepsis.

EPIDEMIOLOGY

There are several well-established risk factors for the development of IE (Table 19–1). The epidemiology of IE has changed over the past several years as rheumatic heart disease has become less common and the incidence of HIV infection and intravenous drug use has increased. Intravenous drug users are especially prone to the development of right-sided IE (infection of the pulmonic or tricuspid valve) secondary to injection of non-sterile material into the venous circulation.

PATHOPHYSIOLOGY

The initial inciting event in the development of endocarditis is bacteremia (bacteria in the bloodstream). Endocarditis results when bacteria adhere to the relatively avascular tissue of the cardiac valves and set up infection. Although endocarditis can occur on healthy valve tissue, it is much more common when the valve tissue has been "roughed up" due to congenital or acquired valve disease. Once the valves are infected, a vegetation slowly develops. Vegetations are friable masses of bacteria, fibrin, and white cells that remain relatively isolated from the immune system due to the avascular nature of valve tissue. Throughout the course of the disease, they seed the bloodstream and cause episodes of transient bacteremia. These masses can also break off and embolize, causing many of the clinical signs and symptoms of IE.

Organisms known to cause IE include *Streptococcus viridans*, *Staphylococcus aureus*, enterococcus, and the HACEK group of organisms (*Haemophilus* spp., *Actinobacillus actinomycetemcomitans*, *Cardiobacterium hominis*, *Eikenella* spp., *Kingella kingae*). For unclear reasons, *Streptococcus bovis* has been associated with inflammatory lesions of the colon including carcinoma and inflammatory bowel disease.

HISTORY

Patients with IE may present in a myriad of ways. Fever, altered mental status, and frank sepsis are common. Patients may complain of dyspnea when acute valve dysfunction results in congestive heart failure. Stroke, gangrenous extremities, or mesenteric ischemia can also be presenting complaints reflecting embolic phenomena. A subset of patients will present in complete heart block due to a perivalvular abscess.

PHYSICAL EXAMINATION

The physical exam in patients with IE should focus on the cardiac dysfunction that results from infection as

TABLE 19–1

Risk Factors for the Development of Infective Endocarditis

1. Intravenous drug abuse
2. Structural heart abnormality such as bicuspid aortic valve
3. Prior history of infective endocarditis
4. Prosthetic heart valve
5. Prior history of rheumatic heart disease
6. HIV infection

TABLE 19–2

Duke Criteria for the Diagnosis of Infective Endocarditis

Major Criteria
1. Persistently positive blood cultures
2. Positive blood cultures for microorganism known to cause endocarditis
   — *Streptococcus viridans*
   — *Streptococcus bovis*
   — HACEK group
   — *Staphylococcus aureus* or *enterococci*
3. Positive echocardiogram for endocarditis
   — oscillating vegetation on a cardiac valve
   — intracardiac abscess
   — valve dehiscence of a prosthetic valve
4. New heart murmur

Minor Criteria
1. Predisposing condition (heart valve abnormality or IVDA)
2. Fever greater than 38.0°C on two separate occasions
3. Vascular phenomena: stroke, Janeway lesions, splinter hemorrhages, mycotic aneurysms, major arterial emboli
4. Immunologic phenomena: Roth's spots, Osler's nodes, positive rheumatoid factor, glomerulonephritis
5. Positive blood cultures not meeting major criteria
6. Positive echocardiogram not meeting major criteria

HACEK: *H*aemophilus spp., *A*ctinobacillus actinomycetemcomitans, *C*ardiobacterium hominis, *E*ikenella spp., *K*ingella kingae
IVDA: Intravenous Drug Abuse

well as evidence of embolic events. Tachycardia and fever are common, except in the case of complete heart block where bradycardia predominates. The fundi should be examined for Roth's spots, which are small white spots on the retina surrounded by hemorrhage. Cardiac exam typically reveals a new murmur of mitral regurgitation or aortic insufficiency depending on the valve involved. Tenderness on abdominal exam may indicate emboli to the viscera. Examination of the extremities classically reveals splinter hemorrhages, Osler's nodes, or Janeway lesions. Splinter hemorrhages are linear hemorrhages under the finger or toenails and represent microemboli. Osler's nodes are small tender lesions that form on the fat pads of the fingers or toes and represent immune complex deposition. Janeway lesions are painless, reddish macular lesions on the hands or feet.

DIFFERENTIAL DIAGNOSIS

- Sepsis
- Tuberculosis
- Congestive heart failure
- Acute myocardial infarction
- Stroke
- Mesenteric ischemia
- Meningitis

DIAGNOSTIC EVALUATION

The diagnosis of IE is based on the findings of persistent bacteremia and endocardial involvement (Table 19–2). Three sets of blood cultures from separate venipuncture sites should be obtained prior to institution of antibiotics. An EKG should be obtained to screen for the presence of conduction abnormalities. Patients with suspected IE should also undergo echocardiography.

TREATMENT

In the acute setting, the treatment of IE should focus on stabilization of the hemodynamic status and institution of appropriate empiric antibiotics. Nafcillin and gentamycin are appropriate first-line empiric agents. Further therapy should be guided by culture results and treatment continued for at least 4 weeks.

◆ KEY POINTS ◆

1. Intravenous drug abuse is associated with right-sided endocarditis.

2. The classic physical findings of IE include Janeway lesions, Roth's spots, Osler's nodes, and splinter hemorrhages.

3. The Duke criteria are used to diagnose suspected cases of IE.

4. At least 4 weeks of antibiotics are required for the treatment of IE due to the relatively avascular nature of cardiac valve tissue.

20 Venous Thromboembolic Disease

Deep venous thrombosis (DVT) is thrombus formation in the deep veins of the pelvis, upper extremities, or lower extremities (e.g., iliac, femoral, or popliteal veins). DVT is a common complication of patients hospitalized with either medical or surgical conditions.

ETIOLOGY

There are three major factors that contribute to the formation of deep venous thromboembolism, known as Virchow's triad:

1. Venous stasis
2. Vessel injury
3. Hypercoagulable states

Table 20–1 summarizes conditions that alter the balance of these factors.

HISTORY

A thorough history is required, including risk factors for DVT (see Table 20–1), family history, and previous episodes. Signs of DVT:

- Pain in extremity
- Swelling or edema in extremity
- Tenderness in extremity
- Discoloration or erythema in extremity

PHYSICAL EXAMINATION

The physical exam in DVT can be completely normal. Common signs of DVT include:

- Palpable venous cord
- Homan's sign (pain behind the knee on forceful dorsiflexion of foot)
- Unilateral edema or swelling (greater than 1.5 cm circumferential difference in extremity is significant)
- Subcutaneous venous distention
- Warmth

DIFFERENTIAL DIAGNOSIS

- Superficial thrombophlebitis
- Cellulitis
- Ruptured Baker's cyst
- Muscle or ligament injury
- Lymphedema
- Bilateral edema (liver, heart, or kidney disease)

TABLE 20–1

Conditions That Alter the Balance of DVT Formation Factors

Etiology	Risk Factors
Stasis	• Prolonged bed rest, paralysis, and/or other immobilization.
	• Long plane or train ride
	• Congestive heart failure
	• Obesity
	• Pregnancy
Vessel injury	• Trauma
	• Surgery
	• Central lines
	• Previous history of DVT or PE
	• Vasculitis
Hypercoagulable state	• Malignancy
	• Deficiency of antithrombin III, protein C, or protein S
	• Increased estrogen: oral contraceptives or pregnancy
	• Antiphospholipid antibodies
	• Ulcerative colitis
	• Nephrotic syndrome
	• Sepsis

DIAGNOSTIC EVALUATION

The clinical exam is unreliable for the diagnosis or exclusion of DVT. The most common method for evaluating a DVT in the emergency department is the Duplex ultrasound, which is noninvasive, highly sensitive, and specific. Venography is considered the gold standard test. However, it is invasive and often not available in the emergency department. Lab studies include CBC, PT, and PTT.

TREATMENT

Treatment of DVT should be initiated as soon as the diagnosis is made, with either IV unfractionated heparin or low molecular weight heparin. The heparin infusion rate is adjusted to maintain the partial thromboplastin time (PTT) at 1.5 to 2.0 times the control.

The benefits of LMWH include the fact that there is no need to monitor the anticoagulation effect, it is easier to administer, it has a longer half-life, and it has a lower incidence of major bleeding complications. Patients will require several months (typically 3 to 6 months) of anticoagulation and are started on warfarin (coumadin) once they are therapeutically anticoagulated with heparin.

An inferior vena caval (IVC) filter should be considered for DVT when there is an absolute contraindication to anticoagulation (active internal bleeding, uncontrolled hypertension, CNS tumor, recent trauma or surgery, or recurrent DVT despite adequate anticoagulation).

In extreme cases, thrombolytic therapy and thrombectomy are indicated for the treatment of DVT.

Most patients with DVT are admitted to the hospital for initial anticoagulation. However, outpatient management of DVT without PE is possible using LMWH.

◆ KEY POINTS ◆

1. Venous stasis, vessel injury, and hypercoagulable states (i.e., Virchow's triad) are the three major factors that contribute to formation of DVT.

2. Signs of DVT include palpable venous cord, Homan's sign, unilateral edema or swelling, and warmth.

3. Duplex ultrasound is the most common method for evaluating DVT in the emergency department.

4. Treatment of proximal DVT may include heparin, warfarin, or low molecular weight heparin.

5. IVC filters are used for patients with recurrent DVT despite adequate anticoagulation or patients with contraindication to anticoagulation.

21

Hypertensive Emergencies

A hypertensive emergency consists of an elevated blood pressure with signs of end-organ damage to the brain, eyes, heart, or kidney (e.g., acute myocardial infarction, unstable angina, acute renal failure, intracranial bleeds, and acute left-ventricular failure). End-organ damage typically occurs when diastolic pressure exceeds 115 to 130 mmHg. Table 21–1 lists the types of hypertensive emergencies.

ETIOLOGY AND PATHOPHYSIOLOGY

Certain factors can predispose patients to hypertensive emergency (Table 21–2). Elevations in blood pressure can cause arterioles to dilate and increase capillary bed pressure, leading to fluid leakage into the tissues. The elevated pressure causes injury to the endothelium leading to fibrin deposition, activation of coagulation mediators, and cell proliferation. Fibrinoid necrosis of small arteries is the pathologic change responsible for end-organ damage. The major organ systems affected are the cardiovascular system, renal system, ophthalmologic system, and central nervous system.

Hypertensive encephalopathy occurs when the normal cerebrovascular autoregulation system is overwhelmed by an acute rise of blood pressure, resulting in vasospasm and brain edema.

In the cardiovascular system, acute elevations in blood pressure cause an increase in left ventricular wall tension leading to myocardial ischemia or infarction. In addition, sudden increase in end-diastolic volume can lead to acute heart failure and pulmonary edema.

In the kidneys, an elevation in blood pressure impairs the protective autoregulation mechanisms and decreases renal perfusion, stimulating the renin-angiotensin system and causing vasoconstriction. The vasoconstriction further reduces renal blood flow leading to acute renal failure, worsening renal function, proteinuria, hematuria, or cast formation.

The eyes are affected by elevations in blood pressure as flame-shaped hemorrhages occur around the optic disk due to high intravascular pressure. In addition, ischemic infarction of the nerve fibers can occur from occlusion of the supplying arterioles (cotton-wool spots). Papilledema is also a common finding from increased intracranial pressure due to acute elevations in blood pressure or due to infarction and hypoxia of the optic disk.

HISTORY

A thorough history is important, especially past history and current medications. Does the patient have a history of hypertension? What is their usual baseline reading?

TABLE 21–1

Hypertensive Emergencies

Type of Emergency	Definition	Symptoms	Signs
Hypertensive encephalopathy	• Abrupt, sustained rise of blood pressure that exceeds the normal cerebrovascular autoregulation and results in brain edema	• Severe headache • Vomiting • Drowsiness • Confusion • Seizures • Visual changes • Blindness • Focal neurologic deficits • Coma	• Blood pressure— diastolic >130 mmHg • Altered mental status • Papilledema

Malignant hypertension	• Severe hypertension associated with evidence of acute and progressive end-organ damage
	• Untreated can lead to:
	  1. Acute renal failure
	  2. Cardiac decompensation
	  3. MI
	  4. Hypertensive cerebral hemorrhage
	  5. Hypertensive encephalopathy
		• Severe headache
		• Blurred vision
		• Dyspnea
		• Chest pain
		• Nocturia
		• Weakness
			• Blood pressure— diastolic >130 mmHg
			• Left ventricular enlargement
			• Rales
			• Retinal findings: Linear hemorrhages, cotton wool spots, papilledema

Are they compliant with their medications? Is there a history of illicit drug use (i.e., cocaine)? Is the patient taking any over-the-counter medications? Are there any symptoms of end-organ damage?

- CNS symptoms: headache, confusion, nausea, vomiting
- Ophthalmic symptoms: blurred vision, diplopia
- Cardiac symptoms: chest pain, dyspnea, palpitations
- Renal symptoms: nocturia, hematuria, oliguria, pedal edema, weakness

PHYSICAL EXAMINATION

Patients with hypertension in the emergency department should have their blood pressure rechecked in both arms to confirm an elevation. The physical exam should focus on signs of end-organ damage.

- Neurologic exam: focal deficits, mental status changes, seizure, coma
- Funduscopic exam: hemorrhages, cotton-wool spots, papilledema
- Cardiovascular exam: carotid bruits, murmurs, extra heart sounds (S3 or S4), tachycardia, rales, jugular venous distention, peripheral edema

DIFFERENTIAL DIAGNOSIS

- Transient hypertension
- Pseudohypertension

TABLE 21–2

Predisposing Factors to Hypertensive Emergencies and Urgencies

Causes	Example
Renal system abnormalities	• Acute glomerulonephritis • Acute renal failure
Cardiovascular abnormalities	• Acute coronary insufficiency • Acute aortic dissection • Accelerated hypertension • Myocardial infarction • Unstable angina
Central nervous system	• Subarachnoid hemorrhage • Intracranial hemorrhage • Thrombotic infarction • Encephalopathy • Head trauma • Transient ischemic attacks
Excessive catecholamine states	• Pheochromocytoma • Monoamine oxidase inhibitor interactions • Antihypertensive medication withdrawal
Drugs	• Cocaine • Amphetamines • Oral contraceptives • Corticosteroids
Pregnancy	• Preeclampsia

- Subarachnoid hemorrhage
- Intracerebral hemorrhage
- Cerebral infarction
- Acute myocardial ischemia or infarction
- Acute pulmonary edema
- Aortic dissection
- Preeclampsia or eclampsia
- Withdrawal syndromes (beta-blockers, clonidine, alcohol)
- Catecholamine excess

DIAGNOSTIC EVALUATION

Most studies are directed for evaluation of end-organ damage, and include:

- ECG: evidence of ischemia, infarction, LVH
- CXR: pulmonary edema or aortic dissection
- Urinalysis: proteinuria, microscopic or gross hematuria, red cell casts
- CBC: microangiopathic hemolytic anemia, thrombocytopenia, and increased fibrin degradation products
- Electrolytes: elevated BUN and creatine, hypokalemia
- Glucose: hypoglycemia can elevate blood pressure
- Head CT in patients with neurologic symptoms to rule out stroke or hemorrhage

TREATMENT

The goal of lowering blood pressure is to prevent end-organ damage. Care must be taken not to lower the blood pressure too quickly, especially in patients with history of poorly controlled hypertension. Treatment usually consists of lowering the blood pressure by 25%. A safe goal is to bring the diastolic blood pressure down to 100 to 110 mmHg over several hours. Reducing blood pressure too quickly can cause cerebral or coronary insufficiency. Nitroprusside is usually the drug of choice for hypertensive emergencies. It is given as an IV drip and titrated to desired blood pressure control. It is contraindicated in pregnancy. Labetalol is commonly used as an alternative agent to nitroprusside. Table 21–3 shows the agents used in hypertensive emergencies.

Hypertension is usually treated with oral medications. Typical agents include beta-blockers, nifedipine, clonidine, and captopril. It is safe to reduce the blood pressure to a diastolic between 105 and 110 mmHg.

All patients with hypertensive emergencies (malignant hypertension or hypertensive encephalopathy) require admission to an intensive care unit.

TABLE 21–3

Agents Used for Hypertensive Emergencies

Agent	Indications	Contraindications
Nitroprusside	• Malignant hypertension • Hypertensive encephalopathy • Aortic dissection (with beta-blocker)	• Pregnancy
Labetalol	• Malignant hypertension • Hypertensive encephalopathy • Aortic dissection	• Beta-blockers
Diazoxide	• Malignant hypertension • Hypertensive encephalopathy • Pregnancy-induced hypertension • Preeclampsia or eclampsia	• Aortic dissection • Acute MI
Phentolamine	• Agent of choice for excess Catecholamine states: 1. Pheochromocytoma 2. MAO inhibitor reactions 3. Cocaine or other stimulants 4. Antihypertensive withdrawal	
Hydralazine	• Eclampsia	
Nitroglycerine	• Myocardial ischemia • Congestive heart failure	

◆ KEY POINTS ◆

1. A hypertensive emergency consists of an elevated blood pressure (DBP >115–130) with signs of end-organ damage.

2. Nitroprusside and labetalol are the treatment of choice in hypertensive emergencies.

3. Hypertension is are typically treated with oral agents such as beta-blockers, clonidine, nifedipine, and ACE inhibitors.

22 Acute Aortic Dissections

An aortic dissection occurs when there is a longitudinal splitting of the arterial wall from a defect in the intimal layer. Dissections can extend distally, proximally, or both.

Complications of aortic dissection include cardiac tamponade, aortic insufficiency, CHF, hemothorax, hemoperitoneum, aortic arterial branch occlusion leading to ischemia (e.g., myocardial infarction or intestinal, renal and lower limb ischemia), and sudden death.

ETIOLOGY AND EPIDEMIOLOGY

Most cases of aortic dissection occur between the ages of 50 and 70. However, they can present in younger age groups with certain predisposing conditions (e.g., Marfan's syndrome). Dissections are twice as common in men as in women. Risk factors for aortic dissection are included in Table 22–1.

PATHOPHYSIOLOGY

Aortic dissections occur from defects in the intimal layer that allow blood under pressure to enter the media and dissect between the layers of the intima and adventitia. The cause of the actual defect in the intima is unclear; however, hypertension is thought to play a significant role. Common sites of tears include fixed areas with a significant amount of stress applied during systole, including the ascending aorta, and between the origin of the left subclavian artery and the ligamentum arteriosum.

The Stanford classification divides dissections into type A (involving ascending aorta) and type B (involving the descending aorta).

HISTORY

The most common presenting symptom of a thoracic aortic dissection is the sudden severe onset of "tearing or ripping" chest pain that radiates to the back or between the scapula. This pain may migrate as the dissection propagates. Patients may also present with:

- Syncope
- Neurologic findings (i.e., hemiplegia, paraplegia, cranial nerve deficits)
- Hoarseness (laryngeal nerve compression)
- Dyspnea with wheezing or stridor (tracheal compression)
- Dysphagia (compression of esophagus)
- Gastrointestinal symptoms (nausea, vomiting, epigastric pain)
- Flank pain
- Lumbar pain

PHYSICAL EXAMINATION

Patients may present with hypertension or hypotension. Check for differences in blood pressures and pulses in

TABLE 22–1

Risk Factors for Aortic Dissection

- Hypertension
- Connective tissue diseases (Marfan's syndrome, Ehlers-Danlos syndrome)
- Bicuspid aortic valve
- Coarctation of the aorta
- Inflammatory diseases of the aorta (syphilitic aortitis, endocarditis, giant cell arteritis, systemic lupus)
- Atherosclerosis
- Smoking
- Pregnancy

the extremities. Look for signs of shock (e.g., cool, diaphoretic skin and decreased level of consciousness) even in the presence of hypertension. On cardiac exam, listen for a diastolic murmur of aortic insufficiency (acute aortic insufficiency indicates dissection into the aortic root), pericardial friction rub, or muffled heart sounds with cardiac tamponade. Look for signs of congestive heart failure (e.g., rales and elevated JVD). On neurologic exam, look for deficits due to involvement of the carotid or spinal arteries. Patients may have hemiplegias, cranial nerve deficits, or a decreased level of consciousness.

DIFFERENTIAL DIAGNOSIS

- Myocardial infarction
- Unstable angina
- Pericarditis
- Pulmonary embolus
- Pneumonia
- Cholelithiasis or cholecystitis
- Pneumothorax
- Esophagitis or esophageal spasm
- Musculoskeletal chest wall pain

DIAGNOSTIC EVALUATION

An electrocardiogram should be obtained to rule out other causes of chest pain, and for signs of preexisting hypertension (i.e., left ventricular hypertrophy). ECG abnormalities consistent with MI can be seen with dissections in 10 to 20% of patients. The most common abnormality seen on chest x-ray is a widened mediastinum. Other chest x-ray abnormalities include obliteration of the aortic knob, deviation of the trachea or esophagus to the right, left hemothorax, and depressed left mainstem bronchus.

Evaluation of an aortic dissection can be performed with CT scan, transesophageal echocardiogram (TEE), MRI, or angiography. CT scan with contrast is commonly used, as it is often the most easily obtainable. TEE can be performed quickly at the bedside, identifying the type of dissection and valvular involvement. MRI is useful, but often limited by availability and hemodynamic instability of the patient. Aortography is still considered the "gold standard" test but is also the most invasive of all the radiographic studies.

TREATMENT

Patients who are hypotensive due to aortic rupture or cardiac tamponade should receive IV fluids and blood transfusions. Unstable patients should receive an immediate vascular surgery consult. For hypertensive patients, the goal of therapy is to maintain systolic blood pressure between 100 and 120 mmHg and limit the progression of the dissection. Control blood pressure with sodium nitroprusside combined with IV beta-blockers. Labetalol is an alternative agent used because it has both alpha and beta blockade properties. In addition, morphine or other narcotics should be given to control pain.

Definitive treatment of ascending aortic dissection (Stanford type A) requires surgical management, while uncomplicated descending aortic dissections (Stanford type B) are usually treated medically (i.e., blood pressure control). However, patients with descending dissections who fail medical management with persistent pain, uncontrolled hypertension, major arterial trunk occlusions (i.e., intestinal, renal, or extremity ischemia) or who develop localized aneurysm require surgical repair.

◆ KEY POINTS ◆

1. Aortic dissection is a longitudinal splitting of the arterial wall from a defect in the intimal layer.

2. Classically, patients present with sudden onset of "tearing or ripping" chest pain that radiates to the back.

3. CXR may show a widened mediastinum.

4. Diagnosis is made by TEE, contrast CT, MRI, or aortogram.

5. Treatment is typically with sodium nitroprusside combined with IV beta-blockers.

23 Abdominal Aortic Aneurysms

An aneurysm is an abnormal dilation of the wall of an artery and is usually twice the normal diameter of the vessel. A true aneurysm involves all three layers of the vessel wall (intima, media, and adventitia). Abdominal aortic aneurysms (AAA) are the most common type and are typically located below the renal arteries.

ETIOLOGY

Risk factors of aortic aneurysms include:

- Atherosclerosis
- Advanced age
- Hypertension
- Smoking
- Connective tissue diseases (Marfan syndrome)
- Familial history of aneurysm
- Hyperlipidemia
- Diabetes

PATHOPHYSIOLOGY

Destruction of the media is an important factor in the pathogenesis of aneurysm formation. Both elastin and collagen are dramatically reduced in the walls of the aneurysm. The combination of risk factors and force on the aorta walls by arterial pressure leads to dilation. As the aorta dilates it creates a greater force on the aortic wall, leading to further dilation. The natural progression of an aneurysm is gradual expansion and eventual rupture.

HISTORY

Most patients with abdominal aneurysms are asymptomatic but may present with a dull constant abdominal, low back, or flank pain. A symptomatic aneurysm typically indicates that the aneurysm has ruptured, is rapidly expanding, or is otherwise complicated by a dissection. Patients with a ruptured AAA often present with syncope and severe, tearing abdominal pain that radiates to the back.

PHYSICAL EXAMINATION

A pulsatile abdominal mass is the classic finding on physical exam of a ruptured AAA. Patients may also have abdominal tenderness or abdominal bruits. Patients may present with hypotension but they can also initially be hemodynamically stable. Blood from a ruptured AAA can also track along the skin and produce ecchymosis in different areas (e.g., flank, scrotum, or anterior abdominal wall).

DIFFERENTIAL DIAGNOSIS

- Renal colic
- Hemorrhagic pancreatitis
- Mesenteric infarction
- Diverticulitis
- Perforated viscus
- Biliary colic
- Bowel obstruction
- Acute MI
- Musculoskeletal back pain
- Lumbosacral disc disease

DIAGNOSTIC EVALUATION

A plain abdominal radiograph may show an arch of calcification of the aortic wall or paravertebral soft tissue mass. An ultrasound is the ideal test, especially in unstable patients, as it is extremely accurate for making the diagnosis of an AAA and measuring its diameter. However, it is not as sensitive in determining whether an AAA has ruptured. An abdominal CT will demonstrate both aneurysmal size and site of rupture, either intraperitoneal or retroperitoneal.

TREATMENT

Patients who present with ruptured AAA who are hemodynamically unstable require immediate surgery and fluid resuscitation. If available, bedside ultrasound should be done to confirm quickly or exclude an aneurysm. In general, hemodynamically unstable patients in whom rupture is confirmed or strongly suspected should go directly to the operating room without waiting for further diagnostic tests or stabilization. An abdominal CT should be used for further diagnostic studies in hemodynamically stable patients when an AAA cannot be identified by ultrasound.

Patients with asymptomatic AAA found on routine exam or radiologic studies should be referred to a vascular surgeon for further evaluation and possible elective repair.

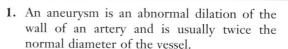

◆ KEY POINTS ◆

1. An aneurysm is an abnormal dilation of the wall of an artery and is usually twice the normal diameter of the vessel.

2. Classic presentation of ruptured abdominal aortic aneurysm (AAA): hypotensive, syncope, back pain, and a pulsatile abdominal mass.

3. Symptomatic, hemodynamically stable patients should have prompt surgical consultation and bedside ultrasound or CT scan.

4. Hemodynamically unstable patients with ruptured AAA require immediate surgical intervention.

24 Pericarditis/ Tamponade

Pericarditis is inflammation of the pericardial sac that surrounds the heart. A pericardial effusion may be present.

EPIDEMIOLOGY AND ETIOLOGY

The most common cause of pericarditis is idiopathic. However, other causes include infectious, neoplastic, connective tissue diseases, cardiac injury, and certain drugs. Table 24–1 contains the causes of acute pericarditis.

PATHOPHYSIOLOGY

The pericardium consists of a visceral layer that surrounds the epicardium and a parietal layer, which surrounds the heart. Normally, the pericardium contains 15–50 ml of fluid. Inflammation can develop in the pericardium due to local and systemic disease processes. Cardiac tamponade is a life-threatening complication of pericarditis.

HISTORY

Patients typically present with sharp, pleuritic (i.e., worsened with cough or inspiration), chest pain that is often positional. The pain is usually worse lying down and relieved sitting up and leaning forward. Other common symptoms include dyspnea, cough, and fever.

PHYSICAL EXAMINATION

On cardiac exam, listen for pericardial friction rub, best heard with patient leaning forward. Look for signs of cardiac tamponade including muffled heart sounds, jugular venous distention, and hypotension (i.e., Beck's triad). Pulsus paradoxus (i.e., fall in systolic BP >15 mmHg with inspiration) may be present with large pericardial effusion or tamponade.

DIFFERENTIAL DIAGNOSIS

- Acute MI
- Cardiac tamponade
- Congestive heart failure
- Pulmonary embolus
- Aortic dissection
- Pneumonia
- Pneumothorax
- Cholecystitis
- Pancreatitis

DIAGNOSTIC EVALUATION

Classic findings seen on ECG include diffuse ST segment elevation in all leads or P-R segment depres-

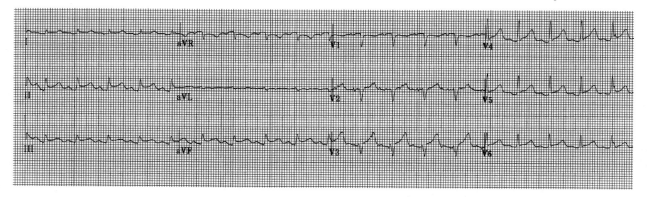

Figure 24–1   Acute pericarditis.

TABLE 24–1

Causes of Acute Pericarditis

Cause	Example
Idiopathic (most common)	
Infectious	• Viral (coxsackievirus, echovirus, HIV) • Bacterial (*Staphylococcus*, *Streptococcus pneumoniae* and beta-hemolytic, *Mycobacterium tuberculosis*) • Fungal (*Histoplasma capsulatum*) • Parasitic
Neoplastic	• Metastatic disease (lung, breast) • Radiation induced • Lymphoma • Leukemia • Melanoma
Connective tissue diseases	• Systemic lupus erythematosus • Scleroderma • Rheumatoid arthritis
Drugs	• Procainamide • Hydralazine • Methyldopa
Cardiac injury	• Post MI-Dressler's syndrome • Post surgical • Post instrumentation • Cardiac trauma • Aortic dissection
Systemic diseases	• Uremia • Amyloidosis • Inflammatory bowel disease • Pancreatitis

sion (Fig. 24–1). Low voltage and electrical alternans (beat to beat change in QRS amplitude) may be seen with large pericardial effusions.

A CXR is often normal but can show an enlarged cardiac silhouette suggestive of pericardial effusion (>250 ml of fluid). It can also help rule out other causes of chest pain including pneumothorax, aortic dissection, or pneumonia.

Echocardiography can help confirm the diagnosis. In tamponade, it may show diffuse hypokinesis with diastolic collapse of the right atrium and ventricle. In addition, pericardiocentesis can be performed and fluid can be sent for gram stain, culture, cytology, glucose, and protein. Lab studies that may be helpful include CBC, electrolytes, ESR (elevated), and cardiac enzymes.

TREATMENT

First assess ABCs. Next, patients should be placed on a cardiac monitor, pulse oximeter, and supplemental oxygen. In addition, IV access, a 12-lead ECG, and CXR should be obtained.

Unstable patients with suspected cardiac tamponade should have ultrasound-guided pericardiocentesis. IV fluids may help while setting up for emergent pericardiocentesis. If ultrasound is not immediately available and patient is hemodynamically unstable, blind pericardiocentesis may be necessary.

Patients with idiopathic, viral, rheumatologic, and post-traumatic pericarditis are usually treated with nonsteroidal antiinflammatory drugs (i.e., aspirin, ibuprofen, or indomethacin). Bacterial pericarditis is treated with drainage and IV antibiotics. Patients with uremic pericarditis usually require dialysis. Patients with neoplastic causes of pericarditis require treatment of the underlying malignancy.

Hemodynamically unstable patients require admission to the ICU for close monitoring. Young patients with mild symptoms who are hemodynamically stable can be safely discharged with close follow-up. An echocardiography should be obtained prior to discharge to evaluate pericardial effusion.

◆ **KEY POINTS** ◆

1. Pericarditis is inflammation, infection, or infiltration of the pericardial sac.

2. Classic symptoms include sharp, pleuritic chest pain that is relieved by sitting up and leaning forward.

3. A pericardial friction rub can be heard on auscultation.

4. Classic ECG findings show diffuse ST elevations in all leads and PR depression.

5. Pericarditis is typically treated with nonsteroidal antiinflammatory drugs.

6. Cardiac tamponade is a complication of pericarditis.

25 Occlusive Arterial Disease

Acute occlusion of an artery by a thrombus or embolus is a true emergency. Immediate therapy is required to save the affected limb.

ETIOLOGY

In approximately 80 to 90% of cases, thromboembolism originating from the heart (e.g., atrial fibrillation) is the cause of acute arterial occlusion. The most frequent location of embolization is lower extremities in areas of bifurcation or vessel tapering. Table 25–1 outlines the etiologies of acute arterial occlusion.

PATHOPHYSIOLOGY

Ischemia is caused by sudden loss of blood supply to meet the metabolic needs of the tissue. If ischemia is prolonged, it eventually leads to irreversible damage and cell death.

HISTORY AND PHYSICAL EXAMINATION

The classic signs and symptoms of patients presenting with acute arterial occlusion include the six "Ps":

- Pain
- Paralysis
- Pallor
- Paresthesia
- Poikilothermia (coolness)
- Pulselessness

DIFFERENTIAL DIAGNOSIS

- Neurologic (nerve entrapment or disc disease)
- Chronic peripheral vascular disease
- Arthritis
- Compartment syndrome
- Diabetic neuropathy pain
- Lumbar spine disorders
- Venous thrombosis
- Frostbite
- Muscle strains
- Fractures and sprains

DIAGNOSTIC EVALUATION

Acute arterial occlusion is predominantly a clinical diagnosis. A hand-held Doppler can document the absence or presence of flow to the affected limb. Other studies include:

- Duplex ultrasound
- ECG (myocardial infarction or atrial fibrillation)

TABLE 25–1

Etiology of Acute Arterial Occlusion

Cardiac Causes of Emboli
- Cardiac arrhythmias (atrial fibrillation)
- Recent myocardial infarction (wall motion abnormality and thrombus formation)
- Tumor emboli from atrial myxomas
- Endocarditis (vegetations from valves)

Noncardiac Sources of Emboli
- Atheromatous plaques
  1. Acute occlusion from plaque rupture, hemorrhage, or thrombus formation.
  2. Cholesterol debris and platelet aggregates usually occlude the microcirculation (i.e., blue toe)
- Thrombi from aneurysms
- Hypercoagulable states
- Vessel injury
- Invasive procedures (i.e., catheters and balloon angioplasty)
- Trauma
- Vasospastic conditions (i.e., Raynaud disease)
- Inflammatory conditions (i.e., collagen vascular diseases: lupus, polyarteritis nodosa)
- Aortic dissection (false lumen can occlude flow in the involved artery)

- Echocardiography (detect intracardiac thrombus or valvular vegetations)
- Angiography

MANAGEMENT

After assessment of ABCs, emergent consultation with a vascular surgeon should be obtained. Next, if there are no contraindications to anticoagulation, start IV heparin to prevent further clot extension or recurrent emboli. For limb-threatening ischemia due to acute occlusion, emergent surgical embolectomy is the treatment of choice. An alternative option to surgery for patients with distal thromboembolic occlusions is intraarterial thrombolysis (i.e., streptokinase, urokinase, or t-PA). Bypass grafting and angioplasty are usually reserved for patients with chronic arterial disease due to atherosclerotic plaques.

 KEY POINTS

1. Remember the "six Ps" of acute arterial occlusion: Pain, Pallor, Paralysis, Poikilothermia, Paresthesia, and Pulselessness.

2. Start heparin in patients without contraindications to anticoagulation.

3. Surgical embolectomy is the treatment of choice for acute arterial occlusion.

26 Pulmonary Embolism

Pulmonary embolism (PE) is the occlusion of pulmonary arteries by the embolization of thrombi, air, fat, or other particulate matter. The most common cause of PE is deep venous thrombosis (95%).

HISTORY

A thorough history is required, including risk factors for DVT (see Table 20–1), family history, and previous episodes. Signs of PE are usually sudden in onset and include:

- Dyspnea
- Chest pain (pleuritic—increased with respiration)
- Cough
- Hemoptysis
- Syncope
- Anxiety

PHYSICAL EXAMINATION

The physical exam in patients with PE can be completely normal. Common signs of PE include:

- Rales or wheezes
- Tachycardia (HR >100)
- Tachypnea (RR >16)

- Low-grade fever (<101°F)
- Loud P2
- S3 or S4 gallop
- Cyanosis
- Diaphoresis

DIFFERENTIAL DIAGNOSIS

- Acute myocardial ischemia or infarction
- Pneumothorax
- Pneumonia
- Rib fracture
- Asthma
- Pericarditis
- Musculoskeletal pain
- Pulmonary edema

DIAGNOSTIC EVALUATION

An electrocardiogram (ECG) should be the first study in patients suspected of having a PE, since it may help rule out other causes of chest pain. The most common finding in patients with PE is sinus tachycardia and nonspecific ST-T wave changes. Other ECG findings in patients with PE include: a right-sided strain pattern with an S wave in lead I, a Q wave and T wave inversion in lead III (S1 Q3 T3), right axis deviation, a new right bundle branch block, T wave inversions in anterior leads (v1–v4).

A chest x-ray may help to rule out other causes of chest pain. Chest x-ray findings suggestive of PE include atelectasis, pleural effusions, elevated hemidiaphragm, Westermark's sign (oligemia in the embolized lung zone), or Hampton's hump (wedge-shaped pleural based density).

Lower extremity ultrasound can be used to evaluate for DVT. An arterial blood gas (ABG) may show hypoxemia, hypocapnia, and respiratory alkalosis. D-dimer, which is a fibrin degradation product, is a serum marker of fibrinolysis (breakdown of blood clots) and may be helpful in combination with other noninvasive tests in evaluating DVT or PE. Echocardiography may show right ventricular dilatation and can be performed in unstable patients at the bedside. A radionuclide ventilation-perfusion (V/Q) scan is used to identify areas of mismatch (ventilated but not perfused) that is suggestive of PE. Spiral computed tomography (CT) can also be used to evaluate for PE.

The gold standard for evaluation of PE is the pulmonary angiogram. A negative PA Gram study excludes the diagnosis of a PE. Pulmonary arteriography should be done when the clinical suspicion for PE is high but other studies are inconclusive.

TREATMENT

Airway, breathing, and circulation should be addressed first. Patients should receive intravenous access, supplemental oxygen, cardiac monitoring, ECG, and a chest x-ray. Hypotensive patients should be treated with IV fluids and pressors as indicated. Unstable patients in shock or significant respiratory distress should be assessed for thrombolytic therapy. Thrombolytic therapy has almost completely replaced embolectomy for the treatment of massive PE with hemodynamic compromise.

Treatment of PE should be initiated once the diagnosis is confirmed. Begin treatment with either IV unfractionated heparin or low molecular weight heparin (LMWH). Patients who have a high clinical suspicion of PE without contraindications for anticoagulation should be started on heparin while awaiting diagnostic tests.

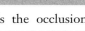

◆ KEY POINTS ◆

1. Pulmonary embolism (PE) is the occlusion of the pulmonary artery. The most common cause of PE is a DVT.

2. Symptoms of PE include dyspnea, chest pain, cough, hemoptysis, and syncope.

3. Signs of PE include rales, tachycardia, tachypnea, and low-grade fever.

4. The gold standard test for pulmonary embolism is the pulmonary angiogram.

5. Anticoagulation with heparin is the mainstay of treatment for PE.

Part IV
Pulmonary
Emergencies

SIGNS AND SYMPTOMS

Dyspnea—The Feeling of Breathlessness:

- Bronchitis/tracheitis
- Upper airway obstruction
- Myocardial infarction
- Congestive heart failure
- Myocarditis
- Pericarditis
- Pericardial effusion
- Pulmonary embolism
- Asthma
- COPD
- Pneumonia

Hemoptysis:

- Tuberculosis
- Bronchiectasis
- Bacterial pneumonia
- Pulmonary aspergillosis
- Lung cancer
- Pulmonary embolism
- Spurious hemoptysis-GI bleeding
- Nasopharyngeal bleeding

27 Pneumonia

Pneumonia is an infection of the lungs by bacteria, virus, or fungus. Despite advances in antimicrobial treatment, pneumonia remains the sixth most common cause of death in the United States and the most common infectious cause of death. Pneumonia is especially deadly in patients at the extremes of age (children and the elderly).

common pathogen in cases of community-acquired pneumonia, causing 20–60% of cases.

Viral causes of pneumonia are influenza A and B, respiratory syncytial virus, adenovirus, parainfluenza 1 and 3, cytomegalovirus, herpes simplex virus, varicella virus, and the hantavirus.

ETIOLOGY

The etiology of community-acquired pneumonia has changed in recent years, reflecting not only an increase in elderly patients, but the effects of HIV (human immunodeficiency virus) and AIDS (acquired immunodeficiency syndrome). Other host factors that impact prognosis are diabetes mellitus, renal failure, chronic obstructive lung disease, alcoholism, congestive heart failure, liver failure, malignancy, and prior antibiotic use.

Bacterial pneumonias have traditionally been divided into "typical" and "atypical" pathogens. Typical organisms include *Streptococcus pneumoniae, Staphylococcus aureus, Haemophilus influenzae,* and *Pseudomonas aeruginosa.* Atypical pneumonias are caused by *Mycoplasma pneumoniae, Chlamydia pneumoniae,* and *Legionella pneumoniae* (Table 27–1). Polymicrobial infections are often seen in cases of aspiration pneumonia. In these instances, oral anaerobes such as *Bacteroides* sp., peptostreptococci, or *Fusobacterium* sp., are the most likely pathogens. *Streptococcus pneumoniae* remains the most

HISTORY

Classically, patients with pneumonia present with fever, chills, cough, sputum production, dyspnea, and pleuritic chest pain. Some pneumonias present with gastrointestinal symptoms such as nausea, vomiting, and abdominal pain. Other useful historical points include sick contacts and travel history, as well as the presence of any of the comorbidities listed above.

PHYSICAL EXAMINATION

Patients with pneumonia frequently are tachypneic (respiratory rate >30), tachycardic, and febrile. These signs combined with hypotension, evidence of extrapulmonary infection (i.e., meningitis), or altered mental status are associated with increased morbidity and mortality. Patients with pneumonia will present with signs of lower respiratory tract infection.

- Tactile fremitus (vibratory tremors felt on palpation of the chest wall)

TABLE 27–1

Characteristics of "Classic" Pneumonia Syndromes

Organism	H&P	Sputum GS	Chest Radiograph	Therapy	Prevention
Streptococcus pneumonia	Extremes of age, rusty sputum	Lancet-shaped gram-positive diplococci	Lobar consolidation	PCN, macrolide, FQ	Pneumovax
Staphylococcus aureus	Post influenza virus, IVDA	Gram-positive cocci in clusters	Lobar consolidation or cavitary	PCN, vancomycin	
Haemophilus influenzae	Smoking, COPD	Encapsulated gram-negative rods	Lobar consolidation	PCN, macrolide, cephalosporin	HiB vaccine
Pseudomonas aeruginosa	Nursing home	Gram-negative rods	Patchy lower lung consolidations	Aminoglycoside, ceftazidime	
Klebsiella pneumoniae	Alcoholics, COPD	Encapsulated gram-negative rods	Lobar consolidation	Aminoglycoside, cefazolin	
Legionella pneumoniae	Cooling systems, COPD, alcoholics	Gram-negative rods	Bilateral patchy infiltrates	Erythromycin, rifampin	
Mycoplasma pneumoniae	Young, healthy	No organisms	Bilateral interstitial infiltrates	Erythromycin, tetracycline	

PCN: penicillin; FQ: fluoroquinolone; IVDA: intravenous drug abuse; COPD: chronic obstructive pulmonary disease

- Dullness to percussion
- Egophony (change in the sound of the spoken letter "e" to an "a" sound over the area of consolidation)
- Rales (crackling sounds in the area of consolidation)

Many patients will have evidence of pleural effusion manifested as decreased breath sounds at the lung bases with dullness to percussion.

DIFFERENTIAL DIAGNOSIS

- Bronchitis
- Pharyngitis
- Sinusitis
- Pulmonary embolism
- Congestive heart failure
- Lung cancer
- Wegener's granulomatosis
- Sarcoidosis

DIAGNOSTIC EVALUATION

Simple chest radiographs are usually sufficient to establish the diagnosis of pneumonia in most cases. Radiographs typically show consolidations or infiltrates in a lobar pattern (typically bacterial infections) or diffuse patchy infiltrates (viral or atypical).

A complete blood count (CBC) typically shows an elevated white blood cell count with either a left shift (predominance of segmented neutrophils and bands) in bacterial pneumonia or a right shift, defined as a lymphocytic predominance, indicating a viral etiology.

Sputum Gram stain is advised in most cases of community-acquired pneumonia and can help guide initial empiric therapy despite the fact that the microbiologic cause is identified in only 50% of cases. Sputum culture is advocated in all hospitalized patients with the caveat that fastidious organisms and oral colonization often make culture results difficult to interpret. Organisms isolated from a sterile site (i.e., blood, pleural fluid, CSF, urine) can be considered etiologic agents in the setting of disease.

TREATMENT

Once a community-acquired pneumonia is diagnosed, the first step in treatment is deciding whether the patient will be admitted to the hospital. Though there are no firm guidelines for which patients require admission, there are well-established historical, physical exam, and laboratory findings that predict a more complicated course.

Historical risk factors that predict an increase in morbidity and mortality from community-acquired pneumonia include:

- Age >65 years
- Coexisting chronic illness
  - Diabetes mellitus
  - End-stage renal disease
  - Congestive heart failure
  - End-stage liver disease
  - History of splenectomy
  - Alcoholism

Physical exam findings that predict an increase in morbidity and mortality include:

- Hypotension
- Fever >101°F
- Respiratory rate greater than 30
- Altered mental status
- Hypoxia (oxygen saturation <90)

Laboratory findings portending a poor outcome include:

- White blood cell less than 4 or greater than 30
- Abnormal renal function (creatinine >1.2 or blood urea nitrogen of >20)
- Multilobar involvement on chest radiograph
- Hematocrit of <30

Initial empiric inpatient therapy for community-acquired pneumonia normally includes a third-generation cephalosporin such as ceftriaxone, a macrolide such as azithromycin and vancomycin if there is concern for penicillin-resistant *Streptococcus pneumoniae*. Outpatient therapy for community-acquired pneumonia usually consists of a macrolide such as clarithromycin or azithromycin or a fluoroquinolone such as levofloxacin.

◆ KEY POINTS ◆

1. Pneumonia remains the leading infectious cause of death in the United States.
2. The most common cause of community-acquired pneumonia is *Streptococcus pneumoniae*.
3. The diagnosis of pneumonia can be made through history, physical exam, and chest radiography.
4. Initial empiric therapy is based on patient characteristics and sputum Gram stain.

28 Pneumothorax

A pneumothorax is an abnormal collection of air in the pleural space. Spontaneous pneumothoraces occur without antecedent trauma. A spontaneous pneumothorax may become a tension pneumothorax if air can enter the pleural space during inspiration but not escape during expiration.

EPIDEMIOLOGY

Classically, spontaneous pneumothoraces occur most commonly in tall, thin men during their 20s and 30s. Height is thought to increase risk for spontaneous pneumothoraces due to an increase in the negative pressure generated at the lung apices. Smokers are almost 20 times more likely to suffer a spontaneous pneumothorax compared with non-smokers. Recurrences are common, with 20–50% of patients suffering a second pneumothorax during their lifetime.

PATHOPHYSIOLOGY

The majority of spontaneous pneumothoraces are caused by rupture of a subpleural bleb resulting in free communication of air between the atmosphere and the pleural space. As air rushes into the pleural space, the lung collapses. Lung collapse results in ventilation-perfusion mismatch as blood flows past the unventilated lung. As the size of the pneumothorax increases, so does the degree of hypoxemia. Activities that increase intrathoracic pressure, such as screaming, coughing, or the Valsalva maneuver (i.e., smoking marijuana), also increase the risk of pneumothorax. Patients with chronic obstructive pulmonary disease (COPD), pneumonia, tuberculosis, asthma, lung cancer, sarcoidosis, and connective tissue diseases such as Marfan's syndrome or Ehlers-Danlos syndrome are at increased risk for pneumothorax.

HISTORY

Classically, pneumothorax presents with the acute onset of dyspnea and ipsilateral pleuritic chest pain. The pain is described as sharp and stabbing and often worsens with inspiration.

PHYSICAL EXAMINATION

Patients with an acute spontaneous pneumothorax may present with tachypnea, tachycardia, and decreased breath sounds on the side of the pneumothorax. The affected hemithorax will be hyperresonant to percussion and subcutaneous air may be palpated in the chest wall in some instances. Hypotension, tracheal deviation, and elevated jugular venous pressure indicate that a simple pneumothorax has progressed to a life-threatening tension pneumothorax.

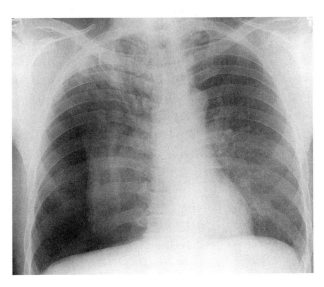

Figure 28–1   Right pneumothorax: there are no visible markings beyond the lung edge.

DIFFERENTIAL DIAGNOSIS

- Myocardial infarction
- Pericarditis
- Aortic dissection
- Pulmonary embolism
- Pleuritis
- Pneumonia
- Herpes zoster
- Costochondritis
- Gastroesophageal reflux disease
- Pancreatitis
- Biliary colic

DIAGNOSTIC EVALUATION

The diagnosis of a spontaneous pneumothorax is made when a suggestive history and physical examination is confirmed by evidence of a pneumothorax on a chest radiograph. Radiographically, a pneumothorax is suggested by hyperlucency and lack of pulmonary vascular markings at the lung periphery (Fig. 28–1). Additionally, a thin line representing the visceral pleura may be visualized. If a standard chest radiograph fails to demonstrate a suspected pneumothorax, expiratory films may be obtained. During expiration, the air in the pleural space cannot be exhaled; thus the affected hemithorax cannot decrease in volume to the same degree as the normal lung.

TREATMENT

Treatment for small pneumothoraces (defined as those involving less than 15% of the volume of a hemithorax) in otherwise healthy patients is conservative. Patients may be admitted to the hospital for observation; the air in the pleura is reabsorbed at a rate of 2% per day. Alternatively, patients may be discharged home with close follow-up and careful instructions. Larger pneumothoraces, or those in patients with underlying comorbidities such as COPD or ischemic heart disease, are usually treated with needle or tube thoracostomy. In needle thoracostomy, a catheter is introduced into the pleural space and air aspirated. If simple aspiration fails, the plastic catheter can be attached to a suction device or water seal and used as a chest tube. Tube thoracostomy is a similar procedure using a chest tube. The tube is left in place until the underlying air leak into the pleural cavity resolves. Most patients requiring needle or tube thoracostomy are hospitalized.

In the event a tension pneumothorax is suspected, immediate needle decompression should occur—even before radiographic studies are obtained. Needle decompression involves inserting a 14-gauge intravenous catheter into the pleural space at the level of the second intercostal space, midclavicular line. This is followed promptly by tube thoracostomy.

Despite adequate treatment, many patients with spontaneous pneumothoraces will suffer a recurrence. Prevention of recurrences is aimed at removal of remaining lung blebs and avoidance of high-risk behaviors.

◆ **KEY POINTS** ◆

1. Spontaneous pneumothoraces occur in tall, thin males in their 20s and 30s and are more common in smokers.

2. Spontaneous pneumothoraces must be rapidly distinguished from the potentially fatal tension pneumothorax.

3. Tension pneumothorax is characterized by hypotension, tracheal deviation, and elevated jugular venous pressures.

4. Treatment of a pneumothorax involves aspiration of air from the pleural cavity by either needle or tube thoracostomy.

29 Asthma

Asthma is a disease of the lower airways characterized by acute exacerbations followed by symptom-free intervals of varying lengths. Although effective treatments for asthma exist, it still is a potentially fatal condition.

EPIDEMIOLOGY

Asthma is a chronic disease occurring in 4–5% of the population. The incidence is highest among African-American males especially those living in Southern inner cities. Over 66% of all new cases of asthma are diagnosed in patients less than 40 years of age.

PATHOPHYSIOLOGY

The hallmarks of asthma are chronic airway inflammation, heightened bronchial reactivity, and mucus production. Asthmatic patients have an exaggerated response to inflammatory stimuli or triggers such as:

- Viral or *Mycoplasma* infections
- Inhaled allergens such as dusts, molds, or pollen
- Perfumes
- Temperature or humidity changes
- Exercise
- Emotional upset
- Drugs, including NSAID (aspirin, ibuprofen), beta-blockers (atenolol, metoprolol), tartazine dye (yellow dye number 5)

These irritants result in the accumulation of inflammatory cells, especially eosinophils, and excess mucous production that results in airway narrowing. The inflammatory response may be so pronounced that luminal plugs form (so-called Curschmann spirals).

HISTORY

The presentation and clinical course of an asthma attack can vary from mild dyspnea (the feeling of breathlessness) to full respiratory arrest. If not in extremis, patients may complain of dyspnea, wheezing, mucus production, and cough, often worsening at night. Important aspects in assessing the severity of an attack include a history of past hospitalizations, ICU admissions, or intubations. The duration of symptoms may also hold prognostic value, as some attacks smolder over days and weeks, while others occur in minutes to seconds.

PHYSICAL EXAMINATION

The acute asthmatic will show signs of respiratory distress with tachypnea and tachycardia. The patient may be hypoxic (room air saturation <90%). Examination of the chest wall may reveal signs of accessory muscle use and retractions. Auscultation of the lungs may reveal wheezes with a prolonged expiratory phase of the respiratory cycle. Due to the inability to completely exhale, the patient may show evidence of hyperinflation with an increased anterior-posterior diameter. Severe asthmatics may show signs of a pulsus paradoxus, which is defined as a greater than 10 mm Hg decrease in the systolic blood pressure during inspiration. A "quiet chest," due to markedly limited air movement, may be a sign of impending respiratory failure.

DIFFERENTIAL DIAGNOSIS

- Chronic obstructive pulmonary disease
- Congestive heart failure
- Pulmonary embolus
- Pneumonia
- Upper airway obstruction

DIAGNOSTIC EVALUATION

The mainstay of diagnostic testing in asthmatic patients is measurement of peak expiratory flow rates or PEFR (L/min). This simple, non-invasive test can be used to measure severity of an asthma attack as well as response to therapy. Hand-held devices are available in most emergency departments and can be given to patients. Reliable measurements require adequate patient effort.

Pulse oximetry is useful in most patients. Arterial blood gas (ABG) analysis should be reserved for only the most severe asthmatic patients. Early in an attack, ABG values may be normal or the patient may exhibit a respiratory alkalosis (hypocapnia) from hyperventilation. As the work of breathing increases and the respiratory muscles begin to tire, a respiratory acidosis with hypercapnia develops. Hypoxia is a late and ominous finding in the asthmatic patient. In the known asthmatic with a mild to moderate attack, routine chest radiographs are unnecessary. If obtained, they will show hyperinflation with concomitant flattening of the diaphragms. Chest radiographs are most useful if the patient has a fever, comorbid disease, or complications of asthma (pneumothorax, pneumomediastinum, or pneumonia) are suspected.

TREATMENT

Treatment of an acute asthma attack is directed at reducing the bronchoconstriction and inflammation that are the hallmarks of the disease. Supplemental oxygen should be given to all patients to maintain oxygen saturations greater than 90%. Beta-2 agonists, such as albuterol, should be given via nebulizer or metered dose inhaler (MDI). These agents produce bronchodilation by acting on beta-2 adrenergic receptors in the airways and provide quick symptomatic relief in most patients.

Aerosolized anticholinergic drugs such as atropine and ipratropium bromide are effective in reversing the vagal mediated bronchoconstriction of the larger central airways. Due to the significant systemic side effects of atropine, ipratropium bromide is now the most widely used nebulized anticholinergic medication.

Corticosteroids are indicated for the control of inflammation. In the acute phase of an asthma attack, steroids should be given orally (prednisone 40–60 mg) or parenterally (methylprednisolone 60–120 mg). Steroids take 6 to 8 hours to reach maximum effectiveness; thus they must be used in concert with beta-2 agonists in the acute setting.

The use of intravenous theophylline, once a mainstay of treatment, has decreased since the advent of the inhaled beta-2 agonists. Magnesium sulfate (1–2 grams IV) is being used frequently for severe asthma flares. Magnesium is helpful due to its bronchodilatory effects.

◆ KEY POINTS ◆

1. Asthma is a chronic inflammatory disease of the lower airways characterized by acute exacerbations.

2. Symptoms of an asthma attack include wheezing, dyspnea, and tachypnea.

3. A "quiet chest" is worrisome for respiratory failure.

4. Peak expiratory flow rates are useful to define the severity of an asthma attack as well as monitor response to therapy.

5. Treatment of asthma revolves around reducing bronchoconstriction with beta-2 agonists and controlling inflammation with corticosteroids.

30 Chronic Obstructive Pulmonary Disease

Chronic obstructive pulmonary disease (COPD) is a term that refers to two clinical conditions, emphysema and chronic bronchitis, whose final common pathway is airway outflow obstruction. Emphysema is a condition defined pathologically as dilation of the air space distal to the terminal bronchiole with destruction of the interalveolar septa. Chronic bronchitis refers to the condition of excess mucus production and productive cough occurring for at least 3 months a year for 2 consecutive years.

EPIDEMIOLOGY

The American Thoracic Society estimates that there are 14 million persons in the United States that are suffering from COPD. The number of patients with chronic bronchitis outnumbers those with emphysema by a factor of 10. Overall, COPD is more common in men than in women, though the number of women with the disease is increasing. Over 80,000 people a year die as a result of COPD, making it the fourth leading cause of death in the United States. Smoking is by far the most important predisposing factor in the development of COPD. Pipe and cigar smokers are more likely to develop COPD than non-smokers, though the rates are less than those of cigarette smokers. Age of starting, total number of pack-years (number of packs of cigarettes per day multiplied by the years of smoking), and current smoking status influence the subsequent risk of developing COPD.

Other less common factors include environmental exposure to asbestos, air pollution, and possibly second-hand smoking. People with cystic fibrosis or a hereditary deficiency of the enzyme alpha-1 antitrypsin are predisposed to the development of COPD, though these conditions cause less than 1% of the total number of cases.

PATHOPHYSIOLOGY

Changes in the lung parenchyma in patients with emphysema occur over the course of years. As the lungs lose their elastic recoil, the normal alveolar architecture is replaced by giant bullae. Pathologically, the emphysematous changes that occur in the lung can be separated into centriacinar, panacinar, and paraseptal varieties. In centriacinar emphysema, lung destruction begins in the respiratory bronchioles and spreads outward towards the periphery. It predominantly affects the upper lung zones and is the type of emphysema associated with cigarette smoking. Panacinar emphysema involves the whole acinus and involves the lower half of the lungs. It is the type associated with alpha-1 antitrypsin disease. Paraseptal emphysema involves the distal airway structures and alveolar sacs and often results in the giant bullae that cause spontaneous pneumothoraces.

Whether due to cigarette smoking or alpha-1 antitrypsin deficiency, the final common pathway in emphysema is a reduction in the elastic recoil of the lung parenchyma resulting in an increase in the physiologic "dead space." In addition, there is an increased propensity of the airway to collapse during expiration causing airway outflow obstruction.

The primary pathologic lesion in chronic bronchitis is hypertrophy of the mucous-producing glands of the lung. These changes are coupled with airway inflammation and hypertrophy of the airway smooth muscle, with the end result being outflow obstruction. Whether emphysema or chronic bronchitis predominates, the physiologic changes that occur are similar. Airflow obstruction leads to chronic ventilation-perfusion mismatch (blood flowing past unaerated lung) and hypoxia. Over time, the vasoconstrictive effects of hypoxia result in pulmonary hypertension. Chronic pulmonary hypertension causes the right ventricle to hypertrophy and eventually dilate and fail, resulting in the clinical condition known as cor pulmonale.

HISTORY

Emphysema presents insidiously with progressive dyspnea, usually without a prominent cough. Shortness of breath occurs first only with exertion but then progresses to dyspnea with minimal exertion and finally to dyspnea at rest. Cyanosis and clubbing (bulbous enlargement of the distal fingers and nails associated with chronic cyanosis) occur as the disease progresses and many patients become dependent on supplemental oxygen. Symptoms of cor pulmonale are late findings.

Patients with chronic bronchitis frequently will give a history of a chronic, productive cough that is worse in the mornings and in the winter months (the so-called "smoker's cough"). Patients may report varying degrees of hemoptysis. As the disease progresses, patients begin to have symptoms year round and often have multiple yearly exacerbations triggered by a viral upper respiratory infection or "chest" cold. Dyspnea, cyanosis, and exercise intolerance occur late in the course of the disease and can significantly limit activity.

PHYSICAL EXAMINATION

The physical examination of a patient with emphysema typically reveals a thin, barrel-chested person in varying degrees of respiratory distress. Tachypnea is prominent and use of accessory respiratory muscles common. If severe hypercarbia is present, the patient may present with altered mental status. The chest is typically hyper-resonant to percussion and may reveal wheezes or basilar rales. The hallmark of emphysema is a prolonged expiratory phase as the patient attempts to exhale against the airway obstruction. Focal lung findings may indicate a superimposed pneumonia. Patients in severe distress often have an ominously quiet chest due to the inability to "move" enough air to auscultate. Heart sounds are distant.

The patient with chronic bronchitis is often obese and the lung exam notable for coarse rhonchi reflecting the inability to clear increased secretions. Examination of the heart may reveal signs of right heart failure (S3 and S4). Heart failure may also present with peripheral edema and signs of fluid overload.

DIFFERENTIAL DIAGNOSIS

- Acute myocardial infarction
- Congestive heart failure
- Cardiogenic shock
- Asthma
- Pneumonia
- Pulmonary embolism
- Foreign body aspiration
- Lung cancer

DIAGNOSTIC EVALUATION

The gold standard for the evaluation of the severity of COPD is spirometry. These measurements serve not only as a diagnostic tool, but can gauge the response to therapy as well. The measurements of interest are the forced vital capacity (FVC), forced expiratory volume in 1 second (FEV_1), and the FEV_1/FVC ratio.

- FVC is the air that can be expired following maximal inspiration.

- FEV_1 is the fraction of the vital capacity that can be exhaled during the first second.

- FEV_1/FVC is the ratio of the two measurements expressed as a percentage.

In the acute setting, FEV_1 is the most useful measurement because it is easily measured and is less variable than other spirometric values. Knowledge of a patient's age, height, and gender allows for the prediction of normal values for comparison. Studies have also shown that FEV_1 values correlate with mortality. Patients with FEV_1 values greater than 1.0 liter have a slightly higher mortality when compared with age- and gender-matched controls. Patients with FEV_1 less than 0.75 liter have a 1-year mortality rate of 30% and a 10-year mortality rate of 95%.

Chest radiographs are generally not useful in un-complicated COPD exacerbations unless complications such as pneumonia or pneumothorax are suspected. If obtained, they classically show hyperinflated lungs with paucity of vascular markings and flattened diaphragms. An electrocardiogram is useful to rule out conditions with similar presenting symptoms or may show evidence of multifocal atrial tachycardia, which is the classic arrhythmia associated with COPD. Arterial blood gas measurements are generally only useful in the critically ill patient. If obtained, they will reveal hypoxemia without hypercarbia early in the disease course. As the patient's clinical condition worsens, hypoxemia becomes more severe and is coupled with varying degrees of hyper-carbia. Complete blood counts may reveal a reactive erythrocytosis or leukocytosis if pneumonia is present.

TREATMENT

Therapy for an acute COPD flare differs depending on the severity of the attack. All patients should be given supplemental oxygen, placed on a monitor and have an IV established. Supplemental oxygen can vary from nasal cannula to endotracheal intubation and mechanical ventilation depending on the clinical presentation.

Beta-2 agonists such as albuterol cause bronchodilation. Care must be taken in patients with COPD and concomitant coronary artery disease because the tachycardia that may result from albuterol administration may precipitate an acute coronary syndrome. Albuterol is often combined with the inhaled anticholinergic medication ipratropium bromide. Ipratropium acts by reversing the vagal mediated bronchoconstriction of the larger central airways.

Oral theophylline has bronchodilatory properties and may enhance respiratory mechanics. Serum levels must be monitored due to the potential for toxicity (nausea, vomiting, palpitations, seizures).

Corticosteroids benefit many COPD patients with acute exacerbations and are given either orally (prednisone 60–80 mg) or parenterally (methylprednisolone 60–120 mg). Due to their delayed onset of action, steroids must be used in concert with other therapies. Finally, if clinical suspicion for pneumonia exists, then appropriate therapy with antibiotics should be initiated based on the most likely pathogens. Specifically, antibiotic coverage should include *Streptococcus pneumoniae*, *Haemophilus influenzae* and *Moraxella catarrhalis*.

 KEY POINTS

1. COPD is a chronic condition that includes two disease entities: emphysema and chronic bronchitis.

2. Smoking is the major risk factor for the development of COPD.

3. The pathologic changes of COPD result in airway outflow obstruction.

4. FEV_1 provides a useful diagnostic tool and also can be used to gauge response to therapy.

Part V
Gastrointestinal Emergencies

SIGNS AND SYMPTOMS

Abdominal Pain:
- Myocardial infarction
- Pneumonia
- Peptic ulcer disease
- Small bowel obstruction
- Mesenteric ischemia
- Pancreatitis
- Biliary colic
- Cholecystitis
- Diverticulitis
- Appendicitis
- Pelvic inflammatory disease
- Ovarian torsion
- Ectopic pregnancy
- Abdominal aortic aneurysm
- Renal colic
- Pyelonephritis

Hematemesis—The Vomiting of Blood:
- Esophageal varices
- Mallory-Weiss tear
- Peptic ulcer disease
- Esophagitis

Melena—Tarry, Black Stools Formed by the Digestion of Blood in the Gastrointestinal Tract:
- Esophageal varices
- Mallory-Weiss tear
- Peptic ulcer disease
- Dieulafoy lesion
- Arteriovenous malformation
- Diverticulosis (including Meckel's diverticulum)

Bright Red Blood Per Rectum:
- Hemorrhoids
- Colon cancer
- Diverticulosis
- Arteriovenous malformation
- Inflammatory bowel disease
- Rectal trauma

31 Gastrointestinal Bleeding

Gastrointestinal bleeding (GIB) is the common clinical endpoint of a myriad of conditions that range from massive hematemesis associated with ruptured esophageal varices to occult blood loss associated with colon carcinoma. The exact etiology of GIB is not always readily apparent and because of the potential for catastrophic results, it should be considered a life-threatening problem.

ETIOLOGY

Lesions that produce GIB can be divided into upper and lower tract processes (Table 31–1). Upper GIB refers to bleeding proximal to the ligament of Treitz while lower GIB occurs distal to this point. Depending on the source of bleeding, patients may present with hematemesis, melena, or hematochezia. Hematemesis is the vomiting of blood. Brisk bleeding of recent onset will be bright red while blood that has been partially digested by stomach acid will have the appearance of coffee grounds. Melena refers to the black, tarry, malodorous stool that occurs when blood has been in the digestive tract for some time. Hematochezia is bright red blood per rectum. Although classic teaching holds that hematemesis and melena indicate an upper source while hematochezia results from lower GIB, brisk upper GIB can cause hematochezia while a slow ooze from a lower source can produce melena.

Risk factors for the development of GIB include use of NSAID (non-steroidal anti-inflammatory drugs), chronic anticoagulation, steroid use, or alcohol abuse.

HISTORY

The history should focus on the circumstances surrounding the episode of bleeding. Severe vomiting prior to bleeding is indicative of a Mallory-Weiss tear. A long history of gastroesophageal reflux that has recently worsened might point towards a gastric or duodenal ulcer. Weight loss and a change in stool caliber are worrisome for colorectal cancer. Complaints of "weakness or lightheadedness" when arising from a lying or seated position may indicate significant GIB. A careful medication history is also essential and should focus on NSAID and anticoagulant use.

PHYSICAL EXAMINATION

Patients with significant GIB will show signs of hypovolemic shock manifested by tachycardia and/or hypotension. Altered mental status, postural drops in blood pressure, or an increase in the pulse rate also indicate significant blood loss. A thorough examination of the nose and throat should be conducted to look for potential sources of swallowed blood that may mimic a GIB. The abdomen should be examined for the presence of a surgical process with emphasis placed on the presence of peritoneal signs (rebound and involuntary guarding). A rectal examination with fecal occult blood testing should be performed on every patient suspected of having a GIB. Examination of the extremities should

TABLE 31–1

Causes of Gastrointestinal Bleeding

Upper Gastrointestinal Bleeding
- Esophageal varices
- Mallory-Weiss tear
- Peptic ulcer disease
- Dieulafoy lesion

Lower Gastrointestinal Bleeding
- Arteriovenous malformation
- Diverticulosis (including Meckel's diverticulum)
- Colon cancer
- Hemorrhoids

focus on signs of shock (cool, clammy extremities indicating peripheral vasoconstriction).

DIFFERENTIAL DIAGNOSIS

- Esophageal varices
- Mallory-Weiss tear
- Peptic ulcer disease
- Dieulafoy lesion
- Arteriovenous malformation
- Diverticulosis (including Meckel's diverticulum)
- Colon cancer
- Hemorrhoids

TABLE 31–2

Common Presentations of Gastrointestinal Bleeding

Condition	Risk Factors	History	Physical Examination	Diagnosis	Treatment
Esophageal varices	Alcoholism	Massive hematemesis	Jaundice, caput medusae, spider angiomata, palmar erythema, asterixis	Upper endoscopy	Sclerotherapy or banding
Peptic ulcer disease	*Helicobacter pylori* infection, NSAID use	Heartburn	Epigastric tenderness	Upper endoscopy	Anti-acid therapy (H2 receptor antagonists, proton pump inhibitors, sucralfate), *H. pylori* eradication (tetracycline, metronidazole, bismuth)
Arteriovenous malformations	Old age	Melena	None	Colonoscopy, tagged red blood cell scan, angiography	Embolization, surgery
Diverticulosis	High fat diet	Fever and abdominal pain	Left lower quadrant abdominal pain	Colonoscopy, CT scan	Surgery

DIAGNOSTIC EVALUATION

A patient with suspected GIB should have intravenous access established (two large-bore 18-gauge or larger catheters), be placed on a cardiac monitor, and given supplemental oxygen. Blood should be sent for baseline chemistries, hematocrit, coagulation studies, and type and crossmatch. In patients with significant GIB, the BUN often will be elevated due to the breakdown and absorption of blood in the gastrointestinal tract. An EKG should be obtained on all patients with coronary artery disease to look for ischemia in the setting of GIB. A nasogastric tube may help differentiate between upper and lower sources if aspiration reveals bright red blood (indicating bleeding proximal to the ligament of Treitz).

Plain radiography is of limited value in acute GIB. Angiography can be used to identify the source of blood loss but requires bleeding rates of 0.5–2.0 mL/min. Technetium-labeled red blood cell scans are more sensitive and can be used to detect bleeding as slow as 0.1 mL/min. Endoscopy is the diagnostic procedure of choice in UGIB, identifying the etiology of bleeding in up to 95% of patients and providing a potential means of treatment with vasopressin infusion. Colonoscopy is less useful in the diagnosis of lower GIB and is rarely used in the acute setting (Table 31–2).

TREATMENT

The initial management of GIB is directed at resuscitation. After assessment of airway and breathing, fluid resuscitation with normal saline or lactated Ringer's solution should be instituted according to the 3-to-1 rule (3 mL of crystalloid for every 1 mL of blood lost). Persistent hypotension despite treatment with three 20 mL/kg fluid boluses mandates blood transfusion. Foley catheter placement is essential to monitor the response to fluid resuscitation. Adequate resuscitation should result in a urine output of at least 30 mL/hr.

Vasopressin and octreotide (a synthetic analogue of somatostatin) has been used in cases of severe variceal bleeding to constrict dilated esophageal vessels, though there has been no proven reduction in mortality. An alternative therapy for the treatment of esophageal varices is balloon tamponade with the Sengstaken-Blakemore tube, a 3-lumen tube that places pressure against the walls of the esophagus and is successful in stopping severe bleeding in almost 75% of patients.

Emergent surgery is reserved for cases of GIB unresponsive to fluid resuscitation and medical management.

◆ KEY POINTS ◆

1. Alcohol, NSAID, steroids, and anticoagulants are risk factors for GIB.

2. Bleeding can be divided into upper (proximal to the ligament of Treitz) and lower (distal to the ligament of Treitz) sources.

3. Crystalloid is the initial resuscitation fluid of choice in cases of GIB.

4. Endoscopy is an accurate diagnostic and therapeutic technique in cases of UGIB.

32 Bowel Obstruction

Intestinal obstruction refers to a mechanical blockage of the alimentary tract preventing the normal passage of bowel contents distal to the site of the obstruction. Conversely, adynamic ileus (also known as paralytic ileus) refers to the cessation of normal intestinal peristalsis and occurs without evidence of a physical obstruction.

ETIOLOGY

The most common causes of small bowel obstruction (SBO) are adhesions and hernias. Adhesions are bands of scar tissue that result from previous abdominal surgery. Hernias can be classified as reducible, incarcerated, or strangulated. Reducible hernias can be manipulated back into the abdominal cavity with manual pressure. When a hernia cannot be reduced, it is termed an incarcerated hernia. Strangulation occurs when bowel edema compromises the blood flow to an incarcerated hernia. Incarcerated and strangulated hernias can give rise to SBO.

Other less common causes of SBO include malignancies, inflammatory bowel disease, bezoars, foreign bodies, gallstones, intussusception, or infection with the *Ascaris* worm.

PATHOPHYSIOLOGY

Obstruction of a hollow viscous leads to increased intraluminal pressure and distension as fluids accumulate in the bowel and are unable to pass distally. Eventually, intraluminal pressure exceeds capillary and lymphatic pressure leading to bowel ischemia. Ischemic bowel rapidly becomes necrotic and intraluminal bacteria spontaneously translocate across the bowel wall leading to bacteremia and sepsis. Obstruction that is allowed to progress to this point has almost a 75% mortality rate.

HISTORY

Typically, patients with SBO present with abdominal pain, nausea, vomiting, and obstipation. Pain is usually described as crampy and colicky with episodes corresponding to the waves of intestinal peristalsis. Depending on the level of obstruction, vomiting may be bilious or feculent. Other important historical points include past abdominal surgeries.

PHYSICAL EXAMINATION

Tachycardia, hypotension, and fever often herald SBO, reflecting fluid losses associated with intractable vomiting. Early in the course of an SBO, the physical examination reveals a distended tympanitic abdomen. Pain is usually diffuse, but signs of peritonitis are absent. Auscultation of the abdomen may reveal high-pitched bowel sounds that occur in rushes associated with peristaltic waves. As the disease process progresses, bowel sounds become hypoactive and signs of peritonitis may

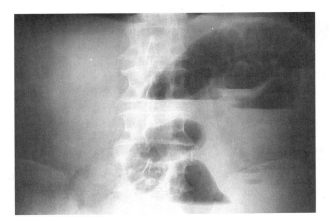

Figure 32–1A Erect film demonstrating multiple small bowel air-fluid levels.

be present. Rectal examination should be performed on all patients suspected of having SBO. Females of child-bearing age should have a pelvic examination performed to rule out gynecologic causes of abdominal pain mimicking the signs and symptoms of obstruction.

DIFFERENTIAL DIAGNOSIS

- Acute myocardial infarction
- Cholecystitis
- Pancreatitis
- Peptic ulcer disease
- Mesenteric ischemia
- Diverticulitis
- Gastroenteritis

DIAGNOSIS

All patients suspected of having an SBO should have intravenous access established, be placed on a cardiac monitor, and given supplemental oxygen. Blood should be sent for chemistries, complete blood counts, and liver function tests. Chemistries may reveal evidence of a hypochloremic metabolic alkalosis due to the loss of large amounts of stomach acid. CBC may reveal an increased white blood cell count and hemoconcentration.

All patients should have a flat plate and upright abdominal radiograph, which in the presence of SBO

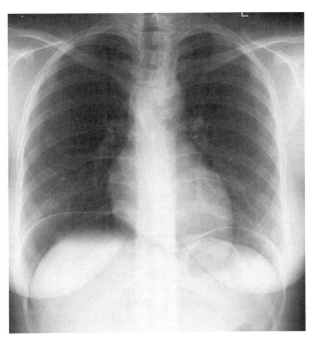

Figure 32–1B Free gas under both diaphragms.

will show dilated loops of small bowel with air-fluid levels (Fig. 32–1A). An upright chest x-ray is essential in order to test for the presence of free air under the diaphragm (Fig. 32–1B). Free intraperitoneal air indicates bowel perforation and is an indication for emergent surgery.

TREATMENT

Surgery is the definitive treatment for bowel obstruction. Prior to transport to the operating room, an attempt should be made to decompress the bowel by nasogastric intubation. Due to the nausea and vomiting that normally accompany SBO, aggressive fluid replacement should be instituted. Broad-spectrum antibiotics (i.e., ampicillin, gentamycin, and metronidazole) are indicated preoperatively.

VOLVULUS

Volvulus of the colon occurs when a segment of large bowel that is mobile twists on its mesenteric attachments and obstructs. For anatomic reasons, volvulus most often occurs in the sigmoid colon or cecum and is responsible for 10% of all large bowel obstructions (LBO). Risk factors for sigmoid volvulus include chronic constipation, and thus it is most common in elderly or debilitated patients. Cecal volvulus most often occurs as a result of a congenital hypermobile cecum. The diagnosis in both cases is made by plain radiographs in up to 90% of patients. Non-operative management of sigmoid volvulus with rectal tube decompression is successful in the majority of cases. All patients with signs of colonic strangulation and infarction, as well as all cases of cecal volvulus, should undergo operative decompression.

◆ **KEY POINTS** ◆

1. Adhesions and hernias cause the majority of SBOs.
2. The hallmarks of obstruction are abdominal pain, vomiting, and obstipation.
3. Plain abdominal radiographs should be the initial radiographs obtained in cases of suspected SBO.
4. Surgery is the definitive treatment of bowel obstruction.

33 Appendicitis

Appendicitis is an acute disease in which inflammation of the appendix leads to ischemia, necrosis, perforation, and eventually peritonitis or abscess formation. Morbidity and mortality can be avoided by a high index of suspicion, early diagnosis, and surgical intervention.

EPIDEMIOLOGY

Appendicitis is more common in males than in females (1.4 to 1) and occurs most commonly in patients aged 10–30. The diagnosis of appendicitis is difficult, especially in patients younger than 3 years of age and older than 60; patients in these age groups have a higher rate of perforation (often as high as 80%). Delay in diagnosis is associated with increased morbidity and mortality. Most surgeons will accept a negative appendectomy rate (surgery for suspected appendicitis in which the appendix is found to be histologically normal) of 15% or more.

PATHOPHYSIOLOGY

The initiating event of appendicitis is obstruction of the appendiceal lumen. Obstruction occurs by a variety of mechanisms. In younger patients, hyperplasia of lymphoid tissue in response to a viral infection is the most common etiology. Appendicitis in older patients typically results after obstruction of the lumen by fecaliths (con-

cretions of stool) or tumor. In certain areas of the world, obstruction can also occur from parasitic infection.

Regardless of the initiating event, obstruction leads to distension as the lumen fills with mucus. Increased luminal pressure eventually results in ischemia and necrosis. Necrosis of the appendix allows for bacterial overgrowth; *Bacteroides fragilis* and *Escherichia coli* are the most common organisms. Eventually, necrosis leads to perforation and peritonitis or abscess formation. Perforation rarely occurs in the first 24 hours of symptoms, making early diagnosis essential.

HISTORY

Classically, appendicitis presents with dull, generalized abdominal pain that slowly settles to the right lower quadrant over the course of 12–24 hours. Poorly localized pain is due to luminal distention while right lower quadrant pain results from irritation of the overlying parietal peritoneum by a necrotic appendix. Nausea and vomiting are common, though they typically follow the onset of pain. Patients with appendicitis are typically anorexic even in the absence of nausea.

PHYSICAL EXAMINATION

Early in the course of appendicitis, the physical exam is often non-specific. Low-grade fever and diffuse abdominal tenderness are present. As the disease progresses,

TABLE 33–1

Physical Examination Signs Associated with Appendicitis

- **Guarding**: May be voluntary or involuntary. Voluntary guarding is contraction of the abdominal musculature to prevent an examiner from depressing the peritoneum and causing pain. Involuntary guarding, also known as rigidity, is a reflex spasm of the abdominal musculature due to peritoneal irritation.
- **Rebound tenderness**: A sign of peritoneal irritation. Pain elicited when manual pressure to the abdomen is rapidly removed.
- **Rovsing's sign**: Associated with rebound tenderness. Manual pressure in the left lower quadrant produces pain in the right lower quadrant.
- **Obturator sign**: Passive flexion and internal rotation of the right hip results in right-sided abdominal pain. A positive test indicates irritation of the obturator muscle.
- **Psoas sign**: Pain elicited in the abdomen with flexion of the right hip against resistance. Indicates irritation of the psoas muscle by an inflamed appendix.

pain becomes localized to McBurney's point (4–6 cm from the iliac crest along a line drawn from the iliac crest to the umbilicus). During pregnancy the clinical presentation of appendicitis may differ due to displacement by the gravid uterus of the appendix from its normal position. Several different physical exam signs are associated with appendicitis (Table 33–1).

DIFFERENTIAL DIAGNOSIS

- Diverticulitis
- Mesenteric ischemia
- Inflammatory bowel disease
- Ectopic pregnancy
- Pelvic inflammatory disease
- Ovarian torsion
- Meckel's diverticulum

DIAGNOSIS

Routine laboratory tests are rarely useful in establishing the diagnosis of appendicitis but they may provide a means of excluding other conditions that present in a similar manner. Early in the course of appendicitis, the white blood cell (WBC) count is mildly elevated with a left shift (predominance of neutrophils). A markedly elevated WBC count is typically associated with perforation. However, up to 30% of patients with appendicitis will have a normal WBC count. A pregnancy test should be performed on all women of childbearing age presenting with abdominal pain.

Plain abdominal radiographs (KUB) are rarely useful in the diagnosis of appendicitis, except in cases of perforation, where free abdominal air is visualized under the diaphragms. Ultrasonography is useful in the diagnosis of appendicitis, especially in children. Findings on ultrasound suggestive of appendicitis include a noncompressible appendix with a thickened wall (>2 mm) and free fluid within the pelvis. Ultrasound has the advantage of potentially diagnosing pelvic pathology that mimics appendicitis, but may be of limited value in patients with a large body habitus.

CT scanning is rapidly becoming the diagnostic procedure of choice for appendicitis. Signs associated with appendicitis include wall thickening (>2 mm), abscess, free fluid, fat stranding in the right lower quadrant, and an appendicolith. Protocols for appendiceal CT scanning include a "standard" approach using oral contrast and a new approach using only rectal contrast. The latter has the advantage of requiring only 15 minutes for preparation as opposed to the 60–90 minutes required when oral contrast is given. Both techniques have sensitivities approaching 98%.

TREATMENT

Treatment for appendicitis is strictly surgical. Preoperative treatment should include intravenous fluids. Without perforation, antibiotics beyond those used for surgical wound prophylaxis (cefazolin) are typically not indicated. In cases of acute appendicitis with perforation, antibiotics should cover anaerobes and enteric gram-negative rods (ampicillin, gentamycin, and metronidazole).

◆ KEY POINTS ◆

1. Appendicitis is difficult to diagnose and a high index of suspicion is essential.

2. Up to 15% of appendectomies may reveal a normal appendix.

3. The diagnosis of appendicitis is most difficult in patients at the extremes of age.

4. Rectal contrast CT scanning is rapidly becoming the diagnostic procedure of choice.

34 Fulminant Hepatic Failure

Fulminant hepatic failure (FHF) is a clinical condition characterized by a decrease in the synthetic capacity of the liver and encephalopathy. To qualify as FHF, the time from onset to liver disease to onset of synthetic dysfunction or hepatic encephalopathy must be less than 2 weeks.

ETIOLOGY

In the United States, hepatitis B, hepatitis D, and acetaminophen overdose cause the majority of the cases of FHF. In over 20% of cases, a specific cause of liver failure is not found. Approximately 10% of the liver transplantations that are done in the United States are for FHF. The major causes of FHF are listed in Table 34–1.

PATHOGENESIS

The clinical manifestations of FHF (hepatic encephalopathy, cerebral edema, coagulopathy, infection, hypoglycemia, and acute renal failure) are the result of a decrease in functional hepatocytes. Encephalopathy is due to increased blood levels of ammonia produced from nitrogenous waste products in the intestinal tract that are normally detoxified by the liver. The mechanism by which cerebral edema develops is poorly understood, though both cytotoxic (due to the effects of ammonia and other nitrogenous waste products) and vasogenic

edema (due to increased permeability of the blood–brain barrier) play a role.

The liver is responsible for the synthesis of many coagulation factors and patients with FHF typically exhibit signs of coagulopathy, most commonly gastrointestinal bleeding.

HISTORY

Patients with FHF will typically give a history of chronic stable liver disease with an acute worsening of their condition. Confusion, coma, gastrointestinal bleeding, and fever may herald the onset of FHF.

PHYSICAL EXAMINATION

Patients with FHF are typically febrile and tachycardic due to infection and hypovolemia. The physical examination may reveal signs of chronic liver disease including ascites, palmar erythema, caput medusa, spider angiomas, Dupuytrene's contractures, jaundice, gynecomastia, and asterixis. Meningismus, rales on lung examination, or abdominal pain may indicate infection.

DIAGNOSTIC EVALUATION

All patients suspected of having FHF should be placed on a cardiac monitor; have an IV established; and have

TABLE 34–1

Major Causes of Fulminant Hepatic Failure

- Hepatitis B, C, D
- Drugs (i.e., acetaminophen, alcohol, carbon tetrachloride, halothane, isoniazid, ketoconazole)
- Toxins (i.e., *Amanita phalloides* mushrooms, Wilson's disease)
- Reye's syndrome
- Heat stroke

blood sent for complete blood counts, prothrombin and partial thromboplastin times, chemistries, ammonia, aminotransferases, acetaminophen levels, and bilirubin. A blood sample should be sent to the blood bank for typing and antibody screening. Blood and urine cultures are indicated if infection is suspected. Computed tomography of the head and abdomen is indicated if intracranial or intra-abdominal pathology is suspected.

TREATMENT

As with all emergencies, management of airway, breathing, and circulation takes precedence over everything else. Patients with profoundly altered mental status require intubation for airway protection. Severe hepatic encephalopathy typically occurs when the intracranial pressure (ICP) is greater than 30 mm Hg and in these cases may benefit from invasive ICP monitoring. Hepatic encephalopathy may be treated with Lactulose. Coagulopathy may be corrected with fresh frozen plasma. Empiric antibiotics after cultures are indicated if infection is suspected and a Foley catheter should be placed to monitor urine output. The definitive treatment is orthotopic liver transplantation, which despite medical advances in immunosuppression, carries a 30–40% mortality rate.

◆ KEY POINTS ◆

1. FHF is defined as a decrease in the synthetic function or onset of hepatic encephalopathy that occurs within two weeks of the onset of liver disease.
2. Acetaminophen and hepatitis B account for the majority of cases of FHF.
3. Hepatic encephalopathy is due to elevated ammonia levels in the blood.
4. Liver transplantation is the definitive treatment of choice.

35 Pancreatitis

Pancreatitis is an acute inflammatory disease of the pancreas characterized by abdominal pain and elevated blood levels of pancreatic enzymes. Hemorrhagic pancreatitis is a sequelae of pancreatitis and is characterized by inflammation, necrosis, and retroperitoneal hemorrhage. Pancreatic pseudocysts are sterile collections of fluid and necrotic debris encased in fibrous tissue. Although typically a self-limited disease requiring only supportive care, a small percentage of cases progress to multi-system organ failure, the systemic inflammatory response syndrome (SIRS), and death.

EPIDEMIOLOGY

The two most common causes of acute pancreatitis are gallstones and alcohol. Elevated blood levels of triglycerides, hypercalcemia, certain prescription drugs, infection (mumps), and trauma also can cause pancreatitis.

PATHOPHYSIOLOGY

The pathophysiology of acute pancreatitis is poorly understood. The normal pancreas secretes digestive enzymes that only become active once they reach the duodenum through the sphincter of Oddi into the gastrointestinal tract. In pancreatitis, these same enzymes are activated inside the pancreas itself, leading to autodi-gestion of the gland. A cycle is then established as autodigestion of pancreatic cells leads to the release of more enzymes, which in turn further attack normal tissue.

HISTORY

Patients with acute pancreatitis present with upper abdominal pain. Typically the pain is centered in the epigastrium, has a characteristic steady "boring" quality, and may be associated with nausea and vomiting. Many patients report that the pain radiates to their back (indicative of the retroperitoneal location of the pancreas).

PHYSICAL EXAMINATION

Fever and tachycardia are common in pancreatitis with shock, coma, and hypoxia heralding more severe cases and the onset of SIRS. Tachypnea, hypoxia, and decreased breath sounds may indicate an associated pleural effusion. The abdomen is typically tender to palpation with hypoactive bowel sounds and guarding (involuntary contraction of the abdominal musculature). Abdominal distension may indicate ileus. Ecchymosis of the umbilical region (Cullen's sign) or the flank (Grey-Turner's sign) is associated with hemorrhagic pancreatitis and a poor prognosis.

TABLE 35–1

Ranson's Criteria for the Prediction of Mortality in Pancreatitis

At Presentation
- Age >55 years
- WBC >16,000/mm^3
- Glucose >200 mg/dL
- LDH >350 IU/L
- AST >250 IU/L

At 48 Hours
- Fall in HCT >10%
- Increase in BUN >5 mg/dL
- Calcium <8 mg/dL
- Arterial PO$_2$ <60 mmHg
- Base deficit >4 mg/L
- Fluid deficit >6 L

WBC: white blood cell, LDH: lactate dehydrogenase, AST: aspartate aminotransferase, HCT: hematocrit, BUN: blood urea nitrogen

DIFFERENTIAL DIAGNOSIS

- Myocardial infarction
- Pneumonia
- Peptic ulcer disease
- Cholecystitis
- Acute cholangitis
- Hepatitis
- Ruptured abdominal aortic aneurysm
- Nephrolithiasis
- Small bowel obstruction
- Appendicitis

DIAGNOSTIC EVALUATION

The laboratory hallmarks of acute pancreatitis are increased blood levels of amylase and lipase. Patients with chronic pancreatitis may not have elevated pancreatic enzymes. Hypocalcemia and leukocytosis may also be seen. Elevated liver function tests may be seen if there is an associated gallstone or the common bile duct is obstructed by edema and swelling. Ranson's criteria is a set of clinical and laboratory values that is used to assess the severity of pancreatitis (Table 35–1). Plain abdominal radiography has little use in the diagnosis of pancreatitis, though it may help to exclude conditions with similar presentations. Ultrasonography and computerized tomography may be useful if complications of pancreatitis such as hemorrhage or pseudocyst formation are suspected.

TREATMENT

The treatment of pancreatitis is supportive in most cases. Due to associated nausea and vomiting, most patients require fluid resuscitation with normal saline. A nasogastric tube should be placed if vomiting persists and the patient should be kept NPO (nothing per os). Narcotic pain medicines are often required. Meperidine is preferred over morphine because the latter has been associated with spasm of the sphincter of Oddi. In more severe cases of pancreatitis when evidence of SIRS is present, intubation and vasopressor therapy may be required.

All patients with acute pancreatitis should be admitted to the hospital and those with evidence of hemorrhagic pancreatitis, shock, or SIRS should be admitted to the intensive care unit.

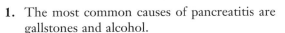

◆ KEY POINTS ◆

1. The most common causes of pancreatitis are gallstones and alcohol.
2. Umbilical (Cullen's sign) and flank (Grey-Turner's sign) ecchymosis are the hallmark of hemorrhagic pancreatitis.
3. Elevated amylase and lipase are diagnostic laboratory abnormalities.
4. SIRS, intra-abdominal hemorrhage, and pseudocyst formation are complications of pancreatitis.

36 Acute Mesenteric Ischemia

Acute mesenteric ischemia is a disease that can have catastrophic consequences including bowel infarction, perforation, sepsis, and death. Despite advances in surgical technique and critical care, the mortality of mesenteric ischemia approaches 70%.

PATHOPHYSIOLOGY

The celiac, superior mesenteric, and inferior mesenteric arteries supply small and large intestines. The celiac axis supplies blood to the stomach and small bowel up to the ligament of Treitz. The inferior mesenteric artery supplies the distal transverse colon to the rectum. The superior mesenteric artery supplies the remainder of the small and large bowel. Mesenteric ischemia results when blood supply to the bowel is insufficient to meet its metabolic demands.

The most common cause (>50%) of acute mesenteric ischemia is an embolism to the superior mesenteric artery from an intracardiac thrombus in the setting of atrial fibrillation. Alternatively, patients with atherosclerotic disease may experience mesenteric ischemia when one of the diseased visceral vessels acutely thromboses. This situation is analogous to myocardial ischemia that occurs with plaque rupture and thrombosis of a coronary artery. Finally, ischemia can occur in the presence of patent artery when a "low-flow" state exists. Cardiogenic shock, cardiopulmonary bypass, and the treatment of hypotension with high-dose vasopressors have all been associated with a low flow state.

Regardless of the cause, ischemia first involves the mucosa, which becomes necrotic. Further ischemia compromises the muscular and serosal layer resulting in transmural infarction. The dead bowel then is no longer able to provide an effective barrier to intraluminal bacteria resulting in generalized peritonitis.

HISTORY

The history typically reveals the acute onset of vague, diffuse abdominal pain in an elderly patient with a history of atrial fibrillation or coronary artery disease. Digoxin is also a risk factor for ischemic bowel due to its potent splanchnic vasoconstrictive effects. Pain is classically described as being out of proportion to the findings on physical exam. Patients presenting late in the course of the disease may present with hypotension, tachycardia, and altered mental status, signaling sepsis.

PHYSICAL EXAMINATION

Depending on when the patient presents, the physical examination can be virtually normal except for vague mid- to lower-abdominal pain without peritoneal signs. Despite the paucity of examination findings, the patient is typically uncomfortable, and may be writhing in agony. The rectal examination may reveal heme positive stools. If the patient presents later in the course of illness and transmural infarction has already occurred, peritoneal signs (rebound tenderness and involuntary guarding) may be present. At this stage, bowel sounds are typically absent and the patient is ill appearing.

DIFFERENTIAL DIAGNOSIS

- Acute myocardial infarction
- Peptic ulcer disease
- Pancreatitis
- Small bowel obstruction
- Volvulus
- Diverticulitis
- Cholecystitis
- Nephrolithiasis
- Ruptured abdominal aortic aneurysm

DIAGNOSTIC EVALUATION

The most important step in the evaluation of mesenteric ischemia is early consideration of the diagnosis. Patients with suspected ischemia should be given supplemental oxygen, placed on a cardiac monitor, and have intravenous access established. The patient should be volume resuscitated, with normal saline or lactated Ringer's if appropriate, and broad-spectrum antibiotics should be initiated. A nasogastric tube should be placed for gastric decompression.

Laboratory results may reveal leukocytosis and evidence of metabolic acidosis. Lactate levels are typically elevated, though this finding is not specific for mesenteric ischemia. Angiography remains the gold standard for diagnosis of intestinal ischemia and may provide a route for infusion of vasodilatory drugs such as papaver-ine that will help restore blood flow to the threatened segment of bowel.

Other less invasive imaging modalities may suggest mesenteric ischemia. Plain abdominal radiographs may show bowel wall thickening or pneumatosis intestinalis (gas in the bowel wall). Pneumatosis and bowel thickening are also evident on CT scanning. CT angiography (using IV contrast) has been shown to be a sensitive and specific modality for the diagnosis of mesenteric ischemia.

TREATMENT

Laparotomy and surgical embolectomy followed by resection of necrotic bowel remains the definitive treatment for mesenteric ischemia. Due to the large sections of bowel involved in most cases, bowel of questionable viability is typically left in place with a "second look" operation 24 hours later to assess the status of the remaining intestine. Postoperative care revolves around intensive hemodynamic monitoring with prompt correction of hypotension and acidosis.

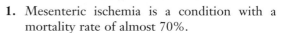

◆ KEY POINTS ◆

1. Mesenteric ischemia is a condition with a mortality rate of almost 70%.
2. Survival of the disease is based on prompt recognition and treatment.
3. Angiography remains the gold standard for diagnosis, although CT also plays a role.
4. Treatment is surgical embolectomy with resection of necrotic bowel.

37 Cholecystitis

Biliary colic is pain resulting from transient obstruction of the gallbladder or common bile duct, usually by a stone (i.e., cholelithiasis). Cholecystitis is inflammation of the gallbladder and usually results from prolonged obstruction by gallstones.

EPIDEMIOLOGY

Table 37–1 contains the risk factors for gallstone formation.

PATHOPHYSIOLOGY

Cholesterol gallstones make up approximately 80% of all stones. They are formed when cholesterol is supersaturated in bile and precipitates out forming solid crystals.

The most common cause of symptomatic cholelithiasis is an obstructing stone. As the gallbladder contracts it may relieve the obstruction, but if it persists, acute cholecystitis can develop. Typical pathogens of cholecystitis include enteric gram-negatives, streptococci, and anaerobes (e.g., *Clostridium* and *Bacteroides fragilis*). A life-threatening complication of gallstones is ascending cholangitis caused by complete obstruction of the common bile duct.

HISTORY

Patients with biliary colic present with an abrupt onset of right upper quadrant (RUQ) pain radiating to the right scapula or epigastrium shortly after eating a fatty meal. However, many patients present with vague, dull epigastric pain that is not well localized. The pain can last between 30 minutes and 6 hours.

Acute cholecystitis may present in a similar manner to biliary colic but is usually more severe, lasts longer than 6 hours, and is usually accompanied by fever. The pain typically becomes sharper and localizes to the RUQ. Associated symptoms include nausea and vomiting. Patients may have a history of similar attacks or known gallstones.

Patients with ascending cholangitis present with fever or chills, jaundice, and RUQ pain (i.e., Charcot triad).

PHYSICAL EXAMINATION

Patients with biliary colic may have RUQ tenderness during the acute episode. The abdomen may also be distended with hypoactive bowel sounds. Patients with cholecystitis may also be mildly icteric, have localized peritonitis, guarding, or a positive Murphy's sign. Ascending cholangitis should be considered in patients with fever, jaundice, RUQ pain, and shock.

DIFFERENTIAL DIAGNOSIS

- Cholangitis
- Gastroesophageal reflux disease

TABLE 37–1

Risk Factors for Cholecystitis and Biliary Calculi

- Increasing age
- Obesity
- Female sex
- Parity
- Diabetes
- Profound weight loss
- Oral contraceptives
- Family history
- Hemolytic anemias
- Cirrhosis
- Infection
- Native American heritage
- Inflammatory bowel disease
- Ileal resection
- Total parenteral nutrition
- Prolonged fasting

- Hepatitis
- Pancreatitis
- Myocardial infarction
- Appendicitis
- Renal colic
- Fitz-Hugh-Curtis syndrome (acute gonococcal perihepatitis)
- Peptic ulcer disease
- Pyelonephritis
- Aortic dissection

DIAGNOSTIC EVALUATION

Lab studies include ECG, CBC, electrolytes, liver function tests, bilirubin, amylase, lipase, urinalysis, and beta

HCG. Patients with biliary colic usually have normal laboratory studies. Patients with acute cholecystitis may have elevations in the white blood count and liver function tests, although these tests can be normal.

A RUQ ultrasound is the diagnostic study of choice and may show gallstones, sludge in the gallbladder, gallbladder distention, gallbladder wall thickening, or pericholecystic fluid. The ultrasound can assess the kidney, liver, or pancreas as other causes of abdominal pain.

TREATMENT

Assess ABCs (airway, breathing, circulation). Biliary colic is usually treated with IV fluids, analgesics, and often antiemetics. Patients can be discharged home, with close follow-up, if their pain has resolved and they can maintain oral hydration. Definitive treatment of symptomatic cholelithiasis is usually an elective cholecystectomy, but medical dissolution therapy and gallstone lithotripsy are other available options.

Patients with acute cholecystitis require prompt surgical consultation. These patients should receive broad-spectrum antibiotics. Definitive treatment of acute cholecystitis is an urgent cholecystectomy usually within 24–72 hours.

Patients with signs of ascending cholangitis who are in shock need emergent decompression of the biliary tree either surgically or endoscopically.

◆ KEY POINTS ◆

1. Cholecystitis is inflammation of the gallbladder.
2. Patients often present with RUQ pain, fever, nausea, and vomiting lasting longer than 6 hours.
3. An RUQ ultrasound is the diagnostic study of choice.
4. Treatment includes IV fluids, broad-spectrum antibiotics, and prompt surgical consultation.

Part VI
Renal and Urogenital Emergencies

Testicular Pain:

- Testicular torsion
- Acute epididymitis
- Orchitis
- Appendicitis
- Testicular or epididymal appendix torsion
- Hernia
- Tumor
- Hydrocele
- Trauma

Nontraumatic Urologic Hematuria:

- Glomerular-glomerulonephritis
- Non-glomerular-infection
- Neoplasm
- Calculus
- Vascular lesions or infarction
- Benign prostatic hyperplasia

Non-Urologic Hematuria:

- Sickle cell disease
- Coagulopathy
- Hematologic anemias
- Iatrogenic drugs—heparin, coumadin
- Catheterization

38

Urinary Tract Infection

A urinary tract infection (UTI) occurs when microorganisms invade a portion of the urinary tract. A lower urinary tract infection involves the urethra or bladder. An upper urinary tract infection involves the kidneys.

ETIOLOGY

Urinary tract infections are more common in women than men. Risk factors for UTIs are outlined in Table 38–1.

Typical microorganisms include *Escherichia coli* (80–90%), *Staphylococcus saprophyticus*, *Klebsiella*, *Proteus mirabilis*, *Enterobacter* spp., *Pseudomonas aeruginosa*, and Group D streptococci.

PATHOPHYSIOLOGY

Urinary tract infections start with colonization of the periurethral area with ascent of microorganisms up the genitourinary tract. Once bacteria reach the bladder, microorganisms grow and can reflux into the ureters and finally infect the renal parenchyma.

HISTORY

Typical symptoms of lower urinary tract infections (i.e., cystitis) include:

- Dysuria
- Increased frequency of urination
- Urgency
- Suprapubic pain
- Hematuria
- Hesitancy

Patients may also present with asymptomatic bacteriuria, especially in pregnant, immunosuppressed, or elderly patients. Typical symptoms of upper urinary tract infections (i.e., pyelonephritis) begin with dysuria and frequency for several days before the onset of:

- Fever or chills
- Flank, back, or abdominal pain
- Costovertebral angle (CVA) tenderness
- Nausea or vomiting
- Malaise

PHYSICAL EXAMINATION

Patients with acute bacterial cystitis usually have a normal physical exam except for mild suprapubic tenderness. Patients with pyelonephritis usually appear ill, have temperatures greater than 38.5°C (101.3°F), and unilateral costovertebral angle (CVA) tenderness. Patients with urosepsis may present with fever, hypotension, tachycardia, tachypnea, and altered mental status.

TABLE 38–1

Risk Factors for UTI

Behavior	• Spermicides (e.g., nonoxynol-9) • Diaphragms • Sexual intercourse • Wiping and local hygiene
Anatomical or functional abnormalities	• Alteration of protective vaginal flora • Short urethra • Urethra trauma (e.g., sexual activity) • Incomplete bladder emptying • Prostatic hypertrophy • Instrumentation or catheterization
Age and gender	• Newborn • Prepubertal girls • Sexually active females • Elderly males and females

Host susceptibility	• Glucose content in urine
	• Host immune factors
	  — renal failure
	  — chronic illness
	  — cancer
	  — drug or alcohol use
	  — pregnancy
	• Increased contamination due to urinary or fecal incontinence
	• Diabetes

Neurologic conditions	• Neurogenic bladder • Spinal cord injury

DIFFERENTIAL DIAGNOSIS OF UTI

- Urethritis (e.g., especially in young males)
- Vulvovaginitis
- Cervicitis
- Pelvic inflammatory disease
- Prostatitis
- Epididymitis

Differential diagnosis of pyelonephritis includes above differential plus:

- Renal abscess
- Nephrolithiasis
- Appendicitis
- Diverticulitis
- Cholecystitis
- Lower lobe pneumonia

DIAGNOSIS

The first test is a urinary dipstick looking for the presence of pyuria (e.g., leukocyte esterase) and bacteriuria (e.g., nitrites). However, symptomatic patients with negative urinary dipstick should have a urinalysis performed. A positive urinalysis is typically greater than 10 WBC/hpf and includes the presence of any bacteria. Hematuria may also be present with upper and lower tract involvement. The specimen should contain no or few epithelial cells.

Urine cultures should be obtained in patients with pyelonephritis, pregnant women, patients who failed recent therapy for UTI, patients with indwelling catheters, or patients with sepsis. A positive culture is defined as 10^2 to 10^5 colony forming units/mL.

Renal imaging is not routinely done for uncomplicated UTI or acute pyelonephritis in healthy patients, but should be considered in elderly, diabetic, or severely ill patients with acute pyelonephritis or complicated UTI. Other indications for imaging include severe or atypical presentations and poor response to initial antibiotic treatment.

TREATMENT

First assess ABCs (airway, breathing, circulation). Patients with urosepsis should have two large-bore IVs, be administered supplemental oxygen, and be placed on a cardiac monitor. These patients require fluid resuscitation with IV crystalloid. In addition, these patients should promptly receive IV antibiotics once a blood and urine culture has been sent. Uncomplicated urinary

TABLE 38–2

Treatment of Urinary Tract Infections

Type of Infection	Microorganisms	Treatment	Disposition
Uncomplicated cystitis	• Escherichia coli • Staphylococcus saprophyticus • Proteus mirabilis • Klebsiella pneumonia	• 3 days • Trimethoprim-sulfamethoxazole • Ciprofloxacin • Norfloxacin • Ofloxacin • Amoxicillin-clavulonate • Levofloxacin	• Home
Uncomplicated pyelonephritis	• Escherichia coli • Staphylococcus saprophyticus • Proteus mirabilis • Klebsiella pneumonia	• 10–14 days • Ceftriaxone • Ampicillin plus gentamicin • Levofloxacin • Ciprofloxacin • Amoxicillin-clavulanate	• First dose of IV antibiotics in ED • If young and healthy, discharge home with oral antibiotics
Uncomplicated cystitis in pregnancy	• Escherichia coli • Staphylococcus saprophyticus • Proteus mirabilis • Klebsiella pneumonia	• 7–10 days • Amoxicillin • Nitrofurantoin	• Home
Complicated urinary tract infection	• Escherichia coli • Staphylococcus saprophyticus • Proteus mirabilis • Klebsiella pneumonia • Enterobacter spp. • Pseudomonas aeruginosa • Group D streptococci • Serratia • Morganella • Staphylococcus aureus • Candida species	• IV antibiotic • Ciprofloxacin • Levofloxacin • Ampicillin plus gentamicin • Cefotaxime • Ceftriaxone • Ticarcillin-clavulanate	• Admission

tract infections in adult women (nonpregnant, nondiabetic) are typically treated with a 3-day course of oral antibiotics. Antibiotics include ciprofloxacin, levofloxacin, or trimethoprim-sulfamethoxazole. All other adult patients will usually require a 7- to 10-day course of antibiotics. These patients are usually discharged home with appropriate follow-up.

Patients with acute pyelonephritis can be discharged home if they can maintain oral medication and hydration. Similar antibiotics are used for pyelonephritis, except these patients require a 10- to 14-day course.

Admit all patients with acute pyelonephritis who are unable to tolerate oral therapy, have intractable nausea or vomiting, known anatomic anomalies, obstruction, indwelling catheter, are pregnant, diabetic, immunosuppressed, elderly, or recently failed outpatient therapy. Table 38–2 outlines the treatment of UTI.

◆ KEY POINTS ◆

1. *Escherichia coli* accounts for 80 to 90% of all UTI.

2. Typical symptoms of lower UTI (i.e., cystitis) include dysuria, frequency, urgency, and suprapubic pain.

3. Typical symptoms of upper UTI (i.e., pyelonephritis) include fever or chills; back, flank, or abdominal pain; costovertebral angle tenderness; and nausea or vomiting.

4. Typical antibiotics include ciprofloxacin, levofloxacin, or trimethoprim-sulfamethoxazole.

39 Testicular Torsion

Torsion of the testis occurs when the testicle twists on the spermatic cord. Testicular torsion causes venous outflow obstruction and arterial occlusion, ultimately leading to infarction of the testicle and impaired fertility.

EPIDEMIOLOGY AND ETIOLOGY

Testicular torsion can occur at any age but is most common during the first year of life and around puberty. The most common deformity that predisposes testicular torsion is a "bell clapper" deformity. Normally the testis and epididymis are anchored to the scrotum by the posterior attachment of the tunica vaginalis. In the "bell clapper" deformity, the tunica vaginalis inserts high on the spermatic cord leaving the testis and epididymis free to rotate within the tunica. "Bell clapper" deformity is usually bilateral.

PATHOPHYSIOLOGY

As the testis and spermatic cord twists, it occludes venous return, and ultimately compromises the arterial supply leading to ischemia. Infarction usually occurs if the blood supply cannot be restored within 6 hours (Fig. 39–1).

HISTORY

The classic presentation of testicular torsion is sudden onset of unilateral testicular pain and scrotal swelling. The pain often radiates to the inguinal canal or lower abdomen. Patients may complain of similar episodes in the past that resolved spontaneously. Nausea and vomiting are common associated symptoms. Torsion can occur after vigorous exercise, trauma, or during sleep.

PHYSICAL EXAMINATION

Common signs of testicular torsion include:

- Testicular enlargement and tenderness
- Erythema and swelling of scrotum
- Horizontal (i.e., transverse) lie instead of the normal vertical orientation
- Elevated, high-riding testis in the scrotum due to twisting and shortening of spermatic cord
- Ipsilateral loss of cremasteric reflex with torsion

DIFFERENTIAL DIAGNOSIS

- Epididymitis
- Orchitis
- Torsion of the appendix testis
- Incarcerated inguinal hernia
- Testicular tumor
- Acute hydrocele or hematocele

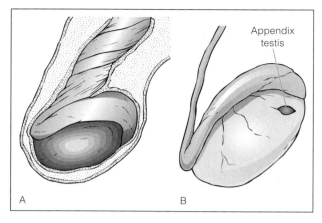

Appendix testis

Figure 39–1   Torsion of the testes (A) is the result of twisting of the spermatic cord, usually within the tunica vaginalis; the appendix testis may also become twisted (B).

DIAGNOSTIC EVALUATIONS

Color Doppler ultrasound is usually the first imaging test. It is considered positive when it shows absent or significantly reduced blood flow to the affected testis as compared to the other side. A urinalysis should be obtained from all patients with testicular pain to help rule out other causes.

TREATMENT

Surgical exploration, detorsion, and bilateral orchiopexy constitute the treatment of testicular torsion. The best results for testicular detorsion involve treatment within 6 hours of onset of pain. An emergent urology consult should be obtained when the history and physical exam are highly suggestive of testicular torsion. In addition, surgical exploration should not be delayed for imaging studies.

If definitive care (i.e., surgical exploration) is delayed, manual detorsion should be attempted. Rotation of the testes during torsion usually occurs from a lateral to medial position; thus, detorsion should be attempted from a medial to lateral fashion. Detorsion is done in a way similar to opening a book (i.e., the right testis should be rotated counterclockwise and the left testis rotated clockwise). The end point is relief of pain. If the pain worsens, then try detorsion in the opposite direction.

All patients who undergo manual detorsion, or patients suspected of having testicular torsion but who have inconclusive imaging studies, require surgical exploration. Patients with normal flow studies can be discharged from the emergency department with appropriate urology follow-up.

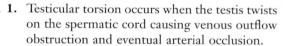

◆ KEY POINTS ◆

1. Testicular torsion occurs when the testis twists on the spermatic cord causing venous outflow obstruction and eventual arterial occlusion.

2. The most common ages are during the first year of life and around puberty.

3. The most common deformity that predisposes testicular torsion is a "bell clapper" deformity.

4. Classic symptoms include sudden onset of unilateral testicular pain with swelling and erythema associated with nausea and vomiting.

5. Color Doppler ultrasound is generally the first imaging study.

6. Surgical exploration is the definitive treatment of testicular torsion.

40 Renal Colic

Renal colic is an acute painful condition caused by the impaction or passing of a calculus (i.e., stone) in the ureter or renal pelvis. The most common types of renal calculi (~75%) are made of calcium salts (e.g., oxalate or phosphate).

EPIDEMIOLOGY AND ETIOLOGY

Urinary stones affect persons of all ages. Males are affected three times more than females. Approximately one-third of patients with a history of kidney stones suffer a recurrence within a year.

PATHOPHYSIOLOGY

The exact mechanism of stone formation is unknown. As stones move through the urinary tract they may become impacted in areas of anatomic bending or narrowing. Common impaction sites include the renal calyx, ureteropelvic junction, and the ureterovesical junction. Kidney stones less than 4 mm have approximately a 90% chance of passing spontaneously, whereas stones greater than 6 mm in diameter have only a 10% chance of passing.

HISTORY

Acute onset of severe, colicky flank pain with radiation to the ipsilateral testicle, labia majora, or groin is the classic presentation of patients with kidney stones. Nausea and vomiting are common associated symptoms. Patients move around "writhing in pain" and are unable to find a comfortable position. Patients may also complain of hematuria. A positive family history or history of previous stones may also be noted.

PHYSICAL EXAMINATION

The physical exam is usually normal. Mild costovertebral angle tenderness may be present. Fever is generally atypical and may suggest infection or a diagnosis other than renal colic.

DIFFERENTIAL DIAGNOSIS

- Aortic dissection or ruptured abdominal aortic aneurysm
- Pyelonephritis
- Renal infarction
- Intestinal ischemia
- Biliary colic
- Appendicitis
- Diverticulitis
- Ruptured ectopic pregnancy
- Ruptured ovarian cyst
- Ovarian or testicular torsion

- Incarcerated or strangulated inguinal hernia
- Lower lobe pneumonia
- Musculoskeletal strain

DIAGNOSTIC EVALUATION

A urinalysis should be the first test ordered when evaluating patients with renal colic. Hematuria supports the diagnosis of renal colic. A beta HCG should be obtained on all women of childbearing age. In addition, CBC, electrolytes, glucose, BUN, creatinine, and urine cultures should be ordered as indicated. Traditionally, intravenous pyelogram (IVP) was the imaging test of choice. However, non-contrast helical computed tomography (CT) is replacing IVP in many institutions. Renal ultrasound is an alternative imaging study. Imaging studies are helpful to determine the size of the stone and the degree of hydronephrosis.

TREATMENT

The mainstay of treatment for renal colic is IV hydration and analgesia. Common analgesics include meperidine (Demerol), morphine, and ketorolac (Toradol). Antiemetics (e.g., prochlorperazine or Vistaril) may be needed to help with associated nausea.

All patients should be admitted with pain refractory to analgesics, persistent nausea and vomiting, ureteral obstruction with infection, or a solitary kidney with complete obstruction. In addition, patients with large (>5 mm) stones, intrinsic renal disease, high obstructions, or significant underlying disease should also be considered for admission. Obstruction in the presence of infection is considered a urologic emergency and requires a prompt urologic consultation.

Patients can be discharged home assuming they have no signs of infection and are able to tolerate oral analgesics and hydration. Follow-up with a urologist or primary care physician should occur within 7 days.

◆ KEY POINTS ◆

1. Renal colic is the acute painful condition caused by the impaction or passing of a calculus in the ureter or renal pelvis.

2. The most common types of urinary stones (~75%) are made of calcium oxalate and calcium phosphate.

3. Helical CT, ultrasound, and IVP are the imaging studies of choice for kidney stones.

4. Stones less than 4 mm have a 90% chance of passing spontaneously.

5. Treatment includes IV hydration, analgesia, and antiemetics.

Part VII
Obstetric and Gynecological Emergencies

SIGNS AND SYMPTOMS

Non-Pregnancy-Related Vaginal Bleeding:

- Malignant neoplasm
- Benign neoplasm
- Trauma
- Ulcerative lesions
- Condyloma acuminata
- Vaginitis
- Foreign body
- Cervical polyps
- Cervicitis
- Endometrial polyps
- Submucous leiomyoma
- Endometrial hyperplasia
- Endometrial carcinoma
- Chronic endometriosis
- Intrauterine device
- Coagulopathy
- Dysfunctional uterine bleeding
- Breakthrough bleeding

Pregnancy-Related Bleeding:

- Ectopic pregnancy
- Abortion (inevitable, incomplete, complete, missed, septic)
- Normal intrauterine pregnancy
- Molar pregnancy
- Vaginal foreign body
- Vulvovaginitis or cervicitis
- Pelvic inflammatory disease
- Placenta previa
- Placental abruption
- Trauma
- Estrogen excess

Postpartum Early Hemorrhage (<24 hours):

- Uterine atony
- Genital tract laceration
- Retained placental products
- Placental accreta
- Hematoma
- Uterine inversion

- Uterine rupture
- Coagulopathy

Postpartum Late Hemorrhage (up to 6 weeks):

- Infection (endometritis)
- Retained placental products
- Delayed placental site involution
- Sloughing of placental site eschar

Pelvic Pain:

- Ovarian cyst
- Menstrual disorders (DUB, dysmenorrhea)
- PID
- Vaginitis or cervicitis
- Nonruptured ectopic pregnancy
- Endometriosis
- Ovarian torsion
- Ectopic pregnancy
- Ovarian cyst rupture
- Hydrosalpinx rupture
- Mittelschmerz

41 Dysfunctional Uterine Bleeding

Irregular vaginal bleeding unrelated to anatomic or organic lesions of the uterus (e.g., malignancy, polyps, and leiomyomas) is referred to as dysfunctional uterine bleeding (DUB). DUB is often excessive, prolonged, and usually related to anovulation (75%).

ETIOLOGY

Tables 41–1 and 41–2 gives the etiology of abnormal vaginal bleeding.

PATHOPHYSIOLOGY

Dysfunctional uterine bleeding (DUB) caused by anovulation is due to estrogen overstimulation of the endometrium. Eventually, the endometrium sloughs off when it outgrows its blood supply. DUB is most likely to occur in association with polycystic ovarian disease, obesity, and adrenal hyperplasia.

HISTORY

Excessive vaginal bleeding is defined as requiring one pad or tampon per hour for several hours. Many women with DUB may complain of delayed menses with onset of heavy, painless vaginal bleeding that is significantly changed from a normal menstrual cycle. Inquire about contraceptive, menstrual history, sexual activity, and prior history of abnormal bleeding.

DIFFERENTIAL DIAGNOSIS

See Tables 41–1 and 41–2.

DIAGNOSTIC EVALUATION

Perform a pelvic exam looking for vulva, vaginal, and cervical lesions. A bimanual exam will evaluate the size and shape of the uterus and adnexal structures. The anus should also be inspected and a rectal exam with guaiac test performed.

Lab studies include a beta HCG, CBC, coagulation studies (PT/PTT). A pelvic ultrasound may be necessary to evaluate for structural abnormalities, especially when masses are felt during the pelvic exam.

TREATMENT

It is important to rule out pregnancy (ectopic pregnancy) in all women of childbearing age with vaginal bleeding. For hemodynamically unstable patients, begin treatment with IV conjugated estrogen. Obtain a gynecology consultation for all hemodynamically unstable patients, as dilation and curettage or operative management may be necessary.

Hemodynamically stable patients with heavy dysfunctional bleeding can usually be controlled with conjugated estrogen and progesterone or combination oral contraceptives. All patients should have follow-up with a gynecologist before completing the course of medication.

TABLE 41–1

Etiology of Abnormal Vaginal Bleeding

Causes	Example
Dysfunction uterine bleeding	• Immature hypothalamic-pituitary-ovarian axis • Perimenopause • Obesity • Polycystic ovarian syndrome
Pregnancy complications	• Threatened, incomplete, or spontaneous abortion • Ectopic or molar pregnancy
Infectious causes	• Pelvic inflammatory disease • Chronic endometritis
Anatomic lesions	• Fibroids • Endometriosis • Polyps • Neoplasms • Endometrial hyperplasia
Medications	• Oral contraceptives • Warfarin • Aspirin • Tricyclic antidepressants • Major tranquilizers
Coagulopathies	• Leukemia • Aplastic anemia • Von Willebrand's disease • Idiopathic thrombocytopenic purpura • Platelet defects • Thalassemia major
Systemic illness	• Adrenal • Thyroid dysfunction • Renal • Hepatic • Diabetes mellitus
Intrauterine device	
Trauma	

TABLE 41–2

Etiology of Abnormal Vaginal Bleeding

Causes	Example
Vaginal	• Trauma • Vaginitis • Malignancy • Foreign body • Condyloma acuminata • Post operative
Vulva	• Trauma • Malignancy • Benign lesions • Urethral caruncle • Ulcerative lesions • Condyloma acuminata
Cervical	• Malignancy • Polyps • Cervicitis • Trauma

◆ KEY POINTS ◆

1. Abnormal vaginal bleeding can occur from uterine or extrauterine causes.
2. Dysfunctional uterine bleeding (DUB) is a diagnosis of exclusion and refers to irregular bleeding in the absence of systemic or structural disease.
3. Gynecology consultation should be obtained in all hemodynamically unstable patients.
4. IV conjugated estrogens should be started in hemodynamically unstable patients.
5. Multiple hormonal treatments are available for outpatient management including estrogen with progesterone, combination oral contraceptives, and medroxyprogesterone.

42

Vaginal Bleeding— First Trimester

There are five types of spontaneous abortion, classified by whether the cervix is dilated or not and whether any or all of the products of conception (POCs) have passed (Table 42–1).

EPIDEMIOLOGY

Approximately 25% of women have bleeding during the first trimester and roughly half (50%) of these women will go on to have spontaneous abortions, 40% will have a viable pregnancy, and 10% will have an ectopic pregnancy.

ETIOLOGY

Bleeding can occur from the site of implantation (e.g., due to ruptured blood vessels in the endometrium) or with marginal separation of the placenta. Risk factors for first trimester bleeding include advanced maternal age, history of previous spontaneous or elective abortion, fibroids, history of infertility, and IUD use prior to pregnancy. Early abortion (<20 wks) is usually due to chromosomal abnormalities. Other causes of spontaneous abortion include fetal malformation from teratogens, maternal infection with viral agents, and fetal exposure to radiation, drugs, or other chemical agents.

PATHOPHYSIOLOGY

Regardless of the etiology, the process of spontaneous abortion is the same. Death of the embryo leads to a decline in placental hormone production, which causes hemorrhage into the decidua and necrosis of adjacent tissue. The blood accumulates between the placenta and decidua basalis leading to detachment of the products of conception. After detachment, the products of conception act as a foreign body stimulating the uterus to contract and expel the products. Uterine bleeding will occur until all of the products have passed. After expulsion is complete the uterus continues to contract, compressing uterine blood vessels and ultimately ceasing the hemorrhage.

HISTORY

Patients present in early pregnancy (<20 wks) with vaginal bleeding and mild to moderate suprapubic or midline lower abdominal pain that may radiate to the lower back. Other symptoms include abdominal cramping, decreased symptoms of pregnancy, passing clots or fetal tissue, lightheadedness and weakness. Establish the date of the last menstrual period (LMP) as well as the quantity, character, and time course of vaginal bleeding.

PHYSICAL EXAMINATION

The abdominal exam may reveal mild to moderate lower abdominal tenderness or peritoneal signs. On speculum exam there may be brisk vaginal bleeding from the cervical os, or evidence of vaginitis, cervicitis, lacerations, or polyps. If tissue is protruding from the cervical os then it is considered dilated. All material in the vaginal vault should be inspected and sent to pathology for analysis.

During the bimanual exam, the length and dilation of the cervix, uterine size, shape, tenderness and consis-

---

TABLE 42–1

Vaginal Bleeding in the First Trimester

Type	History	Internal Cervical Os	Products of Conception (POCs)	Treatment
Threatened	• Early pregnancy, <20 weeks' gestation • Vaginal bleeding • Mild, crampy suprapubic or midline lower abdominal pain • Membranes intact	Closed	• No POCs expelled	• RhoGAM IM to Rh-neg women with at least 7 wks' gestation • Follow closely by OB/GYN • Avoid heavy activity • Pelvic rest • Bed rest
Inevitable	• Moderate to severe crampy lower midline abdominal pain • Significant vaginal bleeding • Membranes ruptured • <20 weeks' gestation	Open	• No POCs expelled	• All specimens should be sent to pathology • OB/GYN consult • Most will have a D&C • RhoGAM for Rh-neg
Incomplete	• <20 weeks' gestation • Uterine bleeding	Open	• Some POCs expelled	• All specimens should be sent to pathology • OB/GYN consult • Most will have D&C • RhoGAM for Rh-neg
Complete	• <20 weeks' gestation • Uterine bleeding	Closed	• All POCs expelled	• RhoGAM for Rh-neg
Septic	• Fever • Abdominal pain • Vaginal bleeding • Infection associated with abortion • Endometritis	Closed or open	• Some POCs retained	• IV antibiotics • OB/GYN consult • Admission • D&C • RhoGAM if appropriate
Missed	• No uterine bleeding • No cardiac activity by US • Uterus small for dates, not growing	Closed	• Retained fetal tissue • Nonviable tissue is not expelled in 4 weeks	• OB/GYN consult • Evacuate uterus, D&C • RhoGAM if Rh-neg

tency, cervical motion tenderness, and adnexal tenderness and fullness need to be evaluated. Unilateral adnexal tenderness or fullness may suggest ectopic pregnancy, ruptured hemorrhagic corpus luteal cyst, or functional corpus luteal cyst of pregnancy.

DIFFERENTIAL DIAGNOSIS

- Ectopic pregnancy
- Ruptured hemorrhagic corpus luteal cyst
- Implantation bleeding
- Trophoblastic disease
- Urethral or rectal hemorrhage
- Cervicitis
- Vaginitis
- Cervical polyps or lacerations
- Cervical carcinoma

DIAGNOSTIC EVALUATION

A CBC, type and screen, Rh status, and quantitative beta-hCG level should be sent. In normal intrauterine pregnancies, the beta-hCG doubles every 36 to 48 hours until it peaks at approximately 100,000 U/mL at 11 weeks. Thus, failure to double suggests an abnormal pregnancy. Hemodynamically unstable patients should be typed and crossmatched. A transvaginal ultrasound should be done to evaluate for intrauterine pregnancy, ectopic pregnancy, or retained products of conception.

TREATMENT

First evaluate ABCs (airway, breathing, circulation). Hemodynamically unstable patients should be placed on a monitor, have supplemental oxygen, two large-bore IVs, and fluid resuscitation. In addition, emergent obstetric and gynecologic consultation should be obtained.

Refer to Table 42–1 for treatment of different types of abortions. All patients discharged home require follow-up with a gynecologist within 48 hours.

Patients who present with endometritis following elective or incomplete abortion require IV antibiotics, OB/GYN consultation, and admission.

All women with first trimester bleeding who are Rho(D)-negative should to be given RhoGAM therapy.

◆ KEY POINTS ◆

1. Spontaneous abortion is defined as non-elective termination of a pregnancy at less than 20 weeks' gestational age or estimated fetal weight of less than 500 g.

2. Transvaginal ultrasound should be performed to evaluate for intrauterine pregnancy, ectopic pregnancy, or retained products of conception.

3. It is important to rule out ectopic pregnancy in all women with first trimester vaginal bleeding.

4. Inevitable, incomplete, and missed abortions are usually completed by a D&C.

5. RhoGAM should be given to all Rh-negative women with first trimester vaginal bleeding.

43

Ectopic Pregnancy

An ectopic pregnancy is defined as implantation of a fertilized ovum outside the uterine cavity. The most common site of ectopic pregnancies is the fallopian tube (~98%). Other sites of implantation include the cervix, the ovary, and the abdominal cavity. An ectopic pregnancy can be life threatening and can lead to intra-abdominal hemorrhage, shock, and death.

EPIDEMIOLOGY AND ETIOLOGY

Overall, 1.7% of all pregnancies will be ectopic. Risk factors for ectopic pregnancies include history of pelvic inflammatory disease (PID), prior ectopic pregnancy, tubal surgery, pelvic surgery, endometriosis, in vitro fertilization, DES exposure in utero, IUD use, and congenital abnormalities of the fallopian tube.

PATHOPHYSIOLOGY

Ectopic pregnancies develop from any factors that prevent or delay the fertilized egg from reaching the uterus (e.g., previous fallopian tube damage from infection).

HISTORY

History should include the patient's reproductive past, menstrual history, and risk factors for ectopic preg-

nancy. Patients may present with symptoms of pregnancy including amenorrhea, nausea, or vomiting. They may also present with abdominal or pelvic pain and abnormal vaginal bleeding. The location of the pain is variable and may be crampy, colicky, steady, or dull. Patients with ruptured ectopics can present with dizziness, syncope, or in shock.

PHYSICAL EXAMINATION

A complete physical exam including pelvic and rectal exams should be done. Patients with ruptured ectopic pregnancies may present in shock with orthostatic hypotension, tachycardia, and generalized abdominal and adnexal tenderness with rebound. On pelvic exam, unilateral adnexal or uterine tenderness or pelvic mass may be present. In addition, patients may also have cervical motion tenderness.

DIFFERENTIAL DIAGNOSIS

- Spontaneous abortion
- Cervicitis
- Intrauterine pregnancy
- Pelvic inflammatory disease
- Ruptured ovarian cyst
- Corpus luteum cyst

- Endometriosis
- Appendicitis
- Ovarian torsion
- Nephrolithiasis
- UTI
- Mittelschmerz
- Gastroenteritis

DIAGNOSTIC EVALUATION

All stable patients with suspected ectopics should have a quantitative beta-hCG, CBC, type and screen and Rh status, and urinalysis. An ultrasound should be obtained to rule out ectopic pregnancy. The gestational sac of a normal intrauterine pregnancy becomes visible with abdominal ultrasound at 6 weeks' gestation (beta-hCG ~ 6000–6500) or by transvaginal ultrasound 1 week earlier (beta-hCG between 1500–2000). Culdocentesis may be performed when ultrasound is not available and the patient is at high risk for an ectopic pregnancy. A test is positive when greater than 5 cc of non-clotting blood is aspirated from the cul-de-sac. Laparoscopy or laparotomy makes the definitive diagnosis of an ectopic pregnancy.

TREATMENT

First evaluate ABCs (airway, breathing, circulation). All unstable patients with ectopic pregnancy require two large, bore IVs, monitor, oxygen, and fluid resuscitation. Blood should be sent for type and crossmatch. Next, obtain an emergent OB/GYN consultation and prepare these patients to go directly to the OR for surgical removal.

Stable patients with ectopic pregnancy, or where one is suspected, require an OB/GYN consult in the emergency department. Surgical treatment may be performed by laparotomy or laparoscopy. Medical treatment with methotrexate is an option for clearly diagnosed, stable, unruptured, ectopic pregnancies.

Women with confirmed ectopic pregnancy require admission, unless they are being treated with methotrexate. In addition, admit women with increased risk factors, no available ultrasound, non-reliable follow-up, beta-hCG greater than 6500 with no evidence of IUP, positive culdocentesis, progressive symptomatology, or physical findings.

Hemodynamically stable women with no evidence of ectopic pregnancy require strict follow-up with OB/GYN in 2 days. All RH-negative women should be given RhoGAM.

◆ KEY POINTS ◆

1. An ectopic pregnancy is defined as any pregnancy outside the uterine cavity, including the abdominal cavity, cervix, and ovary.

2. Symptoms include amenorrhea, nausea, vomiting, abdominal or pelvic pain, or abnormal vaginal bleeding.

3. Transvaginal ultrasound and quantitative beta-hCG are used to help rule out ectopic pregnancies.

4. Treatment options include medical management with methotrexate or surgical removal by laparoscopy or laparotomy.

5. Unstable patients with ectopic pregnancies require IV fluids, blood transfusion, and surgical removal.

44 Preeclampsia and Eclampsia

Preeclampsia is defined as hypertension in pregnancy associated with proteinuria (e.g., >300 mg/day) and nondependent edema (e.g., hands and face). Eclampsia is defined as seizures in a patient with preeclampsia. The HELLP syndrome (Hemolysis, Elevated Liver enzymes, and Low Platelets) is a variant of preeclampsia and eclampsia.

ETIOLOGY

Etiology is unknown, but risk factors include:

- Extremes of reproductive age (<15 or >35)
- Multiple gestations
- Primigravidas or nulliparas
- Black race
- Vascular disease (due to SLE or diabetes)
- Family history of preeclampsia or eclampsia
- Chronic hypertension
- Preexisting renal disease
- Molar pregnancy

PATHOPHYSIOLOGY

Generalized vasospasm is believed to cause preeclampsia. Patients with preeclampsia have an increase in the vasoconstrictor thromboxane and a decrease in the vasodilator prostacyclin leading to vasospasm. Angiotensin II, norepinephrine, and vasopressin levels are also increased. Placental dysfunction appears to be the link in the pathogenesis of hypertension; thus, delivery is the only cure. Major organ systems affected include brain (seizure and stoke), kidneys (renal failure and oliguria), liver (edema and subcapsular hematoma), and small blood vessels (thrombocytopenia and disseminated intravascular coagulation).

HISTORY

Preeclampsia usually occurs during the third trimester of pregnancy. Patients may present with sudden weight gain and notice swelling in their hands and face. Other late findings include headache, epigastric pain, visual disturbances, or oliguria (Table 44–1).

PHYSICAL EXAMINATION

Blood pressure should be measured on two separate occasions or at least 6 hours apart. Visual exam should including funduscopic evaluation looking for papilledema, hemorrhages, or arteriolar spasm. Cardiovascular exam should look for signs of pulmonary edema including jugular venous distention, tachycardia, gallops, tachypnea, and rales. Patients may have right upper quadrant or epigastric tenderness. On neurologic exam, look for hyperreflexia and ankle clonus. Clonus is

TABLE 44–1

Signs and Symptoms of Preeclampsia and Eclampsia

Type	Symptoms	Treatment
Hypertension	• BP >140/90 measured twice at least 6 h apart	• Methyldopa 250 mg every 6 h and titrated for blood pressure control
Mild preeclampsia	• Typically in the third trimester • BP >140/90 or increase in SBP >20 DBP >10 on two separate occasions or at least 6 hours apart • Proteinuria (>300 mg/24 hours) • Nondependent edema (hands, face) or generalized edema or weight gain (>5 lb/wk)	• Delivery: Term or evidence of fetal lung maturity • Admission • Control BP if diastolic is higher than 110 with IV hydralazine: goal DBP 90–100 mmHg • Magnesium sulfate for seizure prophylaxis continued • Obstetric consult
Severe preeclampsia	• SBP >160 or DBP >110 two separate occasions or 6 hours apart • Proteinuria (>5 g/24 hr or >3+dipstick) • Oliguria • RUQ or epigastric pain • Pulmonary edema or cyanosis • IUGR • Cerebral disturbances: headache, somnolence • Visual disturbances: blurred vision, scotomata • Hyperreflexia, clonus • HELLP syndrome	• Expedite delivery regardless of lung maturity • Emergent obstetric consult or transfer to a tertiary care hospital as soon as patient stable • Control BP with IV hydralazine: goal 90–105 mmHg • Magnesium sulfate for seizure prophylaxis
HELLP	• Hemolytic anemia (schistocytes on smear) • Elevated liver enzymes (>2 times normal) • Low platelets (<100,000)	• Expedite delivery regardless of lung maturity • Emergent obstetric consult or transfer to a tertiary care hospital as soon as patient stable • Control BP with IV hydralazine: goal 90–105 mmHg • Magnesium sulfate for seizure prophylaxis
Eclampsia	• Symptoms of preeclampsia • Tonic clonic seizure • Most common symptoms prior to eclamptic seizure include headache, visual changes, and RUQ or epigastric pain	• ABCs • 100% oxygen, maternal cardiac and fetal monitoring • Magnesium sulfate for seizure control and prophylaxis and consider benzodiazepines if poorly controlled • IV hydralazine for BP >160/110 control • Place in left lateral decubitus position • Emergent obstetric consult or transfer to a tertiary care hospital as soon as patient stable • Admission to ICU or delivery room

indicative of impending eclampsia. Fetal monitoring and stress test should be performed.

DIFFERENTIAL DIAGNOSIS

Preeclampsia

- Molar pregnancy
- Essential hypertension
- Renal disease
- Renovascular hypertension
- Primary aldosteronism
- Cushing's syndrome
- Pheochromocytoma
- Thrombocytopenia purpura
- Diabetic nephropathy
- Glomerulonephritis
- Systemic lupus erythematosus

Eclampsia

- Epilepsy
- Encephalitis
- Meningitis
- Cerebral tumors
- Acute porphyria
- Ruptured cerebral aneurysm or intracranial hemorrhage
- Drugs, substance intoxication, or withdrawal
- Electrolyte imbalance

DIAGNOSTIC EVALUATION

Laboratory studies include finger stick glucose, CBC with platelet count, BUN or creatinine, liver function tests, urinalysis, and PT or PTT. Obtain an obstetrical ultrasound to estimate gestational age and fetal viability. Patients with new-onset seizure in the absence of hypertension require a head CT to rule out intracranial bleed or mass, electrolyte studies, and toxicology screen.

Lumbar puncture should be considered for patients with fever and new-onset seizures to rule out meningitis.

MANAGEMENT

First assess ABCs (airway, breathing, circulation). Patients with eclampsia require anticonvulsant therapy and may need airway management. Patients should also be placed on oxygen, continuous blood pressure monitor, maternal cardiac monitoring, and fetal monitoring. Eclampsia seizures are initially controlled with magnesium sulfate. Second line agents include benzodiazepines or barbiturates. Hydralazine is used for blood pressure control. An emergent obstetrical consultation should be obtained.

For patients with severe preeclampsia, control blood pressure with IV hydralazine. Labetalol and diazoxide are other alternatives. Patients should be started on magnesium sulfate for seizure prophylaxis. The definite treatment of preeclampsia is delivery of the fetus. Thus, obtain an emergent OB/GYN consult.

All patients with preeclampsia require admission. Asymptomatic patients without evidence of preeclampsia can be discharged after consultation with the obstetrician.

◆ KEY POINTS ◆

1. Preeclampsia is defined as hypertension in pregnancy associated with proteinuria and nondependent edema.
2. Eclampsia is defined as seizures in a patient with preeclampsia.
3. Delivery is the ultimate treatment for both preeclampsia and eclampsia.
4. Magnesium sulfate for seizure prophylaxis and treatment.
5. Hydralazine is the first-line agent for blood pressure control.
6. Admit all patients with preeclampsia and eclampsia.

45

Vaginal Hemorrhage in Late Pregnancy

The two most common causes of third trimester bleeding are placenta previa and placental abruption. Placenta previa is a placenta that overlaps the cervix to varying degrees. Placental abruption is separation of part of the placenta from the uterine wall prior to the onset of labor. Other causes of vaginal bleeding in late pregnancy include vaginal or cervical trauma, lower genital tract infections, polyps, or hemorrhoids.

EPIDEMIOLOGY

Vaginal bleeding after 20 weeks of gestation occurs in 4% of pregnancies. Placenta previa accounts for approximately 20% of third trimester bleeding. Placental abruption accounts for approximately 30% of vaginal bleeding in the second half of pregnancy.

ETIOLOGY

Risk factors for placenta previa include prior cesarean sections, uterine scars, advanced maternal age, and multiparous women. Risk factors for placental abruption include hypertension, abdominal or pelvic trauma, cocaine or tobacco use, and advanced maternal age.

PATHOPHYSIOLOGY

Placenta previa is caused by abnormal implantation of the placenta near or at the cervical os. Placental abruption is caused by premature separation of a normally implanted placenta before the onset of labor.

HISTORY

History should include prior pregnancy complications, amount of bleeding, passage of clots, character of blood, presence of uterine cramping or pain, history of trauma, or drug use.

Patients with placenta previa typically have bright red, painless vaginal bleeding without fetal distress.

Patients with placental abruption present with dark, painful vaginal bleeding, abdominal pain, uterine hypertonicity, and tenderness. Fetal distress is often present. If bleeding is between the placenta and uterine wall, patients may exhibit signs of shock without evidence of significant external bleeding.

PHYSICAL EXAMINATION

Vaginal exam should not be performed in the emergency department until an ultrasound can be obtained to rule out placenta previa, as digital exam could trigger a hemorrhage. Once ultrasound rules out placenta previa, a cautious vaginal exam can be performed to evaluate for other causes of bleeding. Palpate the abdomen for uterine size and presence of contractions or tenderness. Look for signs of abdominal trauma.

DIFFERENTIAL DIAGNOSIS

- Early labor
- Marginal separation
- Genital tract infections
- Bloody show
- Ruptured vasa previa
- Ruptured uterus
- Cervical carcinoma

DIAGNOSTIC EVALUATION

Use ultrasound to look for rupture or an abnormally positioned placenta. Other tests include type and screen, Rh status, CBC, PT or PTT, urinalysis, and drug screen.

TREATMENT

First assess ABCs (airway, breathing, circulation). Hemodynamically unstable patients need two large-bore IVs, supplemental oxygen, cardiac monitor, and fluid resuscitation. Blood should be sent for type and crossmatch. Check for fetal heart tones with initiation of continuous monitoring to look for signs of fetal distress. An emergent OB/GYN consultation should be obtained.

Hemodynamically stable patients are usually transferred to an obstetrical unit for further evaluation. Patients with placenta previa are often managed expectantly. Patients with placental abruption are admitted to a high-risk prepartum unit. All Rh-negative mothers should be given RhoGAM IM.

 KEY POINTS

1. Placenta previa is an abnormal implantation of the placenta near the cervical os.
2. Placental abruption is a premature separation of a normally implanted placenta.
3. Placenta previa usually presents as painless bright red bleeding.
4. Placental abruption classically presents as painful vaginal bleeding with a firm tender uterus.
5. An ultrasound should be done prior to vaginal exam.
6. OB/GYN consult should be obtained.

Part VIII
Neurologic Emergencies

SIGNS AND SYMPTOMS

Dizziness or Lightheadedness:
- Hyperventilation
- Hypoxia, hypoglycemia
- Dehydration
- Hypotension
- Anemia
- Anesthetics
- Sedatives
- Toxin exposure (e.g., alcohol, inhaled gases)
- Allergic reaction
- Concussion
- Transient ischemic attack
- Stroke
- Cardiac dysrhythmia

Vertigo:
- Labyrinthitis
- Vestibular neuronitis
- Chronic otitis media
- Benign positional vertigo
- Ménière's disease
- Toxins (e.g., salicylates, alcohol, quinine, amino-glycosides)

- Migraine
- Vertebrobasilar vascular insufficiency
- Posterior circulation stroke
- Encephalitis
- Seizure aura
- Migraine
- Malignancy

Headache:
- Muscular headache (e.g., tension)
- Vascular headache (e.g., temporal arteritis, migraine)
- Inflammatory headache (e.g., migraine, carcinoid)
- Hypoxia
- Toxins (e.g., carbon monoxide poisoning)
- Alcohol withdrawal
- Nicotine withdrawal
- Caffeine withdrawal
- Hypotension
- Hypertension
- Sinusitis
- Hemorrhagic stroke
- Ischemic stroke (uncommon)
- Epidural hematoma
- Subdural hematoma
- Subarachnoid hemorrhage

- Meningitis
- Encephalitis
- Cerebral abscess
- Herpetic neuralgia
- Trigeminal neuralgia
- Glaucoma
- Post-lumbar puncture
- Arteriovenous malformation
- Pseudotumor cerebri
- Malignancy

Paresthesias:

- Hyperventilation
- Peripheral neuropathy (e.g., diabetes, thiamine deficiency)
- Varicella zoster
- Peripheral nerve compression (e.g., spinal disc herniation, carpal tunnel syndrome)
- Spinal cord compression (e.g., spinal fracture, spondylolisthesis, disc herniation, abscess, hemorrhage, malignancy)
- Spinal cord ischemia (e.g., dissection, thromboembolism, vitamin B12 deficiency, hypocalcemia, migraine)

Weakness:

- Hypoxia
- Hypoglycemia
- Hyperglycemia
- Hypokalemia
- Hyperkalemia
- Transient ischemic attack
- Stroke
- Subdural hematoma
- Epidural hematoma
- Subarachnoid hemorrhage
- Spinal cord compression (e.g., disc herniation)
- Spinal cord ischemia (e.g., aortic dissection, thromboembolism)
- Peripheral nerve compression
- Transverse myelitis
- Botulism
- Multiple sclerosis
- Guillain-Barré
- Myasthenia gravis
- Amyotrophic lateral sclerosis
- Myopathy
- Migraine

46

Atraumatic Headache

Atraumatic headaches are a common problem, with 64% of the population reporting bothersome headaches at least occasionally. Headache is the ninth most common reason patients seek treatment from their primary physician. Although most headaches are benign in origin, with only 1% resulting from serious disease, life-threatening diagnoses must always be considered.

PATHOPHYSIOLOGY

Not all structures of the head are capable of generating or sensing pain. All extracranial structures (i.e., those outside of the skull) are capable of sensing pain. Although the intracranial venous sinuses and their branches are capable of sensing pain, only the more proximal arteries (e.g., those extending just beyond the Circle of Willis) are capable of sensing and transmitting pain stimuli. Other pain-sensitive intracranial structures include the portion of dura mater overlying the base of the brain, and the vasculature within the dura. Therefore, most of the intracranial stuctures (e.g., brain parenchyma, arachnoid, pia mater, and upper portions of the dura) are incapable of generating or relaying painful stimuli.

Although the ultimate mechanisms leading to headache may still be unclear, headache can be categorized into one of three groups: tension, vascular (via distention, dilation, or traction), or inflammatory. The neuropeptide serotonin is believed to play a significant role. Any specific disease entity may cause headaches by a combination of the above mechanisms.

HISTORY

Due to the paucity of visible signs accompanying most types of headaches, historical information is the most important data in determining the type of headache. The history should include questions about the site, severity, character, and timing of pain, relieving or worsening factors, location and position of the patient during headaches, associated symptoms, past medical history, family history, and occupation. Multiple persons suffering from headache within the same location may point to environmental causes such as carbon monoxide poisoning.

PHYSICAL EXAMINATION

Although the historical information is usually the most important in determining headache origin, a complete physical examination, including a detailed neurologic examination, may reveal further clues. Laboratory and imaging data are not always necessary in the diagnosis of headache pathology, and their utilization must be considered on a case-by-case basis.

DIAGNOSES

Due to the large number of diseases that may cause headache (Table 46–1) the subsequent discussion will

TABLE 46-1

Causes of a Headache

Tension-type headache	Hypercapnia/hypoxia
Migraine/cluster headache	Poisoning (CO, nitrates)
Subarachnoid hemorrhage	Glaucoma
Other intracranial bleed	ENT infection and nasal trauma
Post head-injury	
Intracranial infection	Dental problems
Systemic febrile illnesses	Neck problems
Space-occupying lesion	Cerebrospinal fluid leakage
Temporal arteritis	
Malignant hypertension	Dehydration
Paget's disease	Psychogenic factors, including anxiety and depression

focus on three of the most commonly considered, *atraumatic* causes of headache.

Tension-type Headaches

Tension-type headaches are the most common type of headache, and affect people of all ages. This type of headache may last 30 minutes to 7 days.

Pathophysiology
Tension-type headaches are believed to result from the continuous contraction of head and neck muscles possibly triggered by stress.

History
Tension-type headaches are usually bilateral and originate posteriorly, often described as nonpulsating, tightness of mild to moderate intensity. Tension-type headaches are not typically aggravated by routine physical activity.

Physical Examination
Physical examination may reveal tight, upper, posterior neck musculature. Laboratory and imaging studies are usually normal in patients with a tension-type headache and are generally only ordered to help rule out other headache etiologies.

Treatment
Stress reduction is believed helpful for both treatment and prevention. Non-steroidal, anti-inflammatory drugs (i.e., ibuprofen) and acetaminophen are usually helpful for mild to moderate pain. Narcotics or barbituates are reserved for more severe pain.

Migraine Headaches

Migraine (i.e., "half of the skull" in Greek) headaches are believed to affect approximately 5–10% of the population in the United States. Patients usually present in childhood or adolescence, and rarely begin later in life. Migraines affect women approximately 3 times more than men. Seventy percent of patients with migraine have a family history of the disease. Typical migraines last anywhere from 4 to 72 hours.

Pathophysiology
Migraines are believed to result from vasoconstriction followed by dilation, as well as serotonergic abnormalities leading to neurogenic inflammation.

History
Patients usually describe pain that is unilateral, pulsating in quality, moderate to severe in intensity, and often accompanied by nausea, vomiting, photophobia (light sensitivity), or phonophobia (sound sensitivity). Migraines typically affect the ability of individuals to perform routine activities. Some subtypes of migraines may be preceded by auras such as visual anomalies, or be accompanied by motor deficits such as ophthalmoplegia (e.g., ophthalmoplegic migraine) or hemiplegia (e.g., hemiplegic migraine).

Physical Examination
Physical examination may be unremarkable, or reveal cranial nerve and/or motor abnormalities. New neurologic deficits should prompt the consideration of other, more serious diagnoses. Laboratory and imaging studies are usually normal in patients with a migraine and are only indicated to help rule out other headache etiologies.

Treatment
Phenothiazines (e.g., prochlorperazine) act as an antiemetic as well as an analgesic for migraines. The analgesic mechanism of action for phenothiazines is not fully understood. Ergotomines cause vasoconstriction and stabilize serotonergic neurotransmission. Serotonin, or 5-hydroxytryptamine (5-HT) agonists (e.g.,

TABLE 46–2

Hunt-Hess Classification of Subarachnoid Hemorrhage

Grade	Description
1	Mild headache and slight nuchal rigidity
2	Cranial nerve palsy, severe headache, nuchal rigidity
3	Mild focal deficit, lethargy or confusion
4	Stupor, hemiparesis, early decerebrate rigidity
5	Deep coma, decerebrate rigidity, moribund appearance

sumatriptan), also acts as both an antiemetic and an analgesic agent. Both phenothiazines and 5-HT agonists should be avoided in patients with hypertension, coronary artery disease, or focal neurologic findings. Non-steroidal anti-inflammatory drugs are available in intravenous form (e.g., ketorolac) and may be moderately effective. Steroids are used occasionally after other treatments have been attempted. Narcotics may be helpful for analgesia of severe pain refractory to other interventions. Atypical migraines, or migraines refractory to medications that are usually helpful, should prompt consideration of other headache etiologies.

Subarachnoid Hemorrhage

The incidence of subarachnoid hemorrhage (i.e., SAH) is believed to be 10 cases per 100,000 population. The disease is serious and carries a 40–50% mortality rate. Among survivors, a resulting disability occurs in 30%. The mean age of patients with subarachnoid hemorrhage is 50 year of age and it affects men and women equally. Risk factors include hypertension, smoking, cocaine use, a first-degree relative with the disease, and prior SAH. SAH has been associated with polycystic ovary disease, connective tissue diseases, and coarctation of the aorta. Subarachnoid hemorrhages are commonly graded using the Hunt-Hess classification system (Table 46–2).

Pathophysiology

An arterial aneurysm, usually within or near the Circle of Willis, or an arterial venous malformation dilates and ruptures into the subarachnoid space causing perivascular and dural inflammation perceived as a headache. Dural inflammation may extend down the spine causing neck and back pain.

History

Patients typically report the onset of a severe headache frequently described as "the worst headache of the patient's life" or a "thunderclap" headache. Loss of consciousness, neck pain, back pain, and photophobia may accompany the headache.

Physical Examination

Patients usually appear in moderate to severe distress. Meningismus may be present. Retinal hemorrhage (i.e., "Flare hemorrhage") may also be present on funduscopic exam. Focal neurologic deficits, including cranial nerve abnormalities, may or may not be present.

CT scan of the head is positive for SAH in approximately 90% of cases and is most sensitive within the first 12 hours of hemorrhage. Lumbar puncture is approximately 98% sensitive for SAH and is most accurate after 12 hours of symptoms when xanthochromia (e.g., a breakdown product of blood) may be present. If there is suspicion for SAH, diagnostic evaluation should not stop with a normal head CT; a lumbar puncture should be performed. Angiography and MRI angiography may further define a specific site of aneurysm or hemorrhage.

Treatment

Treatment may require prompt operative resection or embolization of the vascular defect. Temporizing treatments include controlling hypertension and offering analgesics. Nimodipine, a calcium-channel blocker, helps prevent arterial vasospasm, which typically presents a few days after hemorrhage. Anticonvulsants (e.g., phenytoin) are often used prophylactically.

Temporal Arteritis

Temporal arteritis (i.e., Giant cell arteritis) is a form of vasculitis that may cause headache. It is four times more common in women than in men, and it mostly affects people over the age of 50. The disease has been associated with polymyalgia rheumatica. Failure to treat the vasculitis early may result in irreversible neurologic damage.

Pathophysiology

The vasculitis is thought to be autoimmune in origin, affecting medium and small sized arteries. Arteries com-

monly affected include the superficial temporal, vertebral, ophthalmic, internal carotid, and external carotid
arteries. Retinal, basilar, and cerebellar infarcts are
common sequelae.

History
Patients with temporal arteritis are typically older and
complain of sharp, burning, unilateral pain over the
temporal artery that may be worse at night. Occasionally the pain may be bilateral. Patients may report fever,
malaise, weight loss, and visual defects.

Physical Examination
Patients may present with a low-grade fever, a tender
pulseless superficial temporal artery, decreased visual
acuity, optic nerve edema on retinal exam, mild
meningeal signs, and, rarely, other focal neurologic
findings. A nonspecific marker of inflammation, the
erythrocyte sedimentation rate (ESR) is usually elevated. Temporal artery biopsy may show evidence of the
disease, but false-negative biopsies are common.

Treatment
Due to the fact that the vasculitis may progress rapidly,
immediate treatment with steroids to reduce inflammation is warranted. NSAIDs may further aid in analgesia.

Temporal arteritis may cause blindness if not treated
immediately

◆ KEY POINTS ◆

1. Only certain intracranial structures are
capable of sensing and transmitting pain.
2. Tension headaches are typically bilateral and
result from muscle tension secondary to stress.
3. Migraines are usually unilateral and treated
with phenothiazines, ergotomines, 5-HT agonists, narcotics, or NSAIDs.
4. Subarachnoid hemorrhage is a life-threatening,
neurosurgical disease that usually results from
the rupture of an arterial aneurysm within or
adjacent to the Circle of Willis.
5. Temporal arteritis is a vasculitis associated
with headache that may cause blindness if not
treated immediately.
6. New headaches in the elderly are not common
and are more likely to represent underlying
disease.

47

Acute Stroke

Stroke is the disruption of blood flow to a region of brain leading to neurologic dysfunction. Affecting more than 550,000 people annually, stroke is the third leading cause of death and the leading cause of disability in the United States. Transient ischemic attacks (TIAs) are transient periods of neurologic impairment due to cerebral ischemia that last less than 24 hours and resolve completely. Patients who suffer a TIA are at significantly higher risk for developing a stroke and therefore require further evaluation to determine an etiology.

PATHOPHYSIOLOGY

Strokes are divided into ischemic and hemorrhagic types. Ischemic strokes are further classified by their origin as either thrombotic, embolic, or hypoperfusion. Emboli are believed to cause approximately 20% of all strokes. The heart (e.g., thrombi, vegetations, tumor) and arteries (e.g., thrombi, plaque) are the most common sources of emboli. Air, fat, and amniotic fluid may also cause embolic strokes via atrial septal defects. Hypoperfusion usually results from reduced cardiac output (e.g., acute myocardial infarction) or carotid dissection. Hemorrhagic strokes are subdivided by their location as either intracerebral or subarachnoid. Intracerebral hemorrhages usually result from the rupture of small arterioles or arteriovenous malformations often in the setting of hypertension. Subarachnoid hemorrhages are usually due to the rupture of arterial aneurysms or arteriovenous malformations. During a stroke, collateral blood flow may help to maintain perfusion to ischemic regions of brain (Fig. 47–1, Table 47–1).

HISTORY

A complete history should elicit the baseline level of function and how it differs from the current presentation. Family members and close contacts are often invaluable resources. The past medical history frequently suggests a specific stroke etiology (e.g., hypertension, coronary artery disease, atrial fibrillation, cardiac valve replacement, connective tissue disorder). Due to the lack of pain fibers within brain parenchyma, ischemic strokes do not typically cause headache. In contrast, headaches often accompany hemorrhagic strokes. (See the chapter entitled "Atraumatic Headache.") A history of recent neck trauma may suggest carotid dissection.

PHYSICAL EXAMINATION

A complete physical examination should be performed including a detailed neurologic evaluation. Fever may suggest a septic source. Anisocoria (i.e., unequal pupils) and papilladema may represent increased intracranial pressure and brain herniation. A carotid bruit may suggest hypoperfusion, atheromatous emboli, or a carotid dissection. An irregularly, irregular heartbeat

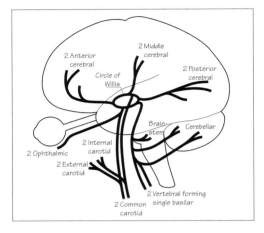

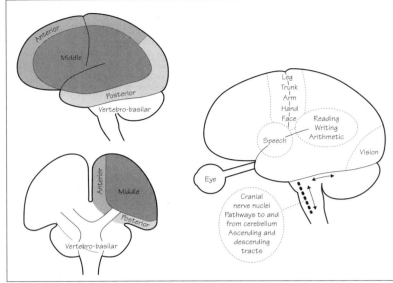

Figure 47–1   A schematic diagram of the arteries supplying the brain. Arterial territories and localization of function within the brain.

TABLE 47–1

Common Manifestations of Stroke Syndrome by Vascular Supply

- Anterior Cerebral Artery
  1. Contralateral extremity weakness (lower > upper)
  2. Altered mentation, reasoning
  3. Bowel and bladder incontinence
- Middle Cerebral Artery
  1. Contralateral face and arm weakness greater than leg
  2. Contralateral sensory deficits
  3. Dysphasia (if dominant brain hemisphere affected)
- Posterior Cerebral Artery
  1. Contralateral visual field deficits
  2. Altered mentation
  3. Cortical blindness
- Vertebrobasilar Arteries
  1. Vertigo or nystagmus
  2. Dysarthria
  3. Dysphagia
  4. Contralateral pain and temperature sensory deficits
  5. Syncope

may represent atrial fibrillation. A thorough neurologic examination should include an assessment of the level of consciousness, language, cognition, cranial nerves, motor function, cerebellar function, sensation, neglect, and, if possible, gait.

DIAGNOSIS

Emergent diagnostic studies in stroke should include a serum glucose, electrocardiogram, and CT scan of the head. Electrolyte, complete blood count, and coagulation studies should also be obtained. The blood sugar should be measured immediately since hypoglycemia is a potentially reversible cause of focal neurologic deficit. CT scanning without intravenous contrast is a very accurate means to differentiate ischemic from hemorrhagic stroke. In general, ischemic strokes are not visible on noncontrast CT imaging of the head until at least 6 hours after brain infarction. MRI is more sensitive for strokes of the posterior fossa as well as those presenting within 6 hours of symptom onset. Imaging with angiography (gold-standard) or ultrasound may help to demonstrate partial or complete occlusion of cerebral and cervical vasculature.

TREATMENT

As with other diseases, a patent airway should be assured. Stroke patients should receive supplemental oxygen and have an intravenous line established. Hypoxia and hypotension should be immediately corrected as they may significantly worsen neurologic outcome. Continuous, intra-arterial blood pressure monitoring may be necessary to accurately monitor blood pressure. Prompt neurology and/or neurosurgical consultation should be sought in all cases of stroke.

In ischemic stroke, the blood pressure is frequently elevated as a result of the brain's autoregulation of cerebral vasculature. Hypertension following ischemic stroke should generally not be treated unless it is severe (i.e., SBP ≥220 or DBP ≥120). Hypertension in stroke is usually treated with intravenous nitroprusside—since it has a short half-life and is easily titratable—or intravenous labetalol. Patients should receive antiplatelet therapy with aspirin if no contraindication exists. Patients with thrombosis, thromboembolic disease, or cervical arterial dissection may benefit from further anticoagulation with heparin as long as the area of brain involved is not extremely large and thus at risk for subsequent hemorrhagic transformation. Intravenous thrombolysis with agents such as TPA (i.e., tissue-plasminogen activator) is a controversial therapy that should only be considered in patients presenting with ischemic strokes of less than 3 hours duration and without evidence of hemorrhage on CT scan of the head. Intra-arterial thrombolysis may be helpful in certain situations and should only be performed by neurologists and interventionalists familiar with the procedure. Patients suffering from an acute ischemic stroke, especially those presenting within 3 hours of symptoms, should be considered for immediate transfer to a local stroke center as such centers offer a morbidity and mortality benefit over other hospitals.

Treatment of hypertension in hemorrhagic stroke is controversial. Elevated blood pressure increases intracerebral bleeding and pressure (ICP). Conversely blood pressure that is too low may reduce the cerebral perfusion pressure (CPP). Most experts support reducing the blood pressure to 140 to 160 mmHg or 80 to 90 mmHg in chronic hypertensive patients, and reducing the blood pressure to normal in patients without previous hypertension. Diuretics (e.g., mannitol, furosemide) may temporarily reduce ICP by fluid shifts and should be considered in patients with signs of significantly elevated ICP and deteriorating neurologic function. Due to the increased risk of seizure in hemorrhagic stroke, most patients should receive a prophylactic anticonvulsant such as phenytoin. Larger and progressively worsening intracerebral hemorrhage may require emergent evacuation by a neurosurgeon.

All patients experiencing an acute stroke should be hospitalized.

 KEY POINTS ◆

1. The origin of strokes is either ischemic or hemorrhagic.

2. Ischemic strokes do not typically cause headache.

3. Hypertension in ischemic stroke may be the adaptive result of compensatory cerebral autoregulation and should not be overtreated.

4. Patients suffering acute ischemic strokes benefit from facilities with stroke centers.

5. Only patients with acute ischemic strokes of less than 3 hours duration should be considered for intravenous thrombolysis.

48 Seizures

A seizure is the clinical manifestation of neurologic dysfunction resulting from abnormal, excessive cortical neuron activity. The origins of seizures are classified as either primary (i.e., recurring without a known cause; epilepsy) or secondary (i.e., resulting from an identified stimulus or disease). Although the incidence of epilepsy within the United States is less than 1%, 10% of the population will experience at least one seizure in their lifetime.

Clinically, seizures are categorized as either generalized or focal (i.e., partial). Generalized seizures are thought to originate from nearly simultaneous activation of both cortical hemispheres resulting in loss of consciousness and usually rhythmic, tonic-clonic, muscle contractions (i.e., convulsions) of all four extremities. Focal seizures initiate from a specific point within one cerebral cortex and manifest symptoms related to the anatomic portion of brain affected. Focal seizures are further subdivided into simple partial and complex partial depending on whether there is loss of consciousness. In simple partial seizures, consciousness is maintained. In complex partial seizures, there is loss of consciousness indicating the spreading or generalizing of aberrant neuronal activity to both cortical hemispheres.

The postictal (post-after; ictus-seizure) period is the variable interval of time immediately following a seizure, usually characterized by transient, impaired consciousness and neurologic function. Most seizures last 1 to 2 minutes. The term *status epilepticus* refers to a potentially life-threatening condition where there is continuous seizure activity for greater than 30 minutes or recurrent seizures without an intervening return to normal, baseline neurologic function. The diagnosis of seizures should be made carefully as the disorder has far-reaching implications related to operating motor vehicles, insurance, and employment. It is important to remember that "not all seizures shake (i.e., nonconvulsive seizures), and not all that shakes is a seizure."

PATHOPHYSIOLOGY

Seizures may result from a large variety of metabolic, infectious, anatomic, and toxic etiologies (Table 48–1). Although the pathophysiology is not completely understood at the neuronal level, neurotransmitters such as acetylcholine (excitatory) and α-aminobutyric acid (GABA; inhibitory) have been proven to exert significant effects. For an individual to be conscious, they must maintain relatively normal function in at least one cortical hemisphere, as well as the reticular activating system (RAS) of the brainstem.

Eye deviation to one side indicates the electrical "overactivity" of the frontal eye field within the opposite frontal lobe and offers a possible site of origin of the seizure. This same circuitry explains why patients "look away from seizures" (electrical overactivity) and "look towards injury" (electrical underactivity). Whether by direct injury, rapid depletion of metabolic substrates (e.g., oxygen and glucose), or some other mechanism,

TABLE 48–1

Common Causes of Seizure

- Metabolic
  1. Hypo-/Hyperglycemia
  2. Hypo-/Hypernatremia
  3. Hypocalcemia
  4. Hyperthermia
- Substance Induced
  1. Isoniazid
  2. Lidocaine
  3. Tricyclic antidepressants
  4. Cocaine
  5. Alcohol withdrawal
  6. Camphor
  7. Carbon monoxide poisoning
  8. Lead poisoning
- Disease-Related (Noninfectious)
  1. Eclampsia
  2. Encephalopathy
  3. Cerebral infarction
  4. Intracranial hemorrhage
  5. Intracranial neoplasm
  6. Epilepsy
- Disease-Related (Infectious)
  1. Meningitis
  2. Encephalitis
  3. Cysticercosis
  4. Malaria (falciparum)
  5. Toxoplasmosis

permanent neuronal injury may ensue within 30 to 60 minutes of continuous seizure activity, even in the absence of apparent convulsions.

HISTORY

Since seizures are relatively short events and usually resolve prior to arriving in the emergency department, historical details are extremely important in the diagnosis and treatment of seizure disorders. Family members and witnesses are often invaluable sources of information. First, it should be determined whether the patient has had previous seizures, and, if so, whether the recent seizure was any different. Obtaining a complete list of current medications is critical and should include recent changes and missed doses. Questions should also illicit information about the individual's location at the time of the seizure, recreational drug abuse, preceding odd sensations (i.e., auras), preceding repetitive movements (i.e., automatisms), time of seizure onset, the progression of physical manifestations, whether or not the patient lost consciousness, and the duration of the seizure. A complete past medical history may suggest possible causes of seizure such as hypo- or hyperglycemia, previous stroke, head injury, or malignancy. In patients with new or atypical seizures, it is important to search for possible causes by questioning the patient about the presence of recent headaches, head trauma, a history of blank spells, staring, unexplained injuries, or developmental delay. The family history may reveal others with seizures or neurologic disorders that may be hereditary and of value in diagnosis. Finally, determining the baseline neurologic function of an individual is critical to know whether the patient has returned to normal.

PHYSICAL EXAMINATION

The physical examination should be comprehensive and include a detailed, complete neurologic evaluation. It is important to look not only for the injuries that may have been caused by the seizure, but for findings that may indicate the origin of the seizure. Seizures may cause fractures, sprains, contusions, dislocations, intra-oral bite injuries, and aspiration. The neurologic examination should evaluate the patient's level of consciousness, cognitive function, cranial nerves, motor function, sensory perception, and cerebellar function. It is common for seizures to cause transient abnormal neurologic findings such as slight anisocoria (i.e., unequal pupil size) or a Babinski sign (i.e., upgoing toes on plantar reflex) that resolve with time. Following a benign seizure, patients should slowly and continually improve. Neurologic deterioration is of great concern, and should signal the clinician to expeditiously search for and treat the disease states that may have caused the seizure.

There are no standard laboratory blood examinations that should be performed on all seizure patients. Rather, laboratory studies should be individualized depending on the clinical context. For example, patients with well-known seizure disorders may warrant anticonvulsant medication levels or no testing at all. In contrast, patients experiencing their first seizure may require more extensive laboratory studies such as electrolytes (e.g., calcium, magnesium, sodium), glucose, and a toxicology screen. Abnormal anticonvulsant drug levels for a particular patient may result from noncompliance, changes in dosing, other medication changes that affect anticonvulsant metabolism, and malabsorption (e.g., vomiting and diarrhea). A creatine kinase may be helpful in cases of prolonged seizure where rhabdomyolysis is of concern. Cerebral spinal fluid (CSF) examination from a lumbar puncture should be performed if infectious etiologies are being considered.

Radiographic imaging of the brain is usually not warranted in patients with recurrent, typical seizures. However, patients experiencing their first seizure, or those with a deteriorating neurologic exam should undergo emergent computed tomography (CT) brain imaging without contrast to assess for bleeding and large structural lesions. CT scan of the brain with contrast may be more sensitive in detecting smaller vascular (e.g., arterial venous malformations, aneurysms) and structural (e.g., metastasis) lesions. However, magnetic resonance imaging (MRI) of the brain is the most sensitive imaging modality for detecting subtle vascular and structural lesions. Since MRI is not always available and requires long scan times, CT is often the initial imaging modality of choice. The ordering of plain film x-rays should be individualized to help diagnose fractures, and certain primary malignancies such as lung cancer when appropriate. Although an electroencephalogram (EEG) may be helpful in the diagnosis, localization, and prognosis of seizures, it is not usually part of the emergency department evaluation.

requiring long-acting paralytics should have their cortical electrical activity monitored continuously with an electroencephalogram (i.e., EEG). Once the airway is secure, reversible metabolic causes of seizure activity should be treated accordingly (e.g., glucose for hypoglycemia, sodium for hyponatremia, and pyridoxime for isoniazid overdose). In most other cases of seizure, benzodiazepines (e.g., diazepam, lorazepam, midazolam) are the first-line pharmacologic treatment. Benzodiazepines are GABA receptor agonists, and are successful in terminating seizure activity in 75–90% of patients. Although the intravenous route of drug administration is preferable, diazepam may be administered rectally, or via the endotracheal tube. Second-line anticonvulsants include phenytoin (i.e., Dilantin) and phenobarbital. Although phosphenytoin may be given faster intravenously than phenytoin, it must be metabolized by the liver for activation, and therefore becomes therapeutic in approximately the same length of time (approximately 20 min) as phenytoin. Similar to benzodiazepines, phenobarbital also acts as a GABA receptor agonist. Adverse reactions to anticonvulsants usually include sedation and hypotension. Phenytoin may also cause cardiac dysrhythmias. Eclampsia should be considered in pregnant and peripartum patients with seizure, and treated with intravenous magnesium.

Patients with seizures refractory to the above interventions should be viewed as critically ill since prolonged seizures lasting longer than 30 to 60 minutes may result in irreversible brain injury. Further anticonvulsant regimens include valproate, barbituate coma, and isoflurane anesthesia.

TREATMENT

The treatment of seizures should first focus on assuring a patent airway. In most cases of seizure, adequate airway protection is achieved by placing the patient on his or her side and suctioning secretions. The area around the patient should be free from hard, immobile objects that may inflict injury to the patient should they be struck during convulsions. In cases of impending airway compromise, including prolonged seizures refractory to initial therapies, definitive airway protection with endotracheal intubation should be established. Long-acting paralytics should generally be avoided if possible since they stop the visible convulsions, but do not terminate cortical seizure activity. Seizing patients

---

◆ KEY POINTS ◆

1. Status epilepticus is continuous seizure activity for greater than 30 minutes or recurrent seizures without an intervening return to the normal, baseline neurologic function.

2. Not all seizures shake, and not all that shakes is a seizure.

3. Permanent neuronal injury may ensue within 30 to 60 minutes of continuous seizure activity, even in the absence of convulsions.

4. Benzodiazepines are the initial treatment of choice for most actively seizing patients.

49 Myasthenia Gravis

Myasthenia gravis (MG) is an autoimmune disease affecting the neuromuscular junction that causes skeletal muscle weakness. The disease affects all age groups. MG is associated with abnormalities of the thymus. Myasthenic crises can be easily triggered by stress (e.g., surgery or infection), rapid corticosteroid withdrawal, overactivity, and many common medications that adversely affect neuromuscular transmission. Complications include respiratory failure, aspiration, and overmedication.

PATHOPHYSIOLOGY

Skeletal muscle stimulation normally occurs when acetylcholine is released from nerve endings and binds to the acetylcholine receptors within the muscle cell membrane. Acetylcholinesterase destroys excess acetylcholine within the neurosynaptic cleft. In patients with MG, antibodies bind and help destroy the acetylcholine receptors making it more difficult for muscle stimulation to occur.

HISTORY

Patients with MG usually first present with oculobulbar complaints of diplopia, blurred vision, or neck weakness that may improve to some degree after rest. Other symptoms may include dysarthria, dysphagia, and occa-

sionally extremity or diaphragm weakness. The disease tends to worsen in hot environments and improve in cold.

PHYSICAL EXAMINATION

Vital signs are usually normal. Examination of the head may reveal ptosis, focal oculomotor weakness, dysarthria, and diplopia. Jaw, neck, and extremity muscles may also be weak. The pupils remain unaffected. Involved muscles groups tend to be easily fatigable. Bedside forced vital capacity testing may be abnormally low suggesting diaphragm involvement. The diagnosis of MG is typically confirmed with the "edrophonium (Tensilon) test," which utilizes a small dose of the short-acting acetylcholinesterase inhibitor intravenously to look for transient improvement of muscle weakness.

TREATMENT

A patent airway must first be assured. Treatment of MG consists of blocking acetylcholinesterase, thereby increasing the available acetylcholine within the neurosynaptic cleft. Pyridostigmine is a commonly used, long-acting acetylcholinesterase inhibitor. Cholinergic crisis (i.e., too much cholinergic activity) may also present with similar weakness making it extremely difficult to differentiate primary myasthenia gravis disease from overmedication. Patients in cholinergic crisis due to overmedication require supportive care. Immuno-suppressive medications such as corticosteroids and aza-thioprine are also effective. Thymectomy may improve the disease and is frequently recommended. During MG crisis due to overmedication, the offending medication should be held. All patients with respiratory compro-mise should be admitted to the hospital for vigilant monitoring.

◆ **KEY POINTS** ◆

1. Myasthenia gravis is an autoimmune disease directed against skeletal muscle acetylcholine receptors causing weakness.

2. The edrophonium (Tensilon) test administers a small dose of the short-acting acetylcholines-terase inhibitor to look for improvement of muscle weakness.

3. In a patient with myasthenic crisis, primary disease must be differentiated from overtreat-ment with cholinergics (i.e., cholinergic crisis).

50 Guillain-Barré Syndrome

Guillan-Barré syndrome (i.e., Landry-Guillain-Barré syndrome and acute inflammatory polyradiculoneuropathy) is believed to be an autoimmune, demyelinating disease that primarily affects the peripheral nervous system causing weakness. In most cases, the weakness starts in the distal lower extremities, ascends to the upper extremities, and occasionally involves the cranial nerves. The degree of the weakness is variable, ranging from small motor deficits to near paralysis that may affect respiration. Most patients experience a short duration of disease and a complete recovery. Complications include respiratory failure, cardiac arrhythmias, labile blood pressure, bladder dysfunction, and diseases associated with immobility.

PATHOPHYSIOLOGY

Microscopy usually reveals peripheral demyelination with associated mononuclear inflammatory infiltrates in the endoneurium and myelin sheath of nerves. Axons are usually spared. The autoimmune response in Guillain-Barré syndrome is frequently preceded by a viral or bacterial infection (e.g., *C. jejuni*) suggesting an infectious trigger.

HISTORY

Patients typically report ascending weakness 2 to 4 weeks following a viral or bacterial illness. Fever is rarely present at the time of weakness. Less commonly, patients may present with cranial nerve abnormalities or dyspnea that may predict a more severe disease course. As many as 30% of patients report significant pain, most commonly manifested in the back.

PHYSICAL EXAMINATION

Patients usually present with weakness in the lower extremities and absent deep tendon reflexes. The most conclusive laboratory test is the cerebral spinal fluid (CSF) analysis that typically reveals a protein level greater than 400 mg/dl and a cell count less than 10/ml. Diminished forced vital capacity measurements may be indicative of imminent respiratory failure. Nerve conduction studies may also be helpful, but are not warranted in the emergency department.

TREATMENT

Due to the high risk of respiratory failure, all patients suspected of having Guillain-Barré syndrome should be hospitalized and carefully monitored. Patients may require endotracheal intubation and mechanical ventilation. Although steroids have been used in the past, no studies have demonstrated a benefit of such therapy. Supportive care, plasma exchange, and intravenous immunoglobulin remain the treatment of choice.

◆ **KEY POINTS** ◆

1. Guillain-Barré syndrome is an autoimmune, demyelinating disease primarily affecting peripheral nerves leading to a pattern of ascending muscle weakness.

2. There is a high risk of respiratory failure.

3. Treatment consists of supportive care, plasma exchange, and intravenous immunoglobulins.

51 Vertigo

Vertigo is the sensation of disequilibrium combined with a sense of movement of one's self or surroundings. Vertigo is divided into peripheral (arising from the inner ear) or central (arising from the brainstem or cerebellum). Peripheral vertigo differs from central vertigo in that it is usually benign in origin, but generates very severe symptoms. Central vertigo frequently results from cerebrovascular or cerebellar disease, and typically causes less intense symptoms.

PATHOPHYSIOLOGY

Spatial orientation results from the central nervous system's integration of stimuli from the eyes, inner ear (semicircular canals), and peripheral proprioceptors. Dysfunction in any of these systems may lead to vertigo.

HISTORY

Patients with peripheral vertigo typically describe the sudden onset of severe vertigo, nausea, and vomiting that is fatigable, aggravated by movement, and occasionally associated with tinnitus or hearing loss. Central disease usually causes the gradual onset of less intense symptoms that are not fatigable, or significantly worsened by movement. Peripheral vertigo tends to last minutes to days, whereas central vertigo usually lasts weeks to months. Headache is unusual in peripheral vertigo and should prompt the consideration of a central disease. Due to frequent brainstem involvement, central vertigo commonly presents with dysphagia, dysarthria, diplopia, ataxia, and facial numbness.

PHYSICAL EXAMINATION

A complete physical examination is important and may be limited by the severity of symptoms. The administration of an anti-vertigo medication (e.g., anticholinergic) will usually not completely resolve the symptoms, but allow for a more accurate examination. Fever may indicate an infectious origin of the vertigo. Fatigable horizontal nystagmus frequently accompanies peripheral vertigo, while nonfatigable horizontal, rotary, or vertical nystagmus is more likely in central disease. Vertical nystagmus usually only occurs in the setting of central vertigo or exposures to dissociative agents such as phencyclidine (PCP) or ketamine. A detailed neurologic exam is mandatory to evaluate for focal neurologic deficits representative of central disease. A thorough neurologic examination should include an assessment of the cranial nerves, motor function, cerebellar function, sensation, and, if possible, gait. The cerebellum, pons, and cranial nerves V–X are especially susceptible to impairment resulting from space occupying intracranial lesions that cause vertigo. Positional vertigo elicited by the Dix-Hallpike test suggests a peripheral source. Emergent diagnostic studies should include a serum glucose, electrocardiogram, and, if central vertigo is suspected, a CT scan of the head. Since MRI is superior to CT at imaging the posterior fossa, as well as detecting demyelinating disease, it may be utilized as an initial imaging study if available for select patients. Additionally, angiography and ultrasound may be useful in detecting vertebrobasilar insuffiency.

TREATMENT

Once determined, the underlying cause of the vertigo should be treated appropriately. Central vertigo typically requires neurology and/or neurosurgical consultation. Symptomatic treatment may be achieved pharmacologically using anticholinergics or antihistamines with anticholinergic activity (e.g., meclizine, diphenhydramine, promethazine, droperidol). Benzodiazepines may also be helpful in mitigating symptoms.

The following are summaries of specific disease entities that are associated with vertigo:

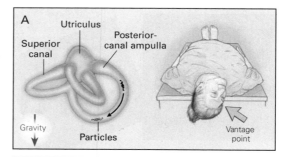

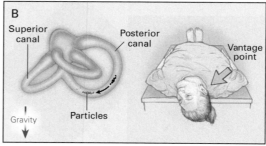

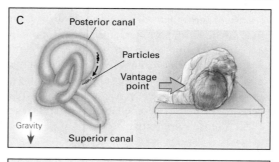

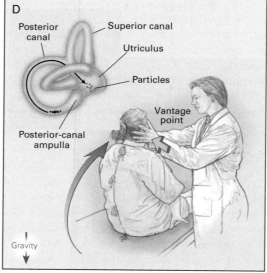

Figure 51–1 Bedside Maneuver for the Treatment of a Patient with Benign Paroxysmal Positional Vertigo Affecting the Right Ear. The presumed position of the debris within the labyrinth during the maneuver is shown in each panel. The maneuver is a three-step procedure. First, a Dix-Hallpike test is performed with the patient's head rotated 45 degrees toward the right ear and the neck slightly extended with the chin pointed slightly upward. This position results in the patient's head hanging to the right (Panel A). Once the vertigo and nystagmus provoked by the Dix-Hallpike test cease, the patient's head is rotated about the rostral-caudal body axis until the left ear is down (Panel B). Then the head and body are further rotated until the head is face down (Panel C). The vertex of the head is kept tilted downward throughout the rotation. The maneuver usually provokes brief vertigo. The patient should be kept in the final, facedown position for about 10 to 15 seconds. With the head kept turned toward the left shoulder, the patient is brought into the seated position (Panel D). Once the patient is upright, the head is tilted so that the chin is pointed slightly downward.

BENIGN POSITIONAL VERTIGO (BPV)

Etiology

Free-floating calcium carbonate crystals (otoliths) within the endolymph of the semicircular canals break free from their attachments causing alterations in endolymphatic pressure and ultimately cupular deflection.

History

BPV most commonly affects the elderly. Patients report fatigable vertigo elicited by head movements.

Physical Examination

Vertigo is elicited by the Dix-Hallpike maneuver, and typically resolves within approximately 30 seconds of head stillness.

Treatment

Symptomatic treatment may be achieved with antivertigo medications. Curative treatment necessitates removal of the free-floating otoliths from the semicircular canals via the Epley maneuver (Fig. 51–1).

LABYRINTHITIS (VESTIBULO-COCHLEAR INFLAMMATION)

Etiology

The most common cause of labyrinthitis is believed to be viral infection. Other causes include toxins (e.g., aminoglycosides, furosemide, NSAIDs) and, rarely, bacterial infection.

History

Patients typically describe the sudden onset of vertigo, nausea, and vomiting accompanied by some degree of hearing loss or tinnitus. Patients may also report current or recent illness such as upper respiratory infection or otitis media.

Physical Examination

Physical examination may reveal fever, otitis media, or hearing loss. Nystagmus is often present at rest and may not significantly worsen by changes in head position.

Treatment

Treatment consists of treating any underlying infection, removing any potentially toxic exposures, and symptom relief with antivertigo medications.

CENTRAL VERTIGO

Specific entities causing central vertigo include cerebrovascular disease, neoplasms, and demyelinating disease such as multiple sclerosis. As described above, a thorough history and physical examination are crucial in the evaluation of a patient with central vertigo. Imaging of the brain with CT or MRI is usually warranted. Further workup should be tailored to the disease entity being considered. Neurologic and/or neurosurgical consultation should be sought early in the diagnosis and treatment of diseases causing central vertigo.

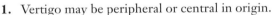

◆ KEY POINTS ◆

1. Vertigo may be peripheral or central in origin.

2. Peripheral vertigo usually begins suddenly with severe symptoms, while central vertigo usually has a gradual onset with milder symptoms.

3. Benign positional vertigo may be elicited by the Dix-Hallpike Test and cured using the Epley maneuver.

4. Labyrinthitis is usually caused by a viral infection, but may also result from bacterial infection or vestibulo-cochlear toxins.

5. Headache is not typically associated with benign vertigo, and should therefore prompt the consideration of more serious disease entities.

6. Cerebellar stroke and vertebrobasilar insufficiency should always be considered in patients with risk factors for vascular disease.

Part IX
Psychiatric
Emergencies

52 Depression and Suicidality

EPIDEMIOLOGY

The lifetime risk of major depression approaches 5 to 20% in the United States with a slight 2:1 female predominance. The incidence of new cases is greatest in the 20–40 age group. Risk factors include a history of depression in first-degree relatives, alcohol and substance abuse, female gender, and prior depression.

PATHOPHYSIOLOGY

Evidence suggests that depression is due to a combination of biologic, genetic, and environmental factors. The biologic theory holds that depression is due to abnormally low circulating levels of norepinephrine and serotonin. Evidence for a genetic basis for depression comes from studies of families and twins of depressed patients.

HISTORY

Major depression is characterized by the following: depressed mood, sleep disturbances, difficulty concentrating, fatigue, anhedonia (decrease in the pleasure derived from previously pleasurable activities), guilt, suicidality, psychomotor retardation or agitation, and a change in appetite (either markedly increased or decreased).

Episodes of major depression typically last from 6 to 12 months. Almost half of patients with major depression die of suicide.

DIFFERENTIAL DIAGNOSIS

- Major depression
- Bipolar disorder
- Dysthymic disorder

TREATMENT

Both pharmacotherapy and psychotherapy have been used in the treatment of depression. There are four major classes of compounds used in the treatment of major depression: selective serotonin reuptake inhibitors (fluoxetine, paroxetine, sertraline), tricyclic antidepressants (desipramine, nortriptyline, imipramine, amitriptyline), monoamine oxidase inhibitors (phenelzine, tranylcypromine), and a mixed group (venlafaxine, bupropion, trazadone, nefazodone). Pharmacotherapy should be continued for at least 6 to 9 months.

SUICIDE

Suicide accounts for over 25,000 deaths a year in the United States with the majority occurring between the ages of 20 and 30. Women are more likely to attempt suicide while men are more likely to succeed. Risk factors for suicide include alcoholism, depression, schizophrenia, or a history of suicide in a first-degree relative. A psychiatrist should evaluate patients with suicidal ideation in order to determine the need for potential hospitalization.

 KEY POINTS

1. Depression is very common.

2. Evidence suggests that depression is due to a deficiency of serotonin and norepinephrine.

3. Treatment of depression involves drug therapy or psychotherapy.

4. Women are more likely to attempt suicide while men are more likely to succeed.

53 Panic Disorder

Anxiety is a common symptom in patients presenting to the emergency department. Though anxiety can be adaptive in certain situations, panic disorder is a maladaptive condition that exists on the continuum of simple anxiety.

DEFINITION

Panic disorder is characterized by recurrent panic attacks. A panic attack is a period of intense anxiety coupled with at least four of the following: chest pain, palpitations, diaphoresis, difficulty breathing, choking sensation, tremors, nausea or abdominal pain, dizziness, fear of dying, fear of being outside of one's body, or fear of going crazy.

EPIDEMIOLOGY

Almost 10% of people report signs and symptoms of panic attacks without meeting the requisite criteria for panic disorder. The lifetime prevalence of panic disorder is between 2% and 5% and occurs more frequently in women.

HISTORY

Patients presenting with a panic attack report signs and symptoms that overlap with many common medical conditions. Patients may complain of cardiac type symptoms such as chest pain, palpitations, or shortness of breath, or gastrointestinal symptoms including abdominal pain, vomiting, or nausea. Neurologic complaints such as weakness, tremors, headaches, or pseudoseizures are also common.

PHYSICAL EXAMINATION

Patients are typically anxious, tachycardic, and tachypneic. They may appear pale and diaphoretic, and may be vomiting. Neurologic examination may reveal sensory or motor deficits.

DIFFERENTIAL DIAGNOSIS

- Generalized anxiety disorder
- Stroke
- Myocardial infarction
- Pulmonary embolism
- Gastroenteritis
- Acute abdominal pain

DIAGNOSTIC EVALUATION

Although a potentially disabling and devastating condition, the diagnosis of panic disorder should be a diagnosis of exclusion in a patient presenting to the emergency department. As the presentation of a panic attack is typically dramatic and mimics that of other potentially life-threatening medical and surgical conditions, the diagnostic evaluation should focus on excluding organic causes of illness, and may include laboratory studies, EKGs, and radiographic studies.

TREATMENT

Once the diagnosis of panic disorder is established, treatment involves use of cognitive therapy or pharmacotherapy. Drugs effective in the treatment of panic disorder include tricyclic antidepressants, monoamine oxidase inhibitors, selective serotonin reuptake inhibitors, and high-potency benzodiazepines such as alprazolam and diazepam. Though effective treatment

exists, panic disorder is typically a chronic and recurrent problem.

 KEY POINTS ◆

1. Panic disorder is common in emergency department populations.

2. The signs and symptoms of panic disorder mimic those of other organic illnesses.

3. Diagnosis hinges on excluding medical illness and keeping panic disorder in the differential diagnosis of patients presenting to the emergency department.

4. Panic disorder can be treated with antidepressant medication and high-potency anxiolytics.

54 Psychosis

Psychosis is defined as loss of contact with reality, characterized by hallucinations and delusions. Hallucinations are false sensory perceptions that have no basis in reality. They may be auditory, visual, olfactory, or gustatory (taste). Delusions are false beliefs that are inconsistent with a person's values and experience. Psychotic patients may experience delusions of control, grandeur, or persecution. Patients with delusions of control are under the mistaken belief that their thoughts and actions are under the control of an external force. Delusions of grandeur are characterized by a false sense of power or invincibility. Persecutory delusions are ones in which the patient believes that everyone is against them. Psychosis is a prominent feature in four clinical disorders that are frequently encountered in the emergency department: schizophrenia, schizophreniform disorder, delusional disorder, and brief psychotic disorder.

SCHIZOPHRENIA

Approximately 1% of the population suffers from schizophrenia with most "first breaks" (first episode of psychosis) occurring in the early 20s for men and late 20s for women. For unclear reasons, children born in the winter months have a higher incidence of schizophrenia. Children who later develop schizophrenia are typically withdrawn, labeled as odd or eccentric, and have behavioral problems at school.

Clinically, schizophrenia is characterized by positive (hallucinations, delusions, disorganized speech and behavior) or negative (catatonia, poverty of speech, flat affect) symptoms that persist for at least 6 months and are associated with a decline in occupational and social functioning. Treatment involves the use of antipsychotic drugs such as haloperidol, chlorpromazine, olanzapine, or risperidone.

SCHIZOPHRENIFORM DISORDER

Schizophreniform disorder is characterized by the same clinical presentation as schizophrenia but is present for less than 6 months. By definition, this is a self-limited disorder.

DELUSIONAL DISORDER

Delusional disorder is characterized by persistent nonbizarre delusions that do not cause impairment of social functioning. Typically, the onset of the delusions occurs in mid-to-late adulthood with women affected more then men. Persecutory delusions, delusions of infidelity on the part of a significant other, or delusions of being ill or having body odor are common. Treatment is typically supportive, though psychotherapy may play a role.

BRIEF PSYCHOTIC DISORDER

Brief psychotic disorder refers to psychosis that lasts from 14 days to 1 month and is typically associated with a stressful life event. Typical precipitants include the death of a loved one or a near death experience. Antipsychotic medication may be required but the disease is typically self-limited.

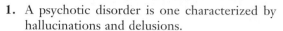

◆ KEY POINTS ◆

1. A psychotic disorder is one characterized by hallucinations and delusions.
2. "First breaks" of schizophrenia typically occur in patients 20–30 years of age.
3. Schizophreniform disorder is characterized by psychosis that lasts less than 6 months.
4. Brief psychotic disorder typically occurs in response to a traumatic life event.

55 Delirium and Dementia

Delirium is an acute confusional state characterized by:

1. Disturbance of consciousness with decreased ability to focus, sustain, or shift attention
2. A change in mental status that cannot be attributed to a pre-existing dementia
3. A waxing and waning pattern to the alteration in consciousness
4. Laboratory evidence of a toxic-metabolic source for the alteration in consciousness

Dementia, unlike delirium, is a more steadily progressive disorder without day-to-day and hour-to-hour fluctuations. The most common types of dementia are Alzheimer's dementia and multi-infarct dementia.

ETIOLOGY

There is an extensive list of substance-related and medical conditions that are associated with acute delirium. Almost any medication can potentially cause delirium but alcohol, benzodiazepines, narcotic pain relievers, and anticholinergic medications, such as diphenhydramine, are the most common. General medical problems that are associated with delirium include urinary tract infections, pneumonia, meningitis, hyponatremia, hypoglycemia, hypoxia, and hypercalcemia.

EPIDEMIOLOGY

Delirium is commonly observed in hospitalized patients especially the elderly. It is estimated that 30 to 50% of elderly, hospitalized patients experience acute delirium at some point during their hospital stay. Risk factors include a history of dementia, Parkinson's disease, cerebrovascular disease, polypharmacy, or infection.

HISTORY

Patients with acute delirium typically have a markedly altered mental status. Psychosis, sleep-wake cycle disturbances, and evening worsening of confusion (sundowning) are common signs and symptoms.

PHYSICAL EXAMINATION

The physical examination should focus on finding treatable causes of delirium. Hypoxia and hypovolemia should be corrected. Kussmaul respirations may be the only indication of hyperglycemia and diabetic ketoacidosis. Careful pulmonary examination may reveal signs of pneumonia.

DIFFERENTIAL DIAGNOSIS

- Dementia
- Psychosis

- Mania
- Meningitis
- Encephalitis
- Stroke
- Substance abuse

DIAGNOSTIC EVALUATION

Blood should be sent for chemistries including calcium, complete blood counts, cultures, and glucose. A urinalysis is necessary to look for signs of infection. A chest radiograph, EKG, and a computed tomography scan of the head may be indicated as part of the diagnostic workup.

TREATMENT

Treatment should be directed at the underlying cause of the acute delirium. Electrolyte abnormalities should be corrected gently, infection treated with appropriate antibiotics, and offending drugs removed. Soft restraints or antipsychotic medication such as haloperidol may be needed in the short term to prevent self-injury during the acute phases of delirium.

◆ KEY POINTS ◆

1. Delirium is characterized by a waxing and waning mental status.
2. Dementia is a chronic progressive disorder most commonly caused by multiple cerebral infarcts or Alzheimer's disease.
3. Delirium is typically caused by infection, electrolyte abnormalities, or drugs.
4. Treatment of delirium is directed at the underlying cause.

Part X
Trauma

56

General Approach to the Trauma Patient

Trauma is primarily a disease of the young, and is the leading cause of death in patients 1 to 37 years of age. It is responsible for more deaths in the 5 to 34 year age group than all other diseases combined. Understanding the mechanism of trauma enables the physician to predict likely injuries. Trauma centers provide unique resources and experience that can benefit trauma patients. Trauma center designations range from level I to level III, with level I facilities offering the highest level of care.

To optimally manage a patient with multiple injuries, a practiced, well-organized team approach is necessary. There should be one team captain, a physician, examining the patient and ordering care, while other specified health care providers perform predetermined tasks.

When evaluating a multiple trauma patient, it is important to identify and treat the most life-threatening injuries first. The identification and treatment of critical injuries (e.g., tension pneumothorax) may be delayed by inappropriately focusing on visibly impressive, less significant injuries (e.g., extremity amputation). Mistakes resulting from "tunnel vision" may be avoided if the approach to the patient is well organized. Systematic primary and secondary surveys help the physician to identify the most critical injuries first. Patients with potential spinal injuries should receive spinal precautions until such injuries are ruled out.

Emergency medical technicians are often invaluable resources for historical patient information. The ideal time to obtain complete historical information from the patient varies depending on the stability of the patient.

Hemodynamically unstable patients require rapid physical assessment and treatment prior to detailed questioning. The following discussion reviews the general sequence for evaluating a multiple trauma patient.

PRIMARY SURVEY

This takes less than 30 seconds; use the mnemonic "ABCDEFG."

Airway

Assure a clear and unobstructed airway by listening to the patient speak and by examining the airway. Patients may require foreign body removal, suctioning, careful repositioning, or endotracheal intubation.

Breathing

The patient's chest should be evaluated for symmetrical wall movement, symmetrical breath sounds, contusions, lacerations, tenderness, and subcutaneous air. Clinically suspected, significant pneumothoraces should be needle decompressed or treated definitively with tube thoracostomy. Sucking chest wounds may require occlusive dressings. Support with mechanical ventilation may be necessary. Patients suffering significant trauma should receive supplemental oxygen.

Circulation

The presence of pulses may help to approximate the systolic blood pressure (e.g., radial pulse present

≥70 mmHg, femoral pulse present ≥60 mmHg, carotid pulse present ≥50 mmHg). Profuse hemorrhage should be controlled. Sternal compressions may be required in a pulseless patient.

Disability

The Glasgow Coma score should be noted. Gross motor function may be quickly assessed by movement of hands and feet.

Exposure

Clothing on victims of significant trauma should be removed to avoid masking significant injuries.

Foley Catheter

The need for a urinary catheter should be determined. Suspected urethral injury is usually a contraindication to the placement of a urinary catheter.

Gastric Tube

The need for an orogastric or nasogastric tube should be determined. **Measured vital signs should now be assessed**.

SECONDARY SURVEY

The survey progresses from head to toe.

Skull

The skull should be evaluated for deformity and lacerations.

Eyes

The pupils should be assessed for symmetry and reaction to light. Extraocular muscles should be assessed for full range of motion and symmetry.

Ears

Tympanic membranes should be assessed for hemotympanum and clear fluid discharge that may represent cerebral spinal fluid.

Face

The face should evaluated for areas of tenderness, deformity, and stability. Racoon's eyes (periorbital ecchymosis) and Battle's sign (ecchymosis over the mastoid) may represent basilar skull fracture.

Nose

The nares should be checked for evidence of obstruction, blood, cerebral spinal fluid, and septal hematoma.

Mouth

The oropharynx should be carefully assessed for broken teeth, foreign bodies, intra-oral soft-tissue injury, and normal mandible occlusion.

Neck

The cervical spine should be palpated for evidence of spinal tenderness or deformity. Evaluation of the cervical spine may require temporary cervical collar removal concurrently with manual cervical spine stabilization. Tracheal deviation and carotid pulse quality should be noted. The jugular veins should be checked for distention.

Chest

The quality of heart and breath sounds should be reassessed. The chest wall may be reevaluated for tenderness, deformity, lacerations, and ecchymoses (e.g., seat-belt sign or steering wheel contusion).

Abdomen

Bowel sounds may be assessed, but their presence or absence adds little in the evaluation of abdominal trauma. The abdomen should be evaluated for ecchymoses, tenderness, and the presence of peritoneal signs (e.g., guarding, shake tenderness, rebound tenderness, and percussion tenderness).

Pelvis

The pelvis should be assessed for tenderness and stability. Stability testing is best performed by simultaneously pressing **down** on both iliac crests, and then **in** on both iliac crests. "Pelvic rocking" adds little information and may worsen fractures as well as hemorrhage.

Genitals

Blood at the urethral meatus, peroneal hematoma, and scrotal hematoma may all represent urethral injury and usually preclude the placement of a urinary catheter.

Rectum

The rectum should be assessed for the presence of gross blood. The position of the prostate should be noted since a high-riding prostate may indicate a urethral injury and preclude urinary catheter placement. During the rectal exam, the sacrum and coccyx may also be internally palpated for fractures.

Extremities

Each extremity should be evaluated for pulses, soft tissue injury, deformity, tenderness, range of motion, strength, and sensation. Pulses are commonly assessed over the femoral, popliteal, dorsalis pedis, posterior tibial, radial, and ulnar arteries.

Back

The back of all supine patients should be considered to harbor life-threatening wounds until adequately examined. Even patients with known spinal injuries require careful, but expeditious assessment of the back. Initially, all patients should be considered to have a spinal injury until proven otherwise. "Log-rolling" patients requires a team approach with careful cervical spine stabilization. The patient's back should be evaluated for soft-tissue injury, deformity, and tenderness.

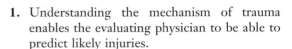

◆ KEY POINTS ◆

1. Understanding the mechanism of trauma enables the evaluating physician to be able to predict likely injuries.

2. Systematic primary and secondary surveys help the physician to identify the most critical injuries first.

3. The back of all supine patients should be considered to harbor life-threatening wounds until proven otherwise.

57

Head Trauma

Head trauma is the leading cause of traumatic death in patients younger than 25 years of age. A concussion is a transient interruption of neurologic function following head trauma. Subarachnoid hemorrhage is the most common abnormality seen on head CT following head trauma.

ANATOMY AND PATHOPHYSIOLOGY

The scalp is composed of five layers. The names of these layers may be remembered by the mnemonic "SCALP": Skin, subCutaneous fascia, galea Aponeurosis, Loose areolar tissue, and Pericranium. The skull is composed of the frontal, ethmoidal, sphenoid, occiptal, temporal, and parietal bones. The cerebral spinal fluid that surrounds the brain provides some cushioning during trauma.

Head trauma may result from direct or indirect injury. Direct injury occurs at the point of contact of a striking object. Indirect injury results when the cranial contents are set in motion by forces other than a contacting object. Contrecoup brain injuries are those that occur at sites distant from the point of impact, and result from the accelerating brain striking against the inner surface of the skull.

Subdural hematomas (SDH) typically occur when bridging veins between the brain and dura tear in the setting of acceleration-deceleration injuries. Brain atrophy, as seen in the elderly and alcoholics, stretches the bridging veins and is a predisposing factor to the for-

mation of subdural hematomas. Epidural hematomas (EDH) form between the dura and skull and usually result from direct trauma over the temporoparietal region of the skull and arterial hemorrhage (primarily from the middle meningeal artery).

The cerebral perfusion pressure (CPP) is a measurement of the blood's pressure gradient across brain tissue, and hence brain perfusion. Intracranial pressure (ICP) results from the enclosure of the cranial contents within the confines of the inelastic skull. Cranial contents include brain parenchyma, blood, CSF, and interstitial fluid. As the total volume of cranial contents increases, so does ICP. CPP may be measured by subtracting the ICP (measured with a transcranial instrument referred to as a "bolt") from the mean arterial blood pressure (MAP) (CPP = MAP – ICP). The brain is able to maintain normal cerebral blood flow (CBF) by "autoregulating" the cerebral vasculature as long as the CPP is consistently between 50 and 160 mmHg.

Increased ICP (>15 mmHg) may result from intracranial swelling or hemorrhage and lead to a reduction in CPP. Brain ischemia results from CPP that is less than 40 mmHg. If the ICP increases out of control, it may result in uncal, transtentorial, or cerebellotonsilar herniation. Uncal herniation is typically evidenced by ipsilateral pupil dilation as it impinges upon the parasympathetic nerve fibers of the third cranial nerve. Transtentorial herniation may initially be subtle, manifesting as mental status changes, but ultimately leads to unconsciousness followed by decorticate posturing, and then decerebrate posturing. Cerebellotonsillar herniation typically causes respiratory and cardiovascular collapse.

HISTORY

Details about the time of injury, mechanism of injury, changes in mental status, and losses of consciousness should be elicited. Patients with subdural hematomas often report progressively worsening headache and other neurologic abnormalities. Patients with epidural hematomas often have had a transient loss of consciousness followed by a lucid interval and ultimately sustained unconsciousness. Subarachnoid hemorrhages typically present with headache and signs of meningeal inflammation.

PHYSICAL EXAMINATION

In addition to the general trauma workup, head injured patients should receive a thorough neurologic examination including a Glasgow Coma Scale (GCS) score. The GCS provides an objective measure of the patient's neurologic function that may be followed over time. In general, a GCS ≤8 constitutes severe head trauma, a GCS of 9 to 13 signifies moderate head trauma, and a GCS of 14 or 15 is considered minor head trauma. Periorbital ecchymosis (i.e., Racoon's eyes) and ecchymosis over the mastoid (i.e., Battle's sign) may represent basilar skull fracture.

Laboratory evaluation of the significantly head injured patient should include glucose, electrolytes, complete blood count, coagulation studies, urine toxicology screen, and a blood alcohol level evaluation. Computed tomography (CT) of the head is indicated in most cases of severe or moderate head trauma. Although CT of the head is controversial in patients with a normal neurologic examination following minor head trauma, it is usually performed if the patient is suspected to have lost consciousness.

On CT, subdural hematomas most commonly manifest as a concave density—adjacent to the skull—that crosses the suture lines (Fig. 57–1). Epidural hematomas usually present as a convex density adjacent to the skull that does not cross the suture lines (Fig. 57–2). Subarachnoid hemorrhage is typically evident as hyperdensity within the subarachnoid space that is most often visible between the cerebral peduncles (Fig. 57–3).

MRI is better than CT at detecting brain infarction as well as posterior fossa and brain stem lesions. Angiography may help to identify vascular thrombosis, or disruption (e.g., dissection).

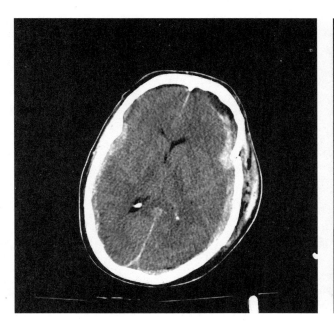

Figure 57–1 Subdural hematoma.

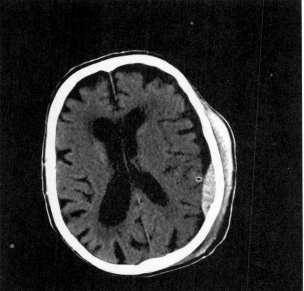

Figure 57–2 Epidural hematoma.

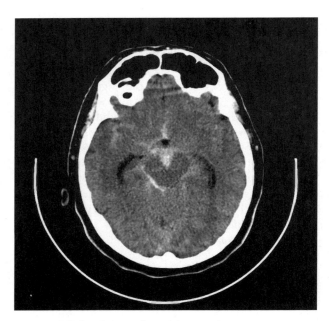

Figure 57–3 Subarachnoid hemorrhage.

TREATMENT

Early neurosurgical consultation is critical in all cases of severe or moderate head injury. Hypoxia and hypotension should be avoided in patients with traumatic brain injury since they are independent predictors of adverse outcome.

The treatment of traumatic injury, as with other trauma, should begin with assuring a patent airway. Combativeness following head trauma may represent significant intracranial pathology requiring sedation and intubation. Hyperventilation to produce a pCO_2 of approximately 30 mmHg may temporarily reduce ICP; however, it should be used with caution since overventilation may lead to vasoconstriction and worsening brain ischemia.

Hypotension is rare and usually a preterminal event in patients suffering traumatic head injury. Intravenous hydration may worsen cerebral edema in the setting of traumatic brain injury, but it should never be withheld from patients with hypovolemic hypotension.

Mannitol, an osmotic diuretic, may help to reduce ICP by pulling edema out of the body's tissues and into the vasculature. Mannitol is thought to improve the CPP by increasing the MAP. It may also improve cerebral blood flow by reducing blood viscosity. Low CPP refractory to resuscitative measures may warrant the administration of intravenous barbiturates to slow brain activity and decrease metabolic demands. Prophylactic anticonvulsants (e.g., phenytoin) are often prescribed to prevent seizures and their associated high metabolic demands. Patients with deteriorating mental status, large intracranial hemorrhage, or severely elevated ICP may require emergent surgical decompression. Steroids have never definitively been proven to benefit patients sustaining traumatic brain injury. Antibiotics should be reserved for patients with heavily contaminated wounds, sinus fractures, and open skull fractures. Galeal lacerations should be repaired with deep absorbable sutures since the muscles adherent to the galea may pull the wound apart if left unclosed.

◆ KEY POINTS ◆

1. Subarachnoid hemorrhage is the most common abnormality seen on head CT following head trauma.

2. Cerebral perfusion pressure (CPP) = mean arterial pressure (MAP) – intracranial pressure (ICP).

3. Epidural hematomas often present as transient loss of consciousness, followed by a lucid interval, and then sustained unconsciousness.

4. Hypoxia and hypotension should be avoided in patients with traumatic brain injury.

58 Facial Trauma

While many facial injuries may not be life threatening, certain injuries may result in ocular and neurologic impairment. Distortions of facial anatomy may also have immeasurable emotional impact. Due to the anatomically distorting effects of locally injected anesthetic fluid, regional anesthesia is often preferable to local anesthesia for soft tissue repair of the face. Severe facial wounds should be repaired by a facial or plastic surgeon if available.

ANATOMY

Lack of tension within certain areas of the skin is natural and results in lines of expression (Fig. 58–1A and B). Most of the face receives and transmits sensory information via the supraorbital, infraorbital, and mental branches of the trigeminal nerve (i.e., fifth cranial nerve) (Fig. 58–2). Knowledge of facial anatomy helps to predict what underlying structures may be at risk given a specific type of injury (e.g., transection of the parotid duct following laceration of the pre-aural soft tissue). The following discussion will focus on specific facial injuries.

LIP LACERATIONS

Lip lacerations require careful repair for optimal cosmetic results. Vermillion border malalignment of just 1 mm is usually apparent from conversational distance. Since local anesthetic injection in the lip swells tissue and blurs the vermillion border, the vermillion border should be marked prior to injection to facilitate accurate reapproximation. Lip tissue revisions that cross the vermillion border should be performed at right angles to the vermillion border. Muscle disruption within the lip should be repaired as a separate layer. Electrical burns to the lip are a matter of concern due to the risk of delayed arterial hemorrhage one week after the initial injury.

ORAL CAVITY INJURIES

Mucosal lacerations of the oral cavity should be closed with 4.0 or 5.0 absorbable sutures. If a through-and-through laceration exists, the muscle and subcutaneous layers should be closed after the mucosa. Deep tongue lacerations should be closed with absorbable synthetic or nonabsorbable silk sutures. Tongue lacerations involving muscle should be closed in layers for optimal results. Although controversial, most significant oral lacerations should be considered contaminated and treated with an antibiotic such as penicillin.

NASAL INJURIES

Nasal injuries may result in septal hematomas that, if left untreated, may lead to septal necrosis as a result of the pressure exerted on the avascular, cartilaginous septum. Anesthesia for nose repairs may be achieved with regional or local anesthesia. Due to the tenuous nature

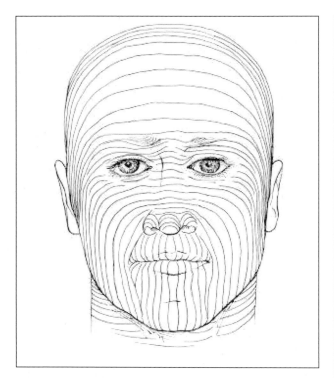

Figure 58–1A   Skin tension lines of the face. Incisions or lacerations parallel to these lines are less likely to create widened scars than those that are perpendicular to these lines. (*Adapted from Simon R, Brenner B: Procedures and techniques in emergency medicine, Baltimore, 1982, Williams & Wilkins, as published in Trott A: Wounds and lacerations, ed 3, St Louis, 1998, Mosby.*)

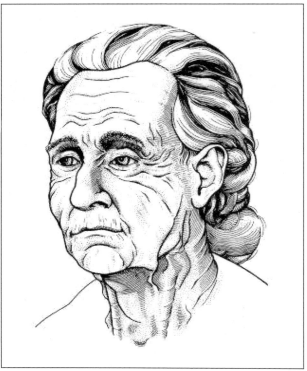

Figure 58–1B   Lines of expression. These natural skin lines represent lines of least tension. Incisions and plasties should, when possible, be made parallel to these lines for minimal scarring and interference with function.

of blood supply to the nose and cartilage, anesthetics should not contain vasoconstrictors such as epinephrine.

Through-and-through nose injuries should be repaired in layers beginning with the mucosa (fine absorbable suture), followed by the cartilage (fine absorbable suture), and skin (fine absorbable or nonabsorbable suture). Significant nasal injuries require antibiotic prophylaxis, and close follow-up with a facial or plastic surgeon.

EAR INJURIES

Similar to the nose, the ear has a tenuous blood supply and is therefore susceptible to necrosis by hematomas

and vasoconstrictors. Complete, regional ear anesthesia may be easily attained by injecting a ring of anesthetic around the base of the ear. Lacerations should be closed in layers beginning with the cartilage (fine absorbable sutures) followed by the skin (fine nonabsorbable or absorbable sutures). Significant ear repairs should be splinted with a compressive dressing to help prevent hematoma formation. Although controversial, antibiotics active against skin flora are generally recommended for most significant ear lacerations.

EYEBROW INJURIES

The key points in repairing eyebrow lacerations are to never shave the eyebrows (they often do not grow back), and to always debride the tissue parallel to the angle of

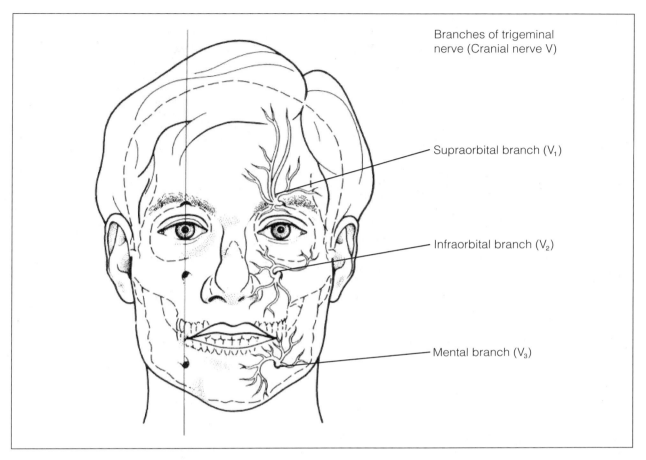

Branches of trigeminal nerve (Cranial nerve V)

Supraorbital branch (V₁)

Infraorbital branch (V₂)

Mental branch (V₃)

Figure 58–2 Sensory innervation of anterior aspect of face (trigeminal nerve). Supraorbital, infraorbital, and mental branches are shown. Note that foramina of bony exit of these nerves lie roughly in straight line passing through pupil and lateral commissure of lips.

the hairs rather than perpendicular to the skin. The eyebrow hairs provide the best landmark for reapproximating the borders of the eyebrow. Debridement of tissue parallel to the angle of the hairs helps to reduce the likelihood of developing a bald spot within the eyebrow.

MAXILLARY FRACTURES

Maxillary fractures should be suspected following trauma that results in significant facial pain, facial swelling, midface mobility, mandible malocclusion, and CSF rhinorrhea. Maxillary fractures may be classified as Le Fort I (maxilla only involving the nasal fossa), Le Fort II (maxilla, nasal bones, medial orbits), or Le Fort III (i.e., craniofacial dysjunction; maxilla, zygoma, nasal bones, ethmoids, vomer, cranial base) (Fig. 58–3). Le Fort fractures may not be symmetrical. CT scan of the face is more sensitive than plain films for detecting facial fractures.

The initial management of facial fractures should focus on assuring a patent airway. Epistaxis may require nasal packing. Both CSF rhinorrhea and intracranial air indicate the presence of an open skull fracture, and typically warrant prophylactic antibiotics to prevent menin-

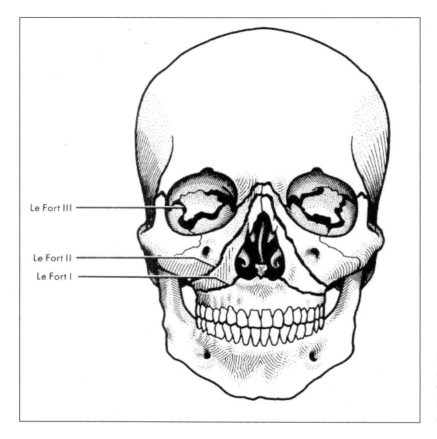

Figure 58–3 Le Fort classification of facial fractures. Le Fort I: palate facial dysjunction. Le Fort II: pyramidal dysjunction. Le Fort III: craniofacial dysjunction.

gitis. Facial or plastic surgery consultation is generally indicated in most cases of facial fracture since the injury may require operative fixation.

ZYGOMA FRACTURES

Zygoma body fractures may result in diplopia, infraorbital (V2 branch of trigeminal nerve) anesthesia, flattening of the cheek, and palpable step-off. CT scan of the face is the most sensitive imaging modality for detecting fractures of the zygoma. Facial or plastic surgery consultation is generally indicated since operative fixation may be required.

ORBITAL FLOOR FRACTURES

The orbital floor is the weakest part of the orbit and is therefore very susceptible to fracture following blunt orbital trauma. Orbital contents, such as the inferior rectus muscle, may herniate into the maxillary sinus through the fracture leading to ocular impingement and diplopia. Massive disruption of the orbital floor may result in the complete displacement of ocular contents in the maxillary sinus ("blow-out fracture"). It is important to note that impaired ocular mobility may result from soft-tissue swelling alone.

A careful ophthalmologic examination and consultation is warranted in significant eye trauma. Corneal abrasions, hyphema (blood in the anterior chamber), retinal detachment, vitreal hemorrhage, orbital emphysema, and orbital hemorrhage are some injuries that may accompany ocular trauma. Facial or plastic surgery consultation within the emergency department is generally indicated if the orbital fracture results in functional ocular impairment. Less significant fractures without functional impairment typically warrant prophylactic antibiotics and outpatient facial or plastic surgery referral.

NASAL BONE FRACTURES

Nasal bone fractures are the most common facial fracture. They typically result in deformity, swelling, crepitance, and nasal bone mobility. The nasal septum should be inspected to check for septal hematomas. Undrained septal hematomas may result in cartilage necrosis. Since most nasal bone fractures are diagnosed clinically, radiologic imaging is usually only necessary if other facial fractures are suspected. Epistaxis is usually self-limiting, but may require nasal packing. Gross deformities may be reduced in the ED. Patients should generally be prescribed analgesics, ice packs, and instructed to follow up with a facial or plastic surgeon within one week for reevaluation.

MANDIBULAR FRACTURES

The mandible forms a ring-like structure and therefore often fractures in two places during trauma. Mandibular fractures typically present with pain, tenderness, and mandible malocclusion. A "panoramic," plain film view of the mandible is the imaging modality of choice for detecting fractures. Anteroposterior and lateral plain film views are indicated if a panoramic view is not available. CT scan of the mandible is the most sensitive imaging modality for detecting fracture, and may be indicated if there is a high clinical suspicion for occult fracture. Patients with mandibular fractures usually require admission and operative fixation. Open fractures, including those associated with intra-oral lacerations, warrant prophylactic antibiotics.

TEMPEROMANDIBULAR JOINT DISLOCATION

Temperomandibular joint dislocation may result from direct trauma, or wider than usual mouth opening (e.g., yawning). Patients often present with joint pain, muscle spasm, and an inability to completely occlude the mandible. Dislocation of the mandibular condyle usually occurs anteriorly and superiorly. Dislocations are more often unilateral than bilateral. Plain film imaging of the mandible is indicated in cases of traumatic dislocation in order to identify fractures prior to reduction.

Mandibular reduction is performed by pressing one's protected thumbs (wrapped in gauze) on top of the third molars, and directing the posterior mandible inferiorly and posteriorly. Conscious sedation may be required to overcome muscle spasms. Facial surgery consultation should be sought in cases accompanied by fracture. Patients without fracture who are successfully reduced may be discharged home with analgesics and instructions for follow-up and limited mouth opening.

◆ KEY POINTS ◆

1. Due to the anatomically distorting effects of locally injected anesthetic fluid, regional anesthesia is generally preferable to local anesthesia for soft tissue repair of the face.

2. Lacerations crossing the vermillion border of the lip require careful reapproximation to avoid noticeable lip line step-offs.

3. Significant intra-oral soft-tissue injuries usually warrant antibiotics.

4. Hematomas of the nasal septum must be drained to avoid cartilage necrosis.

5. Ear splints should be applied following ear repair to avoid hematoma formation and subsequent cartilage necrosis.

6. Facial fractures may cause ocular and neurologic impairment.

59 Spinal Trauma

Approximately half of all spinal injuries result from motor vehicle crashes and another 20% result from falls. Fourteen percent of vertebral injuries result in spinal cord injury. Spinal column injuries are classified by the mechanism of trauma (i.e., flexion, rotation, extension, or vertical compression). Spinal cord injuries are characterized by the degree of damage at a specific level (i.e., incomplete or complete).

ANATOMY

The spine is comprised of 7 cervical vertebrae, 12 thoracic vertebrae, 5 lumbar vertebrae, the sacrum (5 fused vertebrae), and the coccyx (4 fused vertebrae). The vertebrae are separated by cartilage discs, and joined together by a series of ligaments. The spinal cord extends to approximately the level of the second lumbar vertebrae in adults. The cauda equina consists of the peripheral nerve radicles that continue inferiorly within the spinal canal. Spinal cord injury may result from impinging bone fracture fragments, herniated discs, buckling ligaments, hematomas, or vascular disruption. The following discussion will describe specific spinal injuries, including their stability, and then discuss general management principles.

Flexion Injuries of the Spinal Column

Simple Wedge Fractures are **stable** injuries resulting in loss of height, and increased concavity of the anterior aspect of the vertebral body (Fig. 59–1).

A **Teardrop Fracture** is a **potentially unstable** injury that results in a wedge-shaped bone fragment (resembling a "teardrop") being pinched off of the anteroinferior aspect of the vertebral body concurrently with posterior ligamentous injury (Fig. 59–2).

Spinous Process Fractures (Clay Shoveler's Fractures) are **stable** oblique fractures through the base of a spinous process of the lower cervical spine resulting from ligamentous pull (Fig. 59–3). **Subluxation** injuries are **potentially unstable** injuries resulting from ligamentous disruption between vertebrae. They begin posteriorly and extend anteriorly, potentially resulting in disjoined vertebrae and instability without a fracture. Plain films may reveal spinal malalignment, abnormal joint space, and prevertebral soft-tissue swelling.

Bilateral Facet Dislocations are unstable injuries usually associated with neurologic injury. The mechanism of dislocation is similar to subluxation, but more severe. Ligamentous disruption between vertebrae begins posteriorly and extends anteriorly through the anterior ligament, leading to displacement of the vertebra above the injury anteriorly over the vertebra below the injury. The inferior facets of the upper vertebra climb over the superior facets of the lower vertebra and seat anteriorly.

Atlantooccipital (C1/occiput) and Atlantoaxial (C1/C2) Dislocations are very **unstable** injuries that result in disruption and displacement of the atlantooccipital or atlantoaxial joints, and are frequently associated with an odontoid fracture (Fig. 59–4).

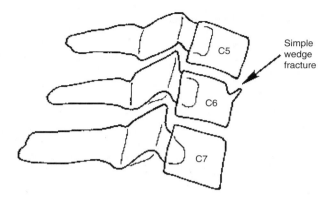

Figure 59–1 Lateral view of simple wedge fracture. Mechanism: flexion. Stability: mechanically stable. Note decrease in height of anterior aspect of C6 vertebral body.

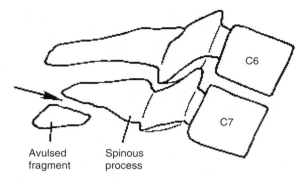

Figure 59–3 Clay shoveler's fracture. Mechanism: flexion. Stability: mechanically stable. Note avulsed fragment off tip of C7 spinous process in coned lateral view.

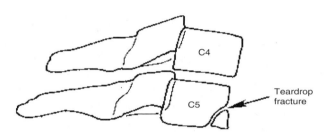

Figure 59–2 Lateral view of teardrop fracture. Mechanism: flexion. Stability: unstable. Fractured fragment off C5 body resembles teardrop.

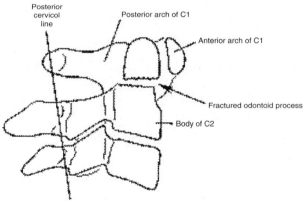

Figure 59–4 Odontoid fracture with anterior dislocation. Mechanism: flexion with shearing. Stability: unstable. Fracture through odontoid with retropharyngeal swelling is demonstrated. Anterior dislocation is confirmed by disrupted posterior cervical line.

Spinal Column Rotational Injuries

Unilateral Facet Dislocations are **stable** injuries that result from ligamentous disruption between vertebrae that begins posteriorly at the same time a rotational force pulls the inferior facet of the upper vertebra anteriorly over the superior facet of the lower vertebra locking the two together. This type of injury is unstable if it occurs at the C1 or C2 level.

Extension Injuries of the Spinal Column

A **Posterior Arch Fracture of C1** is a **potentially unstable** injury that results from forced extension when the posterior arch of C1 gets pinched between the occiput and the spinous process of C2. The ligaments usually remain intact.

Spondylolysis (displacement) **of C2 (Hangman's Fracture)** is an **unstable** injury resulting from forced

extension when the pedicles of C2 fracture with or without vertebral dislocation. Since the pedicle fractures cause the spinal canal to enlarge, neural injury is possible, but usually minimal. For this reason, death from hangings usually results from asphyxiation.

Extension Teardrop Fractures are **potentially unstable** injuries that occur when the strong anterior ligament pulls off the anteroinferior corner piece of a vertebral body. This injury is stable in neck flexion and potentially unstable in neck extension.

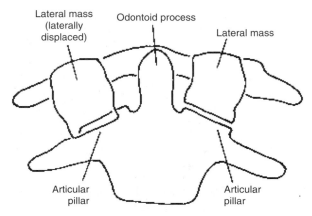

Figure 59–5   Jefferson fracture. Mechanism: vertical compression. Stability: unstable. Unilateral or bilateral lateral displacement of lateral masses of C1 with respect to articular pillars of C2 confirms Jefferson fracture and differentiates this from fracture of posterior neural arch of C1 on AP view.

Compression Injuries of the Spinal Column

Burst Fractures are **potentially unstable** injuries that result when axial loading causes the vertebral end plates to fracture on one another and the vertebral bodies to compress the nucleus propulsus (cartilage disc) so intensely that the vertebral bodies shatter at their center point. Although this is usually a stable fracture, bone fragments may enter the canal and damage the spinal cord.

A **C1 Compression Fracture (i.e., Jefferson Fracture)** is an **unstable** injury caused by the compression and fracture of C1 at its anterior and posterior arches resulting in the lateral displacement of the C1 lateral masses. This injury is typically associated with a disruption of the predental ligament and widening of the predental space (i.e., >3 mm in adults and >5 mm in children) (Fig. 59–5).

Spinal Cord Injuries

Complete spinal cord injuries result in a total loss of motor function and sensation distal to the site of spinal cord injury. If this condition persists for 24 hours or more, the hope of functional recovery is less than 1%.

Incomplete spinal cord injuries spare a portion of the spinal cord, are usually associated with some distal function at the time of injury, and often result in a marked functional recovery.

Incomplete Spinal Cord Injuries

Central Cord Syndrome typically occurs among patients with degenerative arthritis in the setting of cervical hyperextension when the ligamentum flavum buckles into the spinal canal for a fleeting moment and pinches the spinal cord. The primary spinal cord damage occurs in the central gray matter, and usually manifests as weakness that is greater in the upper extremities than the lower extremities. Although a significant amount of functional recovery is expected in central cord syndrome, the ultimate prognosis depends on the severity of the injury.

Brown-Séquard Syndrome occurs when a lateral half of the spinal cord is injured at a specific level. The hemicord injury usually results from penetrating trauma, and presents as ipsilateral motor paralysis and contralateral sensory loss distal to the injury. Although bowel and bladder function is usually maintained, long-term braces are often required to control spastic extremities.

Anterior Cord Syndrome occurs when the anterior aspect of the spinal cord is injured by bone fragment compression, disc herniation, or ischemia resulting from anterior spinal artery compromise. The syndrome manifests as paralysis and loss of pain and temperature sensation distal to the injury. Since the posterior columns are unaffected, position, touch, and vibration sense is usually preserved.

HISTORY

A detailed patient history combined with an understanding of neuroanatomy allows the physician to predict the most likely location and type of spinal cord injury.

PHYSICAL EXAMINATION

A complete examination detailing neurologic function is critical, and should include the evaluation of rectal tone and perirectal sensation. The cervical spine of alert patients may be cleared clinically without radiographic imaging if **none** of the following conditions is present: intoxication, distracting injury, focal neurologic impairment, or midline cervical spine tenderness. If a cervical spine fracture is suspected, plain film imaging of the cervical spine should begin with cross-table lateral, AP, and open-mouth odontoid views. Oblique views may be helpful in visualizing the spinal foramina and pedicles, but are not routinely necessary. Flexion and extension views of the cervical spine may help identify ligamentous injury. Thoracic, lumbar, and sacral AP and lateral views are indicated, respectively, for fractures suspected at these levels. CT scanning of the spine is a more sensitive modality for detecting fracture, especially in the setting of severe degenerative joint disease that may make plain film interpretation difficult. MRI of the spine is the most sensitive imaging modality for detecting spinal cord injury, ligamentous injury, and hematomas.

TREATMENT

Patients suspected of spinal injury should receive spinal immobilization and, if necessary, be moved using logroll precautions. Patients requiring intubation should have their cervical spine stabilized manually and their cervical collar removed prior to attempting intubation. "Spinal shock" secondary to spinal cord injury results from autonomic dysfunction, and usually presents as bradycardia, hypotension, hypothermia, and ileus. Spinal shock should only be considered after the other forms of shock (e.g., hypovolemic shock) have been ruled out. The treatment of spinal shock typically includes intravenous fluids and sympathomimetics. Patients suffering acute, blunt, spinal cord injury may benefit from high-dose, intravenous methylprednisolone if administered within the first 8 hours of injury. Orthopedic or neurosurgical consultation is typically indicated in most cases of spinal injury. Patients with stable fractures may require hospital admission for pain management.

◆ **KEY POINTS** ◆

1. Spinal cord injury may occur in the absence of bony abnormalities.

2. Certain patients can have their cervical spines cleared clinically without radiologic imaging.

3. Spinal shock should only be considered after the other forms of shock (e.g., hypovolemic shock) have been ruled out.

4. Patients suffering acute, blunt, spinal cord injury may benefit from high-dose, intravenous methylprednisolone if administered within the first 8 hours of injury.

60 Chest Trauma

Chest trauma is believed to be responsible for 20% of all traumatic deaths. Significant chest trauma may result in chest wall injury, diaphragm rupture, pulmonary contusion, hemo-pneumothorax, digestive organ disruption, blunt myocardial injury, myocardial rupture, and aortic injury. Chest wall injuries may impair ventilation. Penetrating wounds to the chest should generally not be probed due to the danger of creating a pneumothorax, damaging internal organs, and worsening hemorrhage. The following discussion will focus on specific injuries that result from chest trauma.

RIB FRACTURES

Rib fractures are more common in adults than children following blunt chest wall trauma due to the reduced elasticity of the adult chest wall. Fractures of ribs Nos. 9 through 12 may be associated with intra-abdominal injury. A **flail chest** results when three or more consecutive ribs are fractured at two places creating a free moving segment of the chest wall. Complications of rib fractures include hemo-pneumothorax, internal organ injury, and pneumonia secondary to pain-induced hypoventilation.

History and Physical Examination

Rib fractures usually manifest as worsening pain with deep inspiration, tenderness, swelling, and ecchymosis at the site of injury. Flail chest segments may exhibit paradoxical movement with respiration (in with inspiration and out with expiration) and are highly associated with underlying pulmonary injury. Dedicated rib films are not routinely useful and only indicated if there is suspicion for fractures of ribs Nos. 1–3, Nos. 9–12, or multiple rib fractures. An upright chest x-ray may be useful to identify hemo-pneumothorax.

Treatment

The treatment of rib fractures routinely includes analgesia (e.g., NSAIDs and narcotics) and breathing exercises (e.g., inspirometer). Regional rib blocks with a long-acting local anesthetic may also be helpful. Chest wall wrapping or binding may reduce the pain of rib fractures, but it is no longer prescribed due to the increased risk of hypoventilation and pneumonia. Patients with complications or severe pain refractory to analgesics require hospital admission. Clinically significant flail chests may be internally splinted with endotracheal intubation and positive pressure ventilation.

HEMO-PNEUMOTHORAX

Disruption of air-containing structures (e.g., tracheobronchial tree, lung, and the esophagus) may produce **pneumothorax**, **pneumomediastinum**, or subcutaneous emphysema (air in the subcutaneous tissue). Subcutaneous emphysema in the setting of trauma should be considered to be a result of more significant internal injury until proven otherwise. As air builds up in pressure within the confines of the pleural space or mediastinum, **tension pneumothorax** or **tension pneumomediastinum** may ensue requiring emergent decompression to avoid vascular collapse.

History and Physical Examination

Patients with hemothorax or pneumothorax may present with chest pain, shortness of breath, tachypnea, tachycardia, hypoxia, decreased breath sounds on the affected side, and subcutaneous emphysema. Individuals with tension pneumothorax or tension pneumomediastinum may go on to develop hemodynamic instability and cardiovascular collapse. Although plain film imaging of the chest usually reveals hemo-pneumothorax when present, CT scanning of the chest is more sensitive. Patients with pneumomediastinum usually undergo bronchoscopy (scope of tracheobronchial tree) as well as endoscopy (scope of esophagus) to look for perforations explaining the origin of the air.

Treatment

Patients with a high clinical probability of significant hemo- or pneumothorax should be decompressed with tube thoracostomy (chest tube) prior to imaging. Decompression with needle thoracostomy may provide temporary relief until the definitive placement of a chest tube. Depending on the origin of the air and the severity of symptoms, pneumomediastinum may require decompression, laceration repair, and washout in the operating room. Cases of pneumomediastinum resulting from esophageal perforation usually warrant the administration of broad-spectrum, intravenous antibiotics to help avoid mediastinitis.

PULMONARY CONTUSION

Pulmonary contusion is defined as edema and hemorrhage within lung parenchyma resulting from trauma.

History and Physical Examination

Symptoms and signs of pulmonary contusion include cyanosis, dyspnea, tachypnea, tachycardia, hypoxia, abnormal breath sounds, and chest wall ecchymosis. Lung opacification on chest x-rays evident within 6 hours of trauma usually represents pulmonary contusion. Chest CT scanning is more sensitive than plain films for detecting pulmonary contusion.

Treatment

The treatment of pulmonary contusion is symptomatic and may include ventilatory assistance and pulmonary toilet in more severe cases. Excessive hydration of patients with pulmonary contusion may result in worsening pulmonary edema. Although pneumonia is the most common complication of pulmonary contusion, there is no proven benefit to the administration of empiric antibiotics. Patients with suspected pulmonary contusion may insidiously develop respiratory failure and should therefore be admitted and observed in the hospital.

BLUNT MYOCARDIAL INJURY

Motor vehicle crashes (MVCs) are the most common cause of blunt myocardial injury. The diagnosis of blunt myocardial injury among hemodynamically stable patients is difficult. Complications of blunt myocardial injury include life-threatening dysrhythmias, conduction abnormalities, congestive heart failure, cardiogenic shock, hemopericardium with tamponade, cardiac rupture, valvular injury, coronary artery occlusion, myocardial infarction, ventricular aneurysms, pericarditis, and thromboemboli.

History and Physical Examination

Details about the mechanism of the trauma help in understanding the magnitude of energy involved as well as in formulating the clinical probability of injury. Patients with blunt myocardial injury may present with chest pain, a chest wall contusion, tachycardia, bradycardia, and hypotension.

There is no gold standard test in the diagnosis of blunt myocardial injury. Although electrocardiogram abnormalities (e.g., dysrhythmias, ST segment changes, T wave changes) may represent blunt myocardial injury, the findings are usually nonspecific. Sinus tachycardia is the most common electrocardiographic finding in blunt myocardial injury. The risk of complications is negligible among patients with a completely normal electrocardiogram at presentation.

Other diagnostic modalities for detecting blunt myocardial injury have been studied including cardiac enzymes (e.g., CK-MB and troponin), echocardiography, thallium scintigraphy, angiography, and computed tomography (i.e., CT). Due in part to the fact that the vast majority of blunt myocardial injuries are clinically insignificant, no diagnostic test or combination of tests

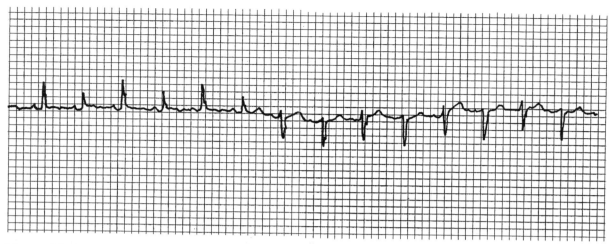

Figure 60–1   Electrical alternans.

has been able to reliably predict which patients will go on to develop complications.

Treatment

The treatment of blunt myocardial injury involves mostly supportive care. In general, asymptomatic patients with a normal ECG do not require further testing or admission. Patients admitted to the hospital for suspected blunt myocardial injury may be safely discharged after 12 hours of observation if no dysrhythmia or other complications occur.

ACUTE PERICARDIAL TAMPONADE

Blunt myocardial injury and cardiac perforation may result in acute pericardial tamponade (blood accumulating within the pericardium and reducing cardiac output). Unlike large, chronic pericardial effusions that stretch the pericardium over time, acute pericardial effusions may lead to pericardial tamponade after accumulating only 50–100 cc of fluid.

History and Physical Examination

Acute pericardial tamponade typically presents with tachycardia, hypotension, and elevated central venous pressure (e.g., jugular venous distention). An elevated "pulsus paradoxus" (change in systolic blood pressure between inspiration and expiration >10 mmHg) may help to identify the presence of a pericardial effusion. However, this value is often difficult to obtain in a noisy

emergency department, and may be elevated in other disease states such as asthma or chronic obstructive pulmonary disease. In acute pericardial tamponade, the heart sounds may be muffled, and the electrocardiogram may reveal "electrical alternans" (Fig. 60–1), which is the beat-to-beat variability in QRS axis that occurs as the heart swings within the accumulated pericardial fluid. Viewing of the cardiac silhouette on chest x-ray is generally not useful in acute tamponade since the pericardium has not had time to stretch and enlarge. Cardiac ultrasound is a noninvasive, sensitive, and specific imaging modality for identifying pericardial effusions and tamponade.

Treatment

The treatment of acute pericardial tamponade should begin with the rapid infusion of intravenous crystalloid via two large-bore intravenous catheters to increase the cardiac output by increasing the preload. Stable patients may be brought to the operating room for pericardial drainage and the repair of a cardiac perforation if present. Unstable patients require emergent pericardial decompression with a pericardiocentesis, or, if necessary, thoracotomy with pericardial window.

TRAUMATIC RUPTURE OF THE THORACIC AORTA

Traumatic rupture of the thoracic aorta has increased in incidence over the years and is likely the result of increasing automobile speeds. Thoracic aortic rupture carries a significant mortality rate believed to be as high as 15%. The vast majority of aortic tears occurs in the descending aorta just distal to the take off of the left subclavian artery. In the past, aortic tears were believed to result from the tethering of the aorta to the thoracic wall by the ligamentum arteriosum. However, more recent data suggests that the injury results from the compression of the aorta between the chest wall and the vertebrae.

History and Physical Examination

Individuals sustaining traumatic rupture of the thoracic aorta may present with chest pain, chest wall contusion, tachycardia, hypotension, and vascular collapse. The most sensitive finding of aortic tear on chest x-ray is widening of the superior mediastinum (sensitivity = 80–90%). Other findings associated with aortic tear on chest x-ray include nasogastric tube deviation to the right, tracheal deviation to the right, blurring of the aortic knob, depression of the left mainstem bronchus, opacification of the apex of the left lung (apical cap), and widening of the peritracheal stripe.

Although aortography remains the gold standard for diagnosing aortic rupture, the sensitivity and specificity of chest CT and transesophageal echocardiography (TEE) now approach that of aortography. Chest MRI is also sensitive at detecting aortic injury, however, it is typically not indicated in the setting of trauma due to the long study times as well as its location outside of the emergency department. Stable patients with a high clinical probability of aortic injury may warrant going straight to aortography. Unstable patients with suspected aortic rupture should have a bedside TEE performed in the resuscitation bay. All other stable patients may undergo CT angiogram of the chest for the evaluation of aortic rupture.

Treatment

The treatment of aortic rupture includes large-bore intravenous access, control of hypertension with short-acting vasodilators (e.g., nitroprusside), as well as short-acting beta-blockers (e.g., esmolol) to mitigate the reflex tachycardia caused by vasodilation. New evidence in aortic rupture suggests that over-resuscitation with intravenous fluids may increase the blood pressure and worsen the mortality by increasing hemorrhage. In general, the systolic blood pressure should be maintained in the 90–120 mmHg range for previously normotensive individuals. Hypotensive patients with aortic rupture require volume resuscitation with blood and crystalloid as well as rapid transport to the operating room for definitive repair.

◆ KEY POINTS ◆

1. Penetrating wounds to the chest should generally not be probed due to the danger of creating a pneumothorax, damaging internal organs, and worsening hemorrhage.

2. Complications of rib fractures include hemopneumothorax, internal organ injury, and pneumonia secondary to pain-induced hypoventilation.

3. Patients with a high clinical probability of significant hemo- or pneumothorax should be decompressed with tube thoracostomy (chest tube) prior to imaging.

4. There is no gold standard test in the diagnosis of blunt myocardial injury.

5. Findings associated with an aortic tear on chest x-ray may include the following: widening of the superior mediastinum, nasogastric tube deviation to the right, tracheal deviation to the right, blurring of the aortic knob, depression of the left mainstem bronchus, opacification of the apex of the left lung (apical cap), and widening of the peritracheal stripe.

61

Abdominal and Genitourinary Trauma

Abdominal trauma may be blunt (e.g., motor vehicle crash) or penetrating (e.g., gunshot wound, stab wound). As a result of frequent multiple organ system involvement and delays in diagnosis, blunt trauma is typically associated with a higher mortality than penetrating trauma.

PATHOPHYSIOLOGY

The spleen and liver are less compressible and, therefore, more susceptible to injury from blunt trauma. Gunshot and stab wounds to the chest are capable of penetrating the peritoneum, depending on their depth and angle of penetration; during expiration, the diaphragm may reach the level of nipple line. Men are more susceptible to urethral injuries than women due to the longer, male urethra. Bladder ruptures may be classified as extraperitoneal (pelvic) or intraperitoneal.

HISTORY

Historical information about the trauma helps to predict the severity and location of injuries. Important data regarding motor vehicle crashes include whether or not the driver was restrained, the condition of the vehicle, air bag deployment, windshield integrity, steering wheel deformity, whether or not the patient lost consciousness, if the patient was ambulatory, and the condition of

the other passengers. Important questions regarding penetrating trauma include the type of weapon, the number of gunshots fired or stabs inflicted, the victim's distance from the weapon, and the position of the patient at the time of injury. General historical questions relating to past medical history, medications, allergies, and recreational drug abuse are important as well.

PHYSICAL EXAMINATION

The examination of patients sustaining abdominopelvic trauma should include assessment of vital signs and a careful evaluation of the chest, abdomen, pelvis, genitals, and back during the secondary survey. Hypotension following significant abdominal trauma should be considered the result of intraperitoneal hemorrhage until proven otherwise. Therapeutic interventions should be simultaneous with the physical examination among hemodynamically unstable patients. The presence of normal bowel sounds does not rule out a serious abdominal injury.

An abdominal ecchymosis inflicted from a seat belt ("seat-belt sign") is associated with an increased incidence of intra-abdominal viscus injury. Although abdominal ecchymosis over the flanks (Gray-Turner's sign) or umbilicus (Cullen's sign) may represent retroperitoneal hemorrhage, these signs usually require at least 12 hours to develop. Similarly, severe abdominal tenderness with peritoneal signs, as seen with intra-abdominal hemorrhage or intestinal perforation, may take hours to develop.

Abdominal wall hematomas may also cause severe focal tenderness. A focally tender right upper quadrant and left upper quadrant may represent splenic and hepatic injuries, respectively. Subcutaneous emphysema and gross blood on rectal examination usually signifies significant intestinal injury.

Signs of urethral injury include blood at the urethral meatus, a high riding prostate, and the presence of a penile, scrotal, or perineal hematoma. The Foley catheter should not be passed in cases of suspected urethral injury. Stab wounds to the abdomen may warrant local exploration to determine if the peritoneum was violated.

Single hematocrit measurements are not typically helpful in the initial management of trauma since plasma volumes have usually not had enough time to equilibrate, and, therefore, measurements may be normal in the setting of significant acute hemorrhage. Serial hematocrits may be of more value in helping to identify internal hemorrhage. Elevated white blood cell counts with a left shift are common following trauma and primarily result from demargination. Pancreatic enzymes (amylase and lipase) should not be routinely sent since normal levels may exist in the presence of severe pancreatic injury, and abnormal levels may result from shock as opposed to direct trauma. Metabolic acidosis, as evidenced by decreased serum bicarbonate, increased base deficit (>−6), or elevated serum lactate may result from hemorrhage and hypovolemia. Elevated liver transaminases may result from hepatic injury, underlying liver disease, or shock.

Grossly bloody urine (i.e., blood in the urine visible with the naked eye) suggests genitourinary injury that requires further investigation. Hemodynamically normal patients who present following blunt trauma rarely (<1%) have significant urinary trauma in the absence of grossly bloody urine. Plain films of the ribs, spine, and pelvis may reveal fractures that are associated with specific intra-abdominal injuries (e.g., right anterior-inferior rib fractures → liver injury). Plain film imaging of the chest and abdomen may reveal free air; however, they are generally insensitive for the detection of intra-abdominal injury following trauma.

Computed tomography (CT) of the abdomen and bedside abdominal ultrasound are currently the imaging modalities of choice for the detection of intra-abdominal injury following trauma. An intravenous

TABLE 61–1

Criteria for Positive Findings on Diagnostic Peritoneal Lavage

Blunt Trauma	
RBCs (per ml)	≥100,000
WBCs (per ml)	≥500
Amylase (IU/L)	≥20
Alkaline phosphatase (IU/L)	≥3
Intestinal contents	Any
Penetrating Trauma	≥
Abdominal stab wound (RBCs/ml)	≥5000
Low chest stab wound (RBCs/ml)	≥5000
Gunshot wound (RBCs/ml)	≥5000

pyelogram (IVP) may be indicated in patients suspected of renal or ureteral injury if CT is not available. Diagnostic peritoneal lavage (DPL) examines the aspirate of an intraperitoneal catheter for the presence of blood and intestinal contents. The DPL catheter is inserted at the bedside under local anesthesia. Once the DPL catheter is in place, aspiration is attempted to evaluate for the presence of gross blood. If the aspiration via the DPL catheter is unremarkable (usually <10 cc of blood and no intestinal contents), then the aspirate is reinjected, 1 liter of normal saline infused, and the fluid recollected by gravity for analysis. Table 61–1 summarizes the interpretation of the DPL fluid cell count.

Abdominal ultrasound is sensitive at detecting greater than 300 cc of free intraperitoneal blood, making it useful in the evaluation of blunt abdominal trauma. The "focused assessment with sonography for trauma" (F.A.S.T.) bedside exam evaluates four regions for the presence of blood: pericardium, perihepatic, perisplenic, and pelvis. Ultrasound has, for the most part, replaced DPL for identifying intra-abdominal blood at the bedside of trauma patients. One of the only indications for ultrasound in penetrating injury is the evaluation of the pericardial space for effusion. Both ultrasound and DPL are generally incapable of detecting retroperitoneal hemorrhage.

Abdominal CT has evolved to be the imaging modality of choice for detecting traumatic visceral and vascular abdominopelvic injuries among stable patients. The administration of intravenous contrast makes abdominal CT imaging of the trauma patient more sensitive at detecting primary vascular and visceral injuries. Although controversial, the oral administration of a water-soluble contrast (e.g., Gastrograffin) may help to identify gastric, duodenal, and rectal perforations. Rectal contrast may be useful if rapid imaging of the lower intestinal tract is necessary.

Pelvic fractures, especially those involving the symphysis pubis, should raise the suspicion for urethral and bladder injuries. Patients suspected of urethral or bladder injury should undergo a retrograde urethrocystogram whereby contrast is injected into the bladder via the urethral meatus. Although failure of the bladder to fill on retrograde urethrocystogram suggests a complete urethral transection, bladder filling does not rule out partial urethral tears. Diagnostic imaging of the abdomen is generally only warranted in cases where the clinical evaluation is inconclusive and there is not an obvious need for laparotomy.

TREATMENT

Treatment should begin with the treatment of other, more life-threatening injuries (e.g., airway). Critically ill patients should be aggressively resuscitated with oxygen, two large-bore intravenous catheters, crystalloid and blood infusions, and frequent hemodynamic monitoring. Surgical consultants should be notified early in cases that may require operative management or admission. Patients with an obvious need for the operating room (e.g., evisceration) should spend a relatively short amount of time in the emergency department and be expeditiously transferred to the operating room for further management.

Patients with profound hypovolemic shock believed to result from intra-abdominal hemorrhage may require emergent thoracotomy and clamping of the descending aorta to control bleeding. The early administration of empiric antibiotics reduces the incidence of intra-abdominal sepsis among patients suspected of gastrointestinal perforation. All patients believed to have sustained gastrointestinal perforation should be taken to the operating room for exploratory laparotomy.

Severely lacerated spleens and livers usually require operative management; however, mild or moderate injuries may be conservatively managed with close monitoring in the surgical intensive care unit. Patients with penetrating wounds that violate the peritoneum are generally taken to the operating room for exploratory laparotomy. However, new evidence suggests that some low-risk abdominal stab wound patients with a normal triple-contrast (oral, rectal, and intravenous) abdominal CT may not require surgery unless they exhibit clinical deterioration during close observation.

The diagnosis of diaphragmatic lacerations typically requires direct visualization in surgery since they are usually very difficult to detect on radiologic abdominal imaging. Due to the risk of future visceral herniation into the chest, most diaphragm injuries are repaired depending on their size and location. High-velocity weapon injuries (e.g., rifles firing bullets greater than 2500 ft/sec) usually require larger areas of debridement due to the tissue damage caused by the shock wave associated with the bullet.

Immediate orthopedic consultation should be sought when caring for patients with unstable pelvic fractures. During pelvic fracture, pelvic veins may be torn and hemorrhage significantly leading to hypotension and shock. Pelvic fractures and subsequent hemorrhage may be treated initially by tying a sheet tightly around the pelvis or applying military antishock trousers (M.A.S.T). However, definitive management of pelvic fractures typically requires external fixation of the pelvis, and possibly embolization of hemorrhaging pelvic veins during angiography.

Urologic consultation should be obtained in all cases of urethral and bladder injury. Careful placement of a Foley catheter may be indicated in patients with a partial urethral tear, however, complete urethral transections often require the placement of a suprapubic catheter to drain the bladder. Sterile, extraperitoneal bladder ruptures are typically treated conservatively with continuous bladder drainage. Most intraperitoneal bladder ruptures require surgical repair. Rupture of the corpus carvernosum (fractured penis), with subsequent hematoma formation, typically follows vigorous intercourse and requires surgical repair. Testicular dislocation (traumatic displacement of a testicle, usually into the abdominal wall) and testicular hematomas generally require surgical management.

◆ KEY POINTS ◆

1. The spleen and liver are less compressible and, therefore, especially susceptible to injury from blunt trauma.

2. Ultrasound has generally replaced DPL as the bedside test of choice for identifying free intraperitoneal blood.

3. Neither ultrasound nor DPL visualizes the retroperitoneum.

4. Abdominal CT has evolved to be the imaging modality of choice for detecting traumatic visceral and vascular abdominopelvic injuries among stable trauma patients.

5. Diagnostic imaging of the abdomen is generally only warranted in cases where the clinical evaluation is inconclusive and there is not an obvious need for laparotomy.

6. Hemodynamically stable patients who present following blunt trauma rarely (<1%) have significant urinary trauma in the absence of grossly bloody urine.

62 General Wound Care

Nearly 10 million patients are seen annually in United States emergency departments for the evaluation of traumatic wounds. Although major wounds may be impressive, minor wounds are much more common and ultimately account for most of the morbidity and disfigurement related to traumatic wounds. The initial care of traumatic wounds in the emergency department has a tremendous effect on the cosmetic result. The risk of infection may be greatly reduced by closing appropriate wounds within 8 to 12 hours of injury.

ANATOMY AND PATHOPHYSIOLOGY

The process of wound healing includes coagulation, inflammation, collagen metabolism, wound contraction, and epithelialization. The activation of fibroblasts and the establishment of the collagen network, upon which tissue restructuring proceeds, is dependent on the presence of lactate, ascorbic acid (vitamin C), and adequate delivery of oxygen to the tissue. Although the tensile strength of a healing wound is markedly improved by 1 week, the wound reaches only 20% of its ultimate strength after 3 weeks and 60% after 4 months. Necrotic tissue or foreign bodies within the wound delay wound healing, increase the risk of infection, and worsen cosmetic results. Normal skin is under constant tension. "Lines of tension" (Fig. 62–1A and B) exist as a result of skin elasticity and the orientation of collagen fiber bundles. Wounds parallel to the lines of expression heal under the least amount of tension and, therefore, produce a smaller, less apparent scar. Wounds perpendicular to the lines of expression often produce a more conspicuous scar.

HISTORY

A complete history should be elicited to help identify patients at risk for poor wound healing (e.g., diabetics), patients with an allergy to local anesthetics, and patients on medications that may react with local anesthetics or antibiotics. Information about a patient's past medical history (e.g., diabetes, HIV) and living conditions (e.g., homeless) may influence initial wound management and follow-up. The patient's tetanus status should also be determined.

PHYSICAL EXAMINATION

In the multiple trauma patient, noncritical wounds should generally not be assessed until the more critical systems have been evaluated and stabilized. The general appearance of a wound should be recorded including its location, size, cleanliness, and bleeding status. A neurovascular examination should evaluate the sensation, motor strength, and blood perfusion of areas potentially affected by the injury.

In most hand injuries, two-point discrimination should be evaluated over both sides (radial and ulnar) of

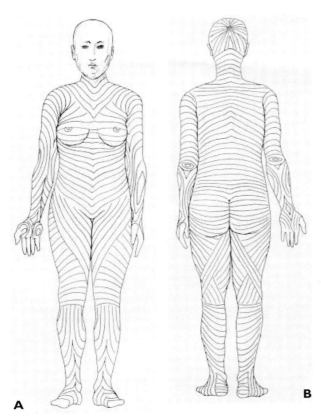

A **B**

Figure 62–1 Skin tension lines of the body surface. *(Adapted from Simon R, Brenner B: Procedures and techniques in emergency medicine, Baltimore, 1982, Williams & Wilkins, as published in Trott A: Wounds and lacerations, ed 3, St Louis, 1998, Mosby.)*

the volar aspect of each distal phalanx. Two-point discrimination is often evaluated using ends of a bent paperclip separated by approximately 4 mm. Circulation to the fingers and toes should be assessed by measuring the capillary refill time (normal <2 sec).

To adequately evaluate a wound, active hemorrhage must be controlled. Hemorrhage control should first be attempted by direct pressure. If direct pressure is unsuccessful, a tourniquet may be used for a short period of time to adequately evaluate and manage the wound. Small lacerations of the skin may be deceiving and actually extend deeply with associated significant internal injuries (e.g., puncture wound).

In general, wounds may be probed carefully to identify their direction and depth. However, the probing of

neck and thoracic wounds is generally contraindicated in the emergency department due to the potential for iatrogenic injury to critical structures. Wound exploration may be painful and typically requires the administration of an anesthetic. In the extremities, it is extremely important to identify injuries to blood vessels, nerves, muscles, tendons, ligaments, and bone. All foreign bodies should be removed and their presence or absence documented on the ED record.

TREATMENT

Anesthesia is usually attained by local or regional nerve blockade with lidocaine. A 1% lidocaine solution contains 10 mg/ml. The anesthesia produced by lidocaine develops within seconds and typically lasts for 20 to 60 minutes. It is usually safe to administer a single dose of locally infiltrated lidocaine in a quantity up to 5 mg/kg not to exceed 300 mg. Lidocaine toxicity may manifest as dysrhythmia, hypotension, or seizure. Due to the vasoconstriction caused by epinephrine, lidocaine solutions containing epinephrine may generally be administered in larger quantities of up to 7 mg/kg. The addition of epinephrine to lidocaine may also help to control wound hemorrhage. Solutions containing epinephrine are generally contraindicated in areas of the body with tenuous blood supply (e.g., fingers, nose, penis, ears, and toes), as well as in wounds with questionable tissue viability. Bupivacaine (Marcaine) is a local anesthetic with an onset of action similar to lidocaine, but the duration of anesthesia is 4 to 8 times longer.

Pain from local anesthetic injection may be reduced by utilizing a small needle (e.g., 27- or 30-gauge), injecting from within the laceration margin, adding sodium bicarbonate to make the solution less acidic, and injecting the anesthetic slowly. The previous belief that a decreased risk of infection was attained by injecting anesthetic through intact skin is unfounded. Topical anesthetic creams (e.g., EMLA) have a much longer onset of action, but may be useful alone or in later combination with injected anesthetic. In areas of the body innervated by a single superficial nerve, it is preferable to attain anesthesia by infiltrating the anesthetic around the nerve at a site distant from the wound (regional block). Regional blocks avoid wound distortion resulting from local anesthetic infiltration, and thus preserve anatomical landmarks for more accurate wound reapproximation.

Wound closures may be classified as primary (closed immediately following the injury), delayed primary (closed after an observation period of 3 to 5 days without infection), or secondary (allowed to remain open and heal-in on its own). Contraindications to wound closure typically include the following: heavy contamination, bites, retained foreign bodies, unresectable devitalized tissue, wounds older than 12 hours, infection, and tissue defects that would require excessive tension if closure were attempted. Prior to closure, wounds should be adequately cleaned and debrided. Scrubbing of the surrounding skin around the wound with antimicrobial cleansers may only be helpful if the areas are heavily contaminated. Most antimicrobial cleansers inhibit wound healing if introduced into the wound. Most wounds should be irrigated under pressure to help cleanse the wound and debride it of foreign bodies and devitalized tissue.

Options for closing wounds include the use of sutures, staples, tissue adhesives (e.g., Dermabond), and surgical tapes. The placement of subcutaneous absorbable sutures in appropriate wounds may help to improve cosmetic outcome by relieving skin tension on the surface sutures, and decreasing deeper pockets of dead space. However, it is important to realize that the placement of subcutaneous sutures (especially in contaminated wounds) is associated with a higher rate of infection.

Following wound closure, patients should be instructed to keep their wounds clean and dry for 24 to 48 hours until there is enough epithelialization to protect the wound from contamination. Bio-occlusive dressings that help the wound to retain some of its natural moisture may speed the rate of healing. After the 24- to 48-hour period, patients may wash their wounds gently with mild soap and water. Topical antibiotic ointments may help reduce the risk of infection and improve cosmesis. Wounds at high risk for infection should be reevaluated within 24 to 48 hours. Erythema, warmth, swelling, drainage, and dehiscence of healing wounds suggest infection. Superficial, nonabsorbable sutures should generally be removed in 3 to 5 days for the face, 7 to 10 days for skin not exposed to significant tension, and 10 to 14 days for skin exposed to significant tension (e.g., over a joint).

Prophylactic antibiotic therapy should not be prescribed routinely, but rather administered judiciously to those at increased risk for infection (e.g., immunosuppressed hosts, poorly perfused tissue, heavily contaminated wounds, bites, intraoral lacerations, open fractures, exposed joints or tendons). Tetanus vaccine and or immunoglobulin should be administered if indicated (see the "Tetanus" chapter). Since exposure to sunlight may worsen the cosmetic appearance of a scar, the topical application (after suture removal) of suntan lotion (SPF ≥15) as well as vitamin E may improve the final wound appearance. Patients should understand that all wounds are subject to infection and scar formation.

◆ KEY POINTS ◆

1. Normal skin is under constant tension.

2. Small lacerations of the skin may be deceiving and actually extend deeply with significant internal injuries.

3. Probing of neck and thoracic wounds is generally contraindicated in the emergency department.

4. Prophylactic antibiotic therapy should not be prescribed routinely, but rather administered judiciously to those at increased risk for infection.

63 Orthopedic Injury of the Extremities

Musculoskeletal complaints represent a large portion of emergency department visits. Complications of ligament and tendon injury frequently include increased joint laxity, weakness, increased susceptibility to reinjury, and tendonitis. Complications of fractures and immobilization may include hemorrhage, vascular injury, nerve injury, compartment syndrome, fracture non-union, avascular necrosis, fat embolism, deep venous thrombosis, thromboembolism, reflex sympathetic dystrophy (i.e., RSD), and loss of function. Delays in the diagnosis and treatment of orthopedic injuries may result in unnecessary complications.

ANATOMY AND PATHOPHYSIOLOGY

The ability to accurately describe orthopedic injuries with pertinent historical and physical examination findings is especially important since significant injuries may warrant orthopedic consultation, but not require the orthopedist to evaluate the patient in the emergency department. A **sprain** is a ligamentous injury resulting from abnormal joint motion. A **strain** is an injury to the muscle-tendon unit that results from stretching or overexertion. **Subluxation** refers to the partial loss of continuity between two articular surfaces. The term **dislocation** indicates a complete loss of continuity between two articular surfaces.

The general anatomy of a bone consists of the following regions: epiphysis, physis, metaphysis, diaphysis (i.e., shaft), and cortex (Fig. 63–1). The following are general types of fractures: transverse (i.e., fracture line perpendicular to the long axis of the bone), oblique (i.e., fracture line oblique to the long axis of the bone), spiral (i.e., fracture line circles the shaft of the bone), and comminuted (i.e., fractures containing more than two fragments), and greenstick (Fig. 63–2).

Fracture descriptions should include information about whether the fracture is open or closed (overlying soft tissue intact or not intact), complete or incomplete (fracture interrupts both cortices of the bone or not), the type of fracture, the fracture location, the percentage and direction of displacement of the distal fragment, the degree and direction of angulation, the percentage of articular surface involved, and any resulting rotational irregularity or loss in height.

Long bone shafts are usually thought of as being divided into proximal, middle, and distal thirds. **Impaction** refers to the forceful collapse of one bone fragment into another. The terms **varus** and **valgus** describe whether the bone segment distal to the fracture angles towards the midline or away from the midline, respectively (Fig. 63–3).

The following is an example of a sentence describing a specific fracture: "The patient has a closed, oblique, complete, midshaft fracture of the right femur with 4 mm of posterior displacement, and 20 degrees of valgus deformity." Specific fractures may require slight variations and additions to the normal description scheme.

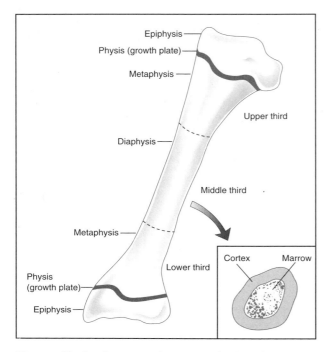

Figure 63–1   Anatomical regions of a long bone.

Greenstick fractures (incomplete angulated long bone fractures) and **Torus fractures** (incomplete fractures appearing as wrinkling or buckling of the cortex) are typically seen in children and are believed to result from increased bone elasticity (Fig. 63–4). In children, the epiphyseal growth plate is generally weaker than the supporting ligaments and tendons, thereby placing children at greater risk for growth plate injuries (Fig. 63–5).

HISTORY

Details about the history of present illness and mechanism of injury make it possible to predict the most likely structures injured. It is important to determine if falls were **mechanical** in origin (e.g., tripped or slipped) or **nonmechanical** (e.g., dysrhythmia). It is easy to miss serious medical conditions by focusing the history and physical examination solely on the injury. The time of the injury is also important and may help determine subsequent management. If an upper extremity is injured, the handedness (right- or left-handed) of the patient should be determined as it may influence management as well as help predict future disability.

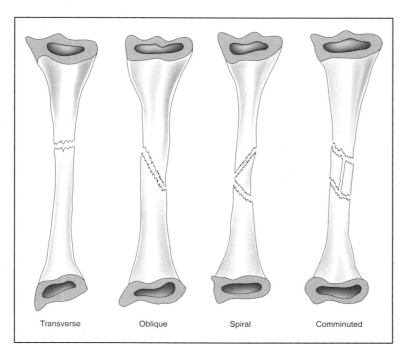

Figure 63–2   Types of fractures.

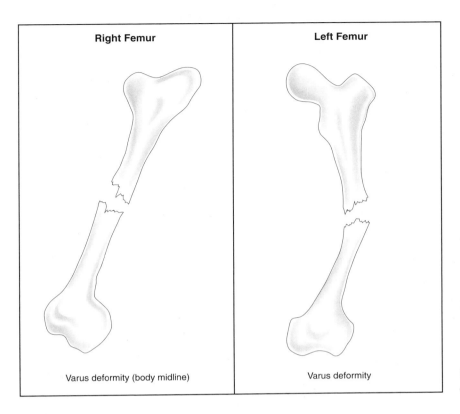

Right Femur

Left Femur

Varus deformity (body midline)

Varus deformity

Figure 63–3 Varus and Valgus deformities.

The past medical history may reveal diseases associated with poor wound and fracture healing (e.g., diabetes, osteoporosis). A complete medication and drug allergy list may help to identify patients at risk for complications such as drug-induced impaired wound healing (e.g., prednisone) and decreased blood clotting (e.g., aspirin and Coumadin). The social history may also help to identify patients at risk for impaired wound healing (e.g., alcoholics, smokers, drug abusers), as well as provide insight into the safety of the home environment. Knowledge of the patient's occupation is usually helpful in weighing the risks and benefits of subsequent treatment.

PHYSICAL EXAMINATION

In a multiple trauma patient, the extremities should not be assessed until other, more critical systems have been evaluated and stabilized. Examination of the extremities should begin by noting the location of the injury as well

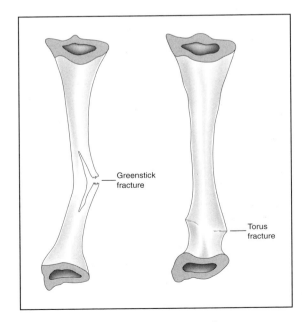

Greenstick fracture

Torus fracture

Figure 63–4 Greenstick and torus fractures.

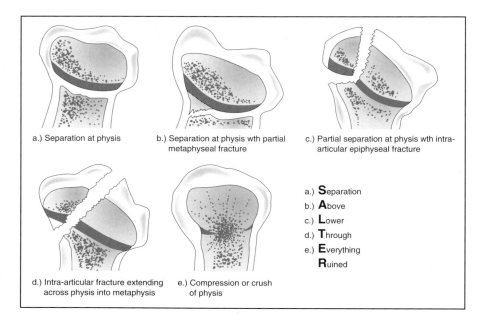

a.) Separation at physis

b.) Separation at physis wth partial metaphyseal fracture

c.) Partial separation at physis wth intra-articular epiphyseal fracture

d.) Intra-articular fracture extending across physis into metaphysis

e.) Compression or crush of physis

a.) **S**eparation
b.) **A**bove
c.) **L**ower
d.) **T**hrough
e.) **E**verything
   Ruined

Figure 63–5 Salter (and Harris) classification of epiphyseal injuries.

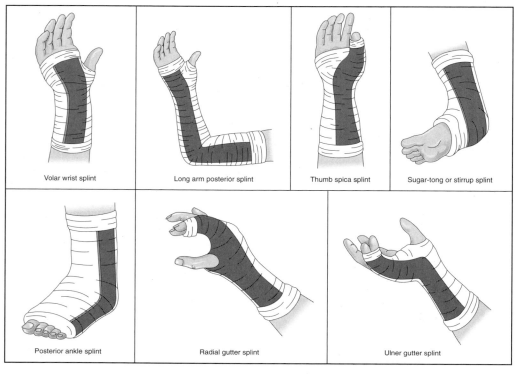

Volar wrist splint

Long arm posterior splint

Thumb spica splint

Sugar-tong or stirrup splint

Posterior ankle splint

Radial gutter splint

Ulner gutter splint

Figure 63–6 Common types of splints.

as the extremity position. The extremity should be assessed for soft tissue injury, loss of length, rotation, and angulation. Since vascular injury may also occur, the presence and character of pulses above and below the site of injury should be evaluated. (A normal pulse is usually described as +2, a weaker pulse as +1, and an absent pulse as 0.)

Evaluation of joint range of motion is important, but may be delayed until after imaging in cases of likely fracture. Joints above and below the site of injury should be evaluated for laxity and range of motion. Deficits in range of motion should be recorded as the number of degrees attainable in any one direction (flexion, extension, abduction, or adduction).

Neurologic testing should include details about sensation as well as motor function. An uninjured, opposite extremity may provide a "normal" comparison. The distribution of sensory deficits may be mapped over a sketch of the involved extremity as well as on the extremity itself for later comparison. Motor deficits should be documented, noting the specific muscle group tested. The inability to move part of a limb may be a sign of muscle or tendon disruption as well as possible neurologic injury.

If a fracture is suspected, plain film radiographs of the area should be performed. In general, a minimum of AP and lateral images should be obtained for improved fracture detection and description. Specific sites of injury may require unique viewing angles. Since the transmission of energy may have injured adjacent structures, it may also be necessary to image the bones above and below the site of injury.

Several imaging decision rules have been derived and validated for specific types of injuries. Decision rules generally have a high sensitivity for detecting fractures, and save millions of dollars by preventing unnecessary imaging. In the setting of normal imaging results, patients highly suspicious for a fracture may indeed have an occult (radiologically undetected) fracture. Computed tomography (CT) or magnetic resonance imaging (MRI) may be warranted in certain cases to help further increase the sensitivity of fracture detection as well

as improve fracture-line delineation. Radionuclide bone scanning (scintigraphy) utilizes the uptake of technetium polyphosphate (TC99) by reactive bone, and may help to identify occult fractures older than 24 hours.

TREATMENT

Orthopedic consultation is typically indicated in complicated cases involving open fractures and joints, as well as at other times when surgical repair may be necessary. In general, treatment should focus on analgesia, swelling reduction, immobilization, appropriate follow-up, and rehabilitation. Significant injuries may require narcotics for analgesia while acetaminophen or ibuprofen may be adequate for a simple sprain. Although reduction of swelling may be initially achieved with anti-inflammatory medications or cooling the site of injury with ice, elevation of the injured extremity above the heart often has a much more profound effect. Reduction of swelling is especially important in patients with splints or casts since the tissue is confined within a closed space. Tissue swelling also makes it more difficult to close an operative wound. Figure 63–6 illustrates several common types of splints. Patients discharged home should be given very clear instructions detailing when and with whom they should be reevaluated, as well as when they should return to the emergency department.

◆ KEY POINTS ◆

1. In children, the epiphyseal growth plate is generally weaker than the supporting ligaments and tendons, placing children at greater risk for growth plate injuries.

2. In general, the management of extremity orthopedic injuries should focus on analgesia, swelling reduction, immobilization, appropriate follow-up, and rehabilitation.

Part XI
Infectious Diseases

64 HIV Infection and AIDS

Human immunodeficiency virus (HIV) infection was first described in the early 1980s after a group of previously healthy homosexual men in San Francisco presented with Kaposi's sarcoma and *Pneumocystis carinii* pneumonia. Initially a rapidly fatal disease, medical advances have turned HIV and AIDS (acquired immunodeficiency syndrome) into a chronic condition.

EPIDEMIOLOGY

Intravenous drug use, unprotected sex (both heterosexual and homosexual), and contact with blood or body fluids are all risk factors for HIV infection. The risk of seroconversion after a hollow bore needle stick injury is approximately 0.2–0.3% (1 in 250–300). The risk of vertical transmission (a neonate acquiring the virus from an infected mother during birth) is approximately 10–30% and is affected by prenatal treatment with zidovudine (AZT). The primary mode of transmission is different in different parts of the world. In the United States, transmission most commonly occurs through homosexual contact or intravenous drug use. In developing countries such as sub-Saharan Africa and parts of Southeast Asia, transmission occurs primarily through heterosexual contact. Worldwide, it is estimated that 30–40 million people are infected with the HIV virus.

PATHOPHYSIOLOGY

The HIV virus is a cytotropic RNA retrovirus that has a high affinity for CD4+ cells of the immune system.

The HIV virus enters the body through the genital mucous membranes or direct exposure to the patient's blood. Once the virus enters a cell, it uses a viral enzyme known as reverse transcriptase to transcribe its RNA genome into a piece of double stranded DNA that is subsequently integrated into the host cell genome. In this way, the virus pirates the host cells' own reproductive mechanisms to replicate.

Two to four weeks after the initial infection, viremia (virus infection of the bloodstream) and systemic dissemination occurs. It is during this time that infectivity is highest and also the time in which standard tests fail to detect infection. The immune system responds vigorously to dissemination resulting in the establishment of a steady-state viral level (viral load). Patients with a higher steady-state level of virus have a poorer prognosis.

CLINICAL MANIFESTATIONS

The natural history of HIV infection can be divided into three stages. Primary HIV infection usually manifests as an acute illness occurring 2–4 weeks after exposure, with symptoms of viremia. Fever, pharyngitis, arthralgias, headache, and a maculopapular rash are the most common manifestations of primary HIV infection. Between 50 and 90% of individuals are symptomatic with primary HIV, with more severe symptoms correlating with more rapid disease progression.

The next stage of HIV infection occurs when a patient becomes symptomatic but does not develop an

TABLE 64–1

AIDS Defining Illnesses

- Esophageal Candidiasis
- Disseminated *Mycobacterium tuberculosis*
- Disseminated histoplasmosis
- Disseminated toxoplasmosis
- Progressive multifocal Leukoencephalopathy
- Kaposi's sarcoma
- *Pneumocystis carinii* pneumonia
- *Mycobacterium avium complex*
- Brain lymphoma
- Herpes simplex virus
- Cytomegalovirus retinitis
- Cryptosporidiosis
- Cryptococcosis
- Invasive cervical cancer
- Coccidioidomycosis
- *Salmonella* septicemia
- HIV wasting
- Recurrent bacterial pneumonia

AIDS-defining illness. Symptoms include peripheral neuropathy, hairy leukoplakia, oral thrush, vulvovaginal candidiasis, cervical dysplasia, or idiopathic thrombocytopenic purpura.

AIDS constitutes the third stage of HIV infection. AIDS is defined as a CD4 count less than 200 regardless of symptoms or the development of an AIDS-defining illness (Table 64–1). The average life expectancy for a patient infected with the HIV virus in the absence of treatment is approximately 10 years, though "long-term survivors" have been identified.

The hallmark of AIDS is the development of opportunistic infection with such organisms as *Pneumocystis carinii* and *Cryptococcus neoformans*. *Pneumocystis carinii* pneumonia (PCP) is one of the pathognomonic illnesses of AIDS and presents as a dry, hacking cough and dyspnea. Chest radiography classically reveals "batwing" perihilar or more diffuse ground glass interstitial infiltrates. The diagnosis of PCP is made by identification of the causative organism in sputum after methenamine silver staining. Treatment of PCP involves either intravenous trimethoprim-sulfamethoxazole or pentamidine.

Cryptococcal meningitis is caused by infection with the fungus *Cryptococcus neoformans*. Patients typically present with fever, meningismus, photophobia and altered mental status. Diagnosis is made by India ink staining of the cerebrospinal fluid or by serum detection of cryptococcal antigen. Both amphotericin B and fluconazole have been used for treatment.

DIAGNOSIS

Most patients infected with HIV will produce antibodies by 6–8 weeks, with the antibody response being almost universal by 6 months. The usual screening test for HIV infection is the ELISA (enzyme-linked immunosorbent assay). The ELISA has a sensitivity approaching 99.7%. All positive ELISA tests must be confirmed with the Western blot, which is highly specific for HIV (99.9%). Once HIV infection is confirmed, most patients will undergo quantitative viral load testing. This is done through HIV RNA PCR. These results can be used to monitor response to therapy.

TREATMENT

Over the past 20 years, research into the viral life cycle has led to several therapeutic options for those infected with the HIV virus. The first agents developed were nucleoside analogues that inhibited the viral enzyme reverse transcriptase and included such agents as zidovudine, didanosine, zalcitabine, stavudine, and lamivudine. Although initially effective in staving off advanced infection, viral immunity to these agents quickly developed, prompting the development of nonnucleoside reverse transcriptase inhibitors such as nevirapine, delavirdine, and efavirenz.

Recently, a new class of drugs has been developed that inhibits HIV viral protease (saquinavir, ritonavir, indinavir, and nelfinavir). Protease is an enzyme that cleaves viral particles during replication, resulting in formation of functional pathogenic virions. This step in viral replication occurs much later than the one targeted by reverse transcriptase inhibitors. Modern HIV treatment involves the use of a "cocktail" of drugs (a nucleoside analogue, non-nucleoside analogue, and a protease inhibitor) that is designed to provide effective inhibition of viral transcription while minimizing the development of resistance. Initiation of therapy is based on a patient's CD4 count and viral load. Current recommendations suggest starting therapy once a patient's CD4 count falls below 500 or the viral load is above 10,000, although these numbers are controversial and some clinicians will begin treating a patient as soon as HIV infection is diagnosed. Serial CD4 counts and measurements of viral load are done to monitor response to therapy.

◆ KEY POINTS ◆

1. Transmission through heterosexual contact is the most common mode of HIV infection.

2. The HIV virus infects CD4 lymphocytes and renders patients functionally immunocompromised.

3. Primary HIV infection is characterized by sore throat, fever, and lymphadenopathy.

4. Treatment of HIV involves a "cocktail" of antiviral drugs.

65

Sepsis and SIRS

Sepsis is the term given to the systemic syndrome that occurs in response to overwhelming infection. It is characterized by widespread release of inflammatory mediators. SIRS (systemic inflammatory response syndrome) refers to the "sepsis-like" syndrome that develops in response to noninfectious conditions such as pancreatitis or trauma. Septic shock refers to hypotension that persists despite adequate fluid resuscitation and evidence of perfusion abnormalities (i.e., altered mental status, oliguria, or metabolic acidosis). Multisystem organ failure (MSOF) is the term for organ dysfunction that occurs in critically ill patients, in which homeostasis cannot be maintained without outside intervention. Several clinical conditions are contained under the umbrella term MSOF, including acute respiratory distress syndrome (ARDS), disseminated intravascular coagulation (DIC), and acute renal failure.

EPIDEMIOLOGY

It is estimated that sepsis and SIRS together cause more than 100,000 deaths per year in the United States. Risk factors for the development of sepsis include bacteremia (bacterial infection of the bloodstream), increasing age, and immunosuppressive comorbidities such as cancer, HIV infection, end-stage renal disease, and diabetes mellitus. The case fatality rate exceeds 50% despite advances in intensive care medicine. Several factors have been identified that influence mortality rate in cases of sepsis (Table 65–1).

PATHOPHYSIOLOGY

Sepsis and SIRS develop in cases where the body's anti-inflammatory mechanisms are overwhelmed by an overly aggressive inflammatory response. Normally, the body's response to infection is a localized inflammatory response that leads to healing (Fig. 65–1). In sepsis and SIRS, the localized inflammatory response spills over and begins to affect normal, uninfected tissue. This generalized response affects primarily the heart, lungs, kidney, and brain.

There are multiple mechanisms by which infection leads to sepsis. In some cases, the cascade leading to sepsis is initiated by exotoxins that are made and released by an organism. Examples include the toxic shock syndrome toxin (TSST-1) produced by *Staphylococcus aureus* and toxin A by *Pseudomonas aeruginosa*. Organisms such as staphylococci (techoic acid) and *Streptococcus pneumoniae* (polysaccharide capsule) each have an antigenic surface component that initiates the sepsis cascade. Gram-negative organisms such as *Escherichia coli* have a distinct endotoxin called lipopolysaccharide (LPS), a component of their cell membrane that is associated with the sepsis syndrome.

CLINICAL MANIFESTATIONS

Clinically, sepsis is characterized by fever (or hypothermia), tachycardia, tachypnea, leukocytosis or leukope-

TABLE 65–1

Associations with Increased Mortality in Sepsis and SIRS

1. Failure to mount a fever in response to infection (indicative of a poor immune response to infection)
2. Development of septic shock
3. Nosocomial (hospital-acquired) infection
4. Source of infection other than urinary tract

TABLE 65–2

Clinical Manifestations in Sepsis and SIRS

1. Temperature >38°C or <36°C
2. Heart rate >90 beats/min
3. Respiratory rate >20 breaths/min or $PaCO_2$ <32 mm Hg
4. White blood cell count >12,000 cells/mm^3, <4000 cells/mm^3, or >10% immature (band) forms

---

Injury→Exposed Endothelium→Aggregation of Polymorphonuclear Cells→Release of Pro-inflammatory and Anti-inflammatory Mediators (Tumor Necrosis Factor, Interferon, Interleukin 1, 2, 6, 8, 10)→Vasodilation/Hyperemia/Increased Vascular Permeability→Healing

Figure 65–1   Normal inflammatory cycle.

---

nia, renal insufficiency, and metabolic acidosis. These clinical parameters are summarized in Table 65–2. Hypotension is the hallmark of septic shock.

DIFFERENTIAL DIAGNOSIS

- Meningitis
- Pneumonia
- Pyelonephritis
- Peritonitis
- Pancreatitis
- Cholangitis
- Cellulitis
- Trauma

DIAGNOSTIC EVALUATION AND TREATMENT

In cases of sepsis, the diagnostic focus is on identifying a cause for the syndrome (infectious versus noninfec-

tious). Blood should be sent for chemistries, complete blood count, and coagulation studies. Two sets of blood cultures should be obtained from two separate venipuncture sites. Urine should be sent for analysis and culture. If evidence of meningitis exists, a lumbar puncture should be performed and the fluid sent for analysis and culture. A chest radiograph may show evidence of pneumonia or ARDS.

The management of sepsis should focus on the ABCs (airway, breathing, circulation). Hypoxia should be corrected by intubation and assisted ventilation. Hypotension should be aggressively treated with intravenous crystalloid infusion if there is no evidence of congestive heart failure. If fluid resuscitation fails to correct hypotension, then consideration can be given to intravenous vasopressors such as phenylephrine, norepinephrine, or dopamine. A urinary catheter should be placed to monitor urine output. A central venous catheter, and in many cases, central venous pressure monitoring with a Swan-Ganz catheter, will help monitor resuscitation. Finally, initiation of antibiotic therapy immediately after fluid is obtained for culture is critically important in cases of sepsis caused by infection.

◆ KEY POINTS ◆

1. Sepsis is the systemic response to overwhelming infection.

2. SIRS is a sepsis-like syndrome that occurs in response to noninfectious conditions.

3. Lipopolysaccharide A is the cell membrane constituent of gram-negative bacteria that causes sepsis.

4. Treatment of sepsis and SIRS involves support of cardiopulmonary systems and an exhaustive search for infectious etiologies.

66 Tuberculosis

Tuberculosis (TB) is a disease known since antiquity that remains a major medical and public health threat. It is caused by infection with the bacterium *Mycobacterium tuberculosis* and remains the most common cause of death in the world due to infectious disease. Although the disease can affect multiple organ systems, the lungs are the most common site (80% of cases) of primary infection.

EPIDEMIOLOGY

The incidence of TB declined between 1900 and 1984 but in 1985, the number of new cases began to rise again, corresponding to the emergence of AIDS and multidrug resistant TB. Risk factors for the development of TB include:

1. Age (higher risk in infants and the elderly)
2. Close contact with a person known to have TB
3. HIV infection
4. Residing in a nursing home
5. Low socioeconomic status
6. Travel to areas with high rates of TB (parts of Asia, Africa, and Latin America)

PATHOPHYSIOLOGY

TB is caused by infection with the bacterium *Mycobacterium tuberculosis*. *M. tuberculosis* is an intracellular, aerobic, acid-fast bacillus (AFB) that is extremely slow growing (generation time of 15–20 hours). Acid-fast organisms resist decolorization with acid alcohol during Gram staining.

TB is spread through respiratory secretions that are transmitted person to person by coughing or sneezing. Droplets with bacteria are inhaled and settle in areas of the lung that are highly ventilated but poorly perfused (i.e., the upper middle or lower upper lung zones). Macrophages respond to the infection and engulf the bacterium. Once intracellular, the bacilli reproduce and more macrophages respond to the infection. Eventually, cell-mediated immunity (via CD4 helper T cells) controls the infection and the bacilli stop multiplying. If the immune response to primary infection is particularly aggressive, cavitation may occur. This process, termed primary TB, can take from 1 to 3 months, during which time the PPD (tuberculin skin test) will turn positive.

In the immunocompetent host, the initial infection is walled off and a granuloma forms. Granulomas are collections of inflammatory cells (particularly Langerhans giant cells) and cellular debris that often have a necrotic, caseous (cheesy) center. A Ghon complex is the term given to a granuloma and its draining lymph node. TB bacilli can survive in a dormant state in the center of these granulomas for years, providing a source of viable bacteria that can escape and cause infection if a patient's cell-mediated immunity weakens (due to cancer, HIV infection, steroid use, or old age). This is termed reactivation or post-primary tuberculosis.

Immunocompromised hosts are also predisposed to disseminated TB. In disseminated or miliary TB, the initial infection is not walled off and bacilli travel hematogenously to distant extrapulmonary sites such as the kidney, pleura, extrapulmonary lymph nodes (scrofula), vertebral bodies (Pott's disease), brain, meninges, or long bones.

HISTORY

Primary TB is often associated only with mild fever and malaise. Symptoms of post-primary TB develop over the course of weeks to months. Patients may complain of fevers, chills, night sweats, weight loss, dyspnea, fatigue, cough, or hemoptysis. Symptoms of miliary TB depend on the site of infection.

PHYSICAL EXAMINATION

Vital signs may reveal fever, and rarely hypoxia. Examination of the lungs may reveal rales or signs of pulmonary effusion. Cavitation is suggested by amphora (hollow sound on auscultation similar to the sound made by blowing across the mouth of a bottle).

DIFFERENTIAL DIAGNOSIS

- Sarcoidosis
- Fungal pneumonia such as histoplasmosis or aspergillosis
- Lung cancer
- Lymphoma

DIAGNOSTIC EVALUATION

The PPD tuberculin skin test is an important diagnostic and screening tool. Five tuberculin units (TU) are injected subcutaneously and the amount of induration surrounding the injection site is measured 48–72 hours later. The current Centers for Disease Control guidelines for the interpretation of PPD tests are given in Table 66–1.

Chest radiographs may reveal calcifications in the lung parenchyma and hilar region representing the Ghon complex. Other patterns suggesting TB include apical pleural scarring or cavitary lesions (Fig. 66–1). It is important to note that approximately 10% of patients with documented TB will have negative chest radiographs.

TABLE 66–1

CDC Guidelines for the Interpretation of PPD Test Results Measuring Maximum Diameter of Induration

Greater than 5 mm of induration is defined as positive in the following instances:
1. Persons who are HIV positive or who have HIV risk factors
2. Persons with recent close contact with a patient with active tuberculosis
3. Persons with a chest radiograph consistent with healed tuberculosis infection

Greater than 10 mm of induration is defined as positive in the following instances:
1. Persons born in foreign countries with high prevalence of tuberculosis
2. Intravenous drug users
3. Low income populations
4. Nursing home residents
5. Children under the age of 4 years
6. Persons with other medical conditions that increase the risk for tuberculosis (diabetes, malignancy, corticosteroid use, immunosuppression, renal failure)

Greater than 15 mm of induration is defined as positive in all other cases.

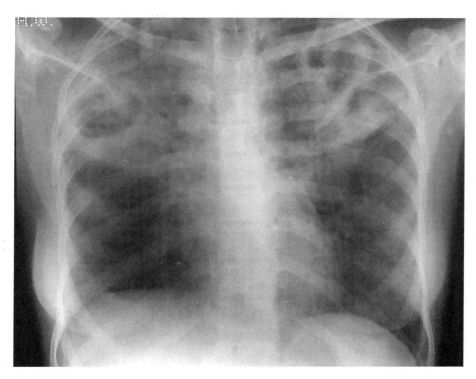

Figure 66–1 Post-primary or reactivation tuberculosis. Bilateral apical cavitary lesions are illustrated on plain chest radiography.

Sputum should be examined for the presence of *M. tuberculosis*. Samples should be stained using the Ziehl-Neelsen technique and examined under direct microscopy. This method is relatively insensitive, as about 10,000 bacilli/ml of sputum are needed for a positive result. In suspected cases of TB with a positive sputum examination, sputum should also be sent for culture to confirm infection. Culture is done in special culture bottles and takes approximately 1 to 2 weeks depending on organism burden.

Routine laboratory investigations are typically non-specific with anemia, hyponatremia, and hypercalcemia being the most common abnormalities.

TREATMENT

Treatment of TB is typically accomplished with a prolonged course of multiple antibiotics. Multiple antibiotics are used due to the high incidence of drug-resistant strains of *M. tuberculosis*. Medications commonly used in the treatment of symptomatic tuberculosis (with major side effects) include:

- Isoniazid (INH)—hepatitis, peripheral neuropathy
- Rifampin (RMP)—gastrointestinal upset
- Pyrazinamide (PZA)—hepatotoxicity
- Streptomycin (STM)—ototoxicity, nephrotoxicity
- Ethambutol (ETH)—oculotoxicity

A standard initial regimen is INH, RMP, and PZA (plus STM or ETH depending on susceptibilities) for 6 to 9 months for uncomplicated pulmonary TB. Extrapulmonary TB is typically treated with longer courses of therapy (i.e., 12–18 months). Due to the profound public health threat that TB poses and due to the fact that many patients with TB (i.e., substance abusers, the homeless, or those with mental illness) are at risk for noncompliance with antituberculosis therapy, the concept of direct observed therapy (DOT) was created. DOT is also recommended for all cases of multidrug resistant TB, regardless of compliance issues.

Prophylactic treatment is used in patients with asymptomatic disease who are identified by PPD screening. Patients with a newly positive PPD test have an approximately 5% chance of developing active, symptomatic disease within the first year. These patients are given 6–9 months of INH. This therapy is controversial in patients over the age of 35 because the incidence of INH-associated hepatitis increases dramatically as age increases.

Perhaps the most important part of the treatment and prevention of TB is isolation of infected patients in closed, negative pressure rooms.

◆ **KEY POINTS** ◆

1. Tuberculosis is an ancient disease that has become a modern public health threat due to HIV and the development of multidrug resistant strains.

2. The most common site of infection in TB is the lungs.

3. Symptoms are generally nonspecific and include fever, chills, night sweats, and hemoptysis.

4. Treatment with multiple antibiotic agents simultaneously increases effectiveness and prevents the development of resistant strains.

67 Tetanus

Tetanus is caused by wound infection with the anaerobic gram-positive rod *Clostridium tetani*. With appropriate immunization, it is a completely preventable disease, though isolated cases still occur with significant morbidity and mortality.

EPIDEMIOLOGY

Tetanus occurs after puncture wounds to an extremity, surgical procedures, or as a result of umbilical cord infections in neonates. Approximately 60 cases of tetanus occur per year, mostly in patients greater than 60 years of age. There is a 25% case fatality rate. Most cases of tetanus occur in the rural South, California, Texas, and Florida.

PATHOPHYSIOLOGY

C. tetani is found in two states: a sporulated and vegetative state. The sporulated form can survive for years in soil and resists destruction. The vegetative form is responsible for the production of an exotoxin called tetanospasmin. Tetanospasmin is responsible for the clinical manifestations of tetanus. The low oxygen tension of a wound favors the transformation of *C. tetani* from the sporulated to the vegetative form and the production of tetanospasmin. The exotoxin then travels by retrograde axonal transport up peripheral nerves to the central nervous system (CNS). Tetanospasmin acts at the motor end plate of skeletal muscle preventing the release of the inhibitory neurotransmitters GABA (α-aminobutyric acid) and glycine. The end result is sustained, unrelenting skeletal muscular contraction.

CLINICAL MANIFESTATIONS

Symptoms of tetanus begin after an incubation period of 1 to 31 days. Localized tetanus is characterized by rigid muscles at the site of the wound that resolves in weeks to months. It may progress to generalized tetanus. Symptoms of generalized tetanus include trismus, risus sardonicus (characteristic facial expression), dysphagia, opisthotonos, flexion of the arms, and extension of the legs. After approximately 2 weeks, a hypersympathetic state of autonomic dysfunction consisting of tachycardia, hypertension, sweating, and hyperpyrexia predominates.

Cephalic tetanus carries a poorer prognosis and is associated with cranial nerve dysfunction. Neonatal tetanus occurs almost solely in underdeveloped countries where maternal immunization is inadequate.

DIFFERENTIAL DIAGNOSIS

* Rabies
* Hypocalcemia

- Meningitis
- Strychnine poisoning

DIAGNOSTIC EVALUATION AND TREATMENT

The diagnosis of tetanus is strictly clinical.

TABLE 67–1

Guidelines for Tetanus Prophylaxis in Wound Management

History of Tetanus Immunizations	Clean, Non-High Risk Wounds	Dirty, Tetanus Prone Wounds
Unknown status or less than 3 doses	Yes Td No TIG	Yes Td Yes TIG
3 or more doses	No Td No TIG	No Td No TIG

Td = tetanus and diphtheria toxoid.
TIG = tetanus immune globulin.

All patients with tetanus should be admitted to the intensive care unit. The offending wound should be cleaned and debrided to decrease the toxin burden. Administration of tetanus immune globulin acts to neutralize circulating toxin but will not reverse the effects of toxin that has already made its way to the CNS. Prophylactic antibiotics (metronidazole) are typically given despite a lack of evidence demonstrating effectiveness. Treatment of autonomic dysfunction is accomplished by intravenous labetalol. Finally, all patients require active immunization because disease does not confer immunity. A guide to tetanus prophylaxis is presented in Table 67–1.

◆ KEY POINTS ◆

1. Tetanus is caused by *Clostridium tetani*, an anaerobic, gram-positive rod.
2. Tetanus is characterized by severe, prolonged muscle contraction (i.e., trismus).
3. The diagnosis is made clinically.
4. Treatment involves administering tetanus immune globulin and establishing active immunity.

68 Meningitis

Meningitis refers to infection of the meninges (lining of the brain and spinal cord). While viral meningitis is common, bacterial meningitis remains the most feared and deadly form. Over 25,000 cases of bacterial meningitis occur yearly, most commonly in adults, with a mortality rate approaching 25% despite treatment.

EPIDEMIOLOGY

The epidemiology of bacterial meningitis has changed over the past 15 years due to the introduction of the *Haemophilus influenzae* type B (HIB) vaccine. Meningitis occurs in neonates by vertical transmission during the birthing process. Group B streptococcus and *Listeria monocytogenes* are the most common pathogens isolated (Table 68–1). In infants (ages 1–3 months), *Streptococcus pneumoniae* and *Neisseria meningitidis* are the most common etiologies. HIB is now a very rare cause of meningitis in this age group, with the incidence decreasing approximately 90% since the introduction of the childhood vaccine. *Streptococcus pneumoniae*, *Neisseria meningitidis*, and *Haemophilus influenzae* are the most common etiologic agents in patients older than 3 months, with *Listeria monocytogenes* becoming more common in patients greater than 60 years of age. Factors predisposing to bacterial meningitis are diabetes mellitus, HIV infection, pneumonia, otitis media, and alcohol abuse.

Viral or "aseptic" meningitis can be caused by a number of organisms including HIV, the Epstein-Barr virus, cytomegalovirus, enterovirus, varicella-zoster virus, and herpes simplex virus. Other organisms, such as *Cryptococcus neoformans*, *Treponema pallidum*, and *Mycobacterium tuberculosis*, are all known to cause meningitis in immunocompromised hosts.

PATHOPHYSIOLOGY

Meningitis begins with bacterial invasion of the cerebrospinal fluid (CSF). The brain is normally protected from infection by three layers of meninges (pia mater, arachnoid, and dura). Once any one of the layers is breached, infection of the CSF can occur. As the bacteria begin to flourish in the CSF, the host response results in an influx of white blood cells and a proliferation of inflammatory mediators that lead to a disruption of the blood-brain barrier. The clinical manifestations of meningitis are due to systemic infection combined with meningeal irritation and cerebral edema that result from the host response to infection.

HISTORY

Patients with meningitis may present in a myriad of ways depending on the age and the offending organism. Viral meningitis typically presents in a less fulminant manner than bacterial infection. Patients may complain of fever, headache, seizures, or photophobia. Family members may relate a history of altered mental status

TABLE 68–1

Age-Based Etiologic Agents and Empiric Antibiotic Therapy in Bacterial Meningitis

Age	Most Common Etiologies	Empiric Antibiotic Therapy
Neonates	Group B strep, *Escherichia coli*, *Listeria monocytogenes*	Ampicillin and cefotaxime
Ages 1–3 months	*Streptococcus pneumoniae*, *Neisseria meningitidis*, *Haemophilus influenzae*	Ampicillin, ceftriaxone or cefotaxime, and dexamethasone
Ages 3 months–50 years	*Streptococcus pneumoniae*, *Neisseria meningitidis*, *Haemophilus influenzae*	Ceftriaxone or cefotaxime, vancomycin, and dexamethasone
Age >50 years or alcoholic	*Streptococcus pneumoniae*, *Listeria monocytogenes*	Ampicillin, ceftriaxone or cefotaxime, and dexamethasone

or confusion. Although clusters of cases have been reported, especially in army barracks and college dormitories, a history of contact with another infected individual is rarely elicited. Neonates or infants may present with nothing more than irritability and decreased feeding. A high index of suspicion is required in these cases.

PHYSICAL EXAMINATION

Fever, tachycardia, and hypotension are commonly seen with fulminant meningitis. Nuchal rigidity is a sign of meningeal irritation. Meningeal irritation may be revealed by examining for Kernig's or Brudzinski's sign. Kernig's sign refers to pain in the neck or back that occurs when a patient with meningitis attempts to extend the leg at the knee while the thigh is held in 90 degrees of flexion. Brudzinski's sign refers to spontaneous flexion of the hips during attempted passive flexion of the neck. Both signs are suggestive of meningitis, but are neither sensitive nor specific for the disorder.

A complete neurologic examination should be conducted to look for signs of CNS infection. The fundoscopic examination (looking for papilledema) and evaluation of cranial nerve function are particularly important to assess for evidence of increased intracranial pressure (ICP) or herniation. The skin should be carefully examined for the presence of a petechial rash. Petechia or purpura has been reported to occur in

60–80% of patients with meningitis secondary to *N. meningitidis* and in a smaller proportion of patients infected with other organisms.

DIFFERENTIAL DIAGNOSIS

- Subarachnoid hemorrhage
- Encephalitis
- Brain abscess
- Epidural abscess
- Infective endocarditis
- Carcinomatous meningitis

DIAGNOSTIC EVALUATION

All patients suspected of having meningitis should be placed on a monitor in an isolation room and have intravenous access quickly established. In cases of suspected meningitis, blood should be sent for complete blood count with differential, coagulation studies (looking for evidence of DIC), and culture.

Preparations should be made for a lumbar puncture (LP), which is the definitive gold standard diagnostic test for meningitis. All patients with focal neurologic deficit, papilledema, or alteration in mental status should undergo computed tomography of the head to rule out mass lesion prior to LP. If there is to be any delay in performing an LP, empiric antibiotics must be started

TABLE 68–2

Cerebrospinal Fluid Characteristics in Bacterial and Viral Meningitis

Parameters	Bacterial Meningitis	Viral Meningitis
Opening pressure	>300 mm Hg	<200 mm Hg
WBC	>1000/microliter	<1000/microliter
Differential	>80% polymorphonuclear	<50% polymorphonuclear
Glucose	<40 mg/dL	>40 mg/dL
Protein	>200 mg/dL	<200 mg/dL
Gram stain	Positive	Negative
Culture	Positive	Negative

immediately, ideally within 30 minutes of the patient's arrival in the emergency department. An opening pressure should be measured prior to collection of any CSF. CSF should be sent for cell counts and white blood cell differential, Gram stain and culture, protein, and glucose. Gram stain provides a rapid means of pathogen identification in up to 90% of patients. The CSF characteristics of viral and bacterial meningitis are listed in Table 68–2. If an "atypical" organism such as cryptococcus, tuberculosis, or syphilis is suspected on the basis of clinical grounds (HIV infection or other immunocompromise), extra CSF should be drawn off for serologic testing.

TREATMENT

Bacterial meningitis is a life-threatening emergency and can be fatal in a matter of hours. Due to the fulminant nature of the disease, antibiotic therapy must begin within 30 minutes of a patient's arrival in the emergency department. If lumbar puncture is to be delayed in any way, therapy should begin prior to collection of CSF. If the time between initiation of antibiotics and LP is less than 2 hours, culture of CSF will not be adversely affected.

For a list of the recommended empiric antibiotic therapies based on age and likely pathogen, see Table 68–1. Ceftriaxone, or another third-generation cephalosporin, plus vancomycin is an excellent choice for empiric coverage of *S. pneumoniae* and *N. meningitidis*. The incidence of

penicillin resistant *S. pneumoniae* is rising and approaches 33% of isolates in some areas and, therefore, empiric penicillin G is no longer recommended for treatment of meningitis. Ampicillin should be added to cover for *L. monocytogenes* in older patients. Once results of the Gram stain and culture and sensitivities become available, the antibiotic regimen can be narrowed.

Due to the fact that many of the pathologic manifestations of bacterial meningitis are caused by the overwhelming inflammatory host response to infection, corticosteroids may be considered prior to initiation of antibiotic therapy in patients greater than 1 year of age. Steroids, particularly dexamethasone, are thought to block the deleterious effects of the severe CNS inflammation that occurs with bacterial meningitis.

Patients with proven or suspected meningitis, whether it is bacterial or viral, should be admitted to the hospital on intravenous antibiotics until culture results return. If the culture is negative and the patient has improved clinically, then a diagnosis of viral meningitis can be made and the patient safely discharged home. Patients with evidence of septic shock need to be closely monitored in an intensive care unit setting.

Prophylactic antibiotics should be offered to all close household contacts of patients with bacterial meningitis to prevent subsequent infection. Rifampin (1 dose per day for 4 doses) is the recommended drug for postexposure prophylaxis (PEP). PEP is recommended only for household contacts or those exposed to respiratory droplets from the index case. Routine daily contact does not require PEP.

◆ KEY POINTS ◆

1. The HIB vaccine has dramatically altered the epidemiology of bacterial meningitis.

2. Group B streptococcus causes the majority of neonatal meningitis, while *S. pneumococcus* and *N. meningitidis* are more common in older patients.

3. Culture of CSF is the gold standard for the diagnosis of bacterial meningitis.

4. Due to the high morbidity and mortality of untreated bacterial meningitis, antibiotics should not be delayed for diagnostic testing in patients in the emergency department.

69

Tick-Borne Illnesses

Ticks are ubiquitous pests that are found on every continent except Antarctica and serve as an important vector for human disease. Ticks are blood-sucking parasites that belong to three separate families, of which only Ixodidae (hard bodied ticks) and Argasidae (soft bodied ticks) cause human disease. A full list of tick-borne illnesses is found in Table 69–1.

LYME DISEASE

Epidemiology

Lyme disease is the most common tick-borne illness in the United States. It was initially described in the late 1970s after a cluster of patients with oligoarticular arthritis was identified in Lyme, Connecticut. Since 1982, the number of cases has been steadily increasing with approximately 12,500 cases a year occurring between 1993 and 1997. The majority of cases occurs in the late spring and early summer in the Northeast United States.

Clinical Manifestations

Lyme disease is a multisystem disease that occurs in three stages. All stages need not occur, and stages may overlap. Stage 1 is characterized by localized infection at the site of the tick bite. Approximately 1 week after the bite, an annular, "target" lesion known as erythema chronicum migrans develops and spreads out in a concentric fashion. Fever, chills, fatigue, headache, stiff neck, and arthralgias may accompany the rash. The rash and systemic symptoms typically resolve in 4 to 5 weeks. Stage 2 (disseminated infection) occurs weeks to months after the initial infection and is characterized by cardiac, neurologic, and ocular findings. Cardiac involvement is uncommon (approximately 5% of cases). Manifestations of Lyme carditis include myocarditis, pericarditis, and atrioventricular block. The most common neurologic manifestation of Lyme disease is meningoencephalitis, though cranial neuropathies (Bell's palsy) and peripheral nervous system involvement occur frequently. The third stage is characterized by chronic arthritis, nervous system dysfunction, and fatigue.

Diagnostic Evaluation and Treatment

Diagnosis of Lyme disease is based primarily on the clinical presentation in a patient from an endemic area. A history of tick bite can be elicited in only 33% of cases. Routine laboratory examinations are typically non-specific and unhelpful. Serologic testing for antibodies to *Borrelia burgdorferi* by means of ELISA (enzyme-linked immunosorbent assay) is helpful. Treatment of mild Lyme disease can be accomplished by oral doxycycline while severe disease (carditis, meningoencephalitis) is usually treated by intravenous ceftriaxone.

TULAREMIA

Epidemiology

Tularemia is caused by *Francisella tularensis*, a small gram-negative coccobacillus. It was first described in the

TABLE 69–1

Major Tick-Borne Illnesses Found in the United States

Disease	Pathogen	Classification	Tick Vector	Geographic Region
Lyme disease	Borrelia burgdorferi	Bacteria (spirochete)	Ixodes scapularis, Ixodes pacificus	Northeast, Upper Midwest, California
Relapsing fever	Borrelia hermsii	Bacteria (spirochete)	Ornithodoros hemsii	West
Tularemia	Francisella tularensis	Bacteria	Dermacentor variabilis, Amblyomma americanum	South
Rocky Mountain spotted fever	Rickettsia rickettsii	Rickettsia	Dermacentor andersoni, Dermacentor variabilis	Southeast, West, South Central
Q fever	Coxiella burnetii	Rickettsia	Dermacentor andersoni	Ubiquitous
Ehrlichiosis	Ehrlichia chaffeensis	Rickettsia	Rhipicephalus sanguineus	South, East
Babesiosis	Babesia microti	Protozoa	Ixodes scapularis	Coastal New England
Colorado Tick fever	Orbivirus	Viral	Dermacentor andersoni	West
Tick paralysis	Salivary Neurotoxin	Toxin	Dermacentor andersoni, Amblyomma americanum	Ubiquitous

1800s when a group of people developed a febrile illness with generalized lymphadenopathy after eating rabbit meat. Most cases in the United States occur in the south central states of Arkansas, Oklahoma, Texas, Louisiana, and Mississippi. Person-to-person transmission is extremely rare and most cases are associated with exposure to rodents, rabbits, handling infected skins, or tick-borne transmission occurring from May to August.

Clinical Manifestations

Clinical manifestations of tularemia depend on the site of inoculation and can be separated into six distinct syndromes. The most common form is the ulceroglandular form (80% of cases) and is characterized by ulceration at the inoculation site followed by tender local lymphadenopathy. Glandular tularemia is similar in presentation (tender lymphadenopathy) but is not associated with ulcer formation. Oculoglandular tularemia is relatively rare (1% of cases) and presents with unilateral conjunctivitis, photophobia, and pre-auricular lymphadenopathy. Pharyngeal tularemia is characterized by exudative pharyngitis and cervical lymphadenopathy. Systemic symptoms such as fever, chills, diarrhea, and abdominal pain are common with typhoidal tularemia (10% of cases). Finally, pulmonary tularemia occurs as a result of inhalation of organisms and presents with symptoms indistinguishable from other bacterial pneumonias.

Diagnostic Evaluation and Treatment

The diagnosis of tularemia is based on characteristic clinical findings and confirmed by serologic testing. Antibody titers are performed on presentation and 2 weeks later (acute and convalescent titers). A fourfold rise in the antibody titers between the acute and convalescent specimens is considered positive. The drug of choice for the treatment of all forms of tularemia is streptomycin for 2 weeks.

ROCKY MOUNTAIN SPOTTED FEVER (RMSF)

Epidemiology

RMSF is caused by infection with *Rickettsia rickettsii*, a small, intracellular coccobacillus. It occurs primarily in the southern, western, and central United States and has a mortality of 25% if left untreated. The most significant factor in case fatalities is delay in diagnosis. Most cases occur between the months of April and September.

Clinical Manifestations

RMSF affects multiple organ systems and can present in a myriad of ways. The period from tick bite to the onset of symptoms is typically 1 to 2 weeks. The disease typically presents with nonspecific, systemic complaints such as fever, malaise, severe headache, myalgias, or gastrointestinal upset. Three to five days after the onset of symptoms, most patients (85–90%) develop the characteristic maculopapular rash of RMSF. As the disease progresses, the rash spreads from the extremities to the trunk, sparing the face, and becomes petechial. Cardiopulmonary manifestations of RMSF include left ventricular dysfunction, noncardiac pulmonary edema, and interstitial pneumonitis. The central nervous system is also commonly affected in RMSF. Clinical symptoms range from confusion and altered mental status to frank coma. Death is typically due to septic shock and the acute respiratory distress syndrome (ARDS).

Diagnosis and Treatment

The diagnosis of RMSF is established by serology or by immunofluorescent staining of skin biopsy specimens. Culture of the organism responsible for RMSF is rarely undertaken due to the hazards this practice poses for laboratory personnel. Treatment is with doxycycline or chloramphenicol for 7 to 14 days.

EHRLICHIOSIS

Epidemiology

Ehrlichiosis is a tick-borne illness caused by the rickettsial organism *Ehrlichia chaffeensis*. It occurs most commonly in the early summer months in the South Central and South Atlantic states.

Clinical Manifestations

Almost 75% of patients recall a tick bite in the weeks preceding the onset of illness. The incubation period is 1 to 3 weeks and the initial presentation is nonspecific and includes fever, headaches, and malaise. A maculopapular rash develops in a subset of patients while severe complications such as renal failure, disseminated intravascular coagulation (DIC), and death have been reported. Common laboratory abnormalities include leukopenia, thrombocytopenia, elevated liver enzymes, and perhaps CSF pleocytosis.

Diagnosis and Treatment

The diagnosis of ehrlichiosis depends mainly on the clinical presentation with confirmatory serology. Doxycycline, tetracycline, and chloramphenicol can all be used for treatment.

BABESIOSIS

Babesiosis is caused by an intraerythrocytic protozoan that is transmitted by the tick *Ixodes scapularis*, the same vector responsible for transmission of Lyme disease. Most cases occur in coastal New England. Common symptoms include malaise, fever, anorexia, fatigue, and myalgias. Hepatosplenomegaly may be found. Evidence of hemolytic anemia (due to the lysis of red blood cells by the intracellular parasite), thrombocytopenia, and elevated liver enzymes may be found on laboratory analysis. Symptoms last from weeks to over a year and are more severe in patients with prior splenectomy. Diagnosis is by thick smear of the peripheral blood. Therapy with quinine and clindamycin is reserved for severe cases.

◆ KEY POINTS ◆

1. The target lesions of erythema chronicum migrans suggest Lyme disease.
2. Tularemia is associated with exposure to rabbits or other lagamorphs.
3. Rocky Mountain spotted fever is characterized by fever, headache, and petechial rash.
4. Babesiosis is caused by a protozoan that infects erythrocytes.

70 Rabies

EPIDEMIOLOGY

Rabies is a uniformly fatal disorder that causes between 25,000 and 50,000 deaths per year worldwide. Due to an effective national campaign to immunize domestic animals, there have been less than 20 cases of human rabies in the United States since 1980. Rabies is caused by an RNA-containing, bullet-shaped rhabdovirus that is transmitted to humans by the bite of an infected carnivorous animal or bat. Skunks, foxes, raccoons, bats, and less commonly dogs and cats can carry the rabies virus, while rodents and lagamorphs (rabbits) rarely are infected. Wildlife is the natural reservoir for the rabies virus and rabid animals can be found in the mid-Atlantic, Southern, and Midwest regions of the United States. Rabies is rare in the Ohio River Valley and the Rocky Mountain region.

PATHOPHYSIOLOGY

Virtually all cases of animal-to-human transmission of the rabies virus have occurred after a bite, though cases of non-bite exposures (abrasions, scratches, mucous membrane contact with infected material) causing the disease have been reported. The rabies virus is excreted in the saliva of infected animals and behavioral changes that are induced by infection (lability and aggressiveness) promote the spread of the disease by making infected animals more likely to bite. Once the virus is transmitted from a rabid animal to a human, the initial infection and viral replication occurs in the myocytes at the site of inoculation. The virus then travels across the motor end plate into a peripheral nerve. Once inside the peripheral nervous system, the virus ascends towards the central nervous system (CNS). Symptoms of the disease correlate with the arrival of the virus in the CNS. The time required to reach the CNS depends on the site of inoculation as the virus moves approximately 3 mm/hr. Bites on the head or neck have incubation periods as short as 15 days while symptoms from lower extremity bites can take as long as 3 to 6 months to manifest.

CLINICAL MANIFESTATIONS

The most common presentation is a patient who has traveled to a region of the world where rabies is endemic and sustained a bite wound. After an incubation period of 1 to 3 months or longer (clinical disease after an incubation period of 7 years has been documented), the patient typically develops fever, malaise, headache, sore throat, and paresthesias at the wound site. These symptoms last 2–10 days, and then evidence of CNS dysfunction becomes evident. The CNS manifestations of rabies can be grouped into two separate syndromes. In the "furious" or encephalitic form (80% of cases), bulbar and peripheral muscle spasms and opisthotonus occur in conjunction with restlessness, agitation, and altered mental status. The paralytic form of rabies (20%) is char-

TABLE 70-1

Guidelines for Rabies Post-Exposure Prophylaxis

Agent	Dose	Site	Timing
HRIG	20IU/kg	1/2 dose at the exposure site, 1/2 dose intramuscular	Day 0
HDCV	1 ml	Intramuscular	Day 0, 3, 7, 14, 28

acterized by a symmetric, ascending flaccid paralysis. Hydrophobia refers to the bulbar and laryngeal spasm that occurs when an infected patient attempts to drink water. Untreated, the disease progresses to seizures, coma, apnea, and death in approximately 4 to 7 days.

DIFFERENTIAL DIAGNOSIS

- Viral encephalitis
- Polio
- Tetanus
- Meningitis
- Brain abscess
- Guillain-Barré syndrome

DIAGNOSTIC EVALUATION

The premortem diagnosis of rabies relies on the detection of rabies virus antigen or antibody in body fluids by fluorescent antibody testing. Brain biopsy may reveal Negri bodies, which are the pathognomonic histologic finding in rabies infection. Negri bodies are small eosinophilic intracellular inclusions that are thought to be the site of CNS viral replication.

TREATMENT

There is no known treatment for rabies. Supportive care and aggressive support of circulatory and respiratory function is essential. Only three cases of recovery have ever been reported.

PREVENTION

Prevention of rabies is possible after infection, but is successful only if it is administered prior to CNS involvement. Prevention involves the administration of post-exposure prophylaxis (PEP), which is the combination of human rabies immune globulin (HRIG) and human diploid cell vaccine (HDCV). HRIG offers passive immunity, while HDCV confers active immunity. Prior to PEP, aggressive local wound care (scrubbing, debridement, tetanus prophylaxis) should occur. The decision to offer PEP is based on the species of attacking animal, the nature of the exposure (bite versus other exposure), whether the animal is available for observation and testing, and whether the animal has been immunized against the rabies virus. Most cases of PEP in the United States occur after a bite wound by an uncaptured dog or cat in an endemic area or a bite wound by an uncaptured bat or other high-risk carnivore. Guidelines for the administration of HRIG and HDCV are given in Table 70-1.

◆ KEY POINTS ◆

1. Rabies is a rare disease transmitted by the bite of an infected animal.
2. Rabies travels from wound site to the central nervous system via peripheral nerves.
3. Clinically, rabies occurs in two forms, encephalitic and paralytic.
4. Postexposure prophylaxis involves treatment with human rabies immune globulin and human diploid cell vaccine.

71

Infectious Diarrhea

Infectious diarrhea is the second leading cause of death worldwide and the leading cause of death in children. Although diarrhea alone rarely poses a health threat to healthy individuals in developed countries, it has significant morbidity and mortality in poorer countries without access to adequate medical care.

ETIOLOGY

Infectious diarrhea can be caused by bacteria, viruses, or protozoa (Table 71–1).

Bacterial

Salmonella

The genus *Salmonella* contains several pathogenic gram-negative rods that cause diarrhea. Infection with *Salmonella* typically occurs after ingestion of contaminated eggs, dairy products, or poultry. The clinical manifestations of *Salmonella* infection range from simple acute gastroenteritis to severe septicemia due to the propensity of *Salmonella* to directly invade the colonic mucosa. Diarrhea is typically bloody and is accompanied by tenesmus, fever, and abdominal pain. Symptoms resolve spontaneously in 10 to 14 days.

Shigella

Shigella is a genus of gram-negative rods belonging to the family Enterobacteriaceae. *Shigella* is highly pathogenic and as few as 10 organisms can cause disease.

Typically spread by fecal-oral contact or contaminated foods, *Shigella* causes a severe form of dysentery (bloody, profuse diarrhea).

Campylobacter

Campylobacter jejuni infection is acquired from eating undercooked poultry or contaminated natural water sources ("backpacker's diarrhea"). Direct invasion of the colonic mucosa is responsible for the symptoms of *Campylobacter* infection. After an incubation period of 2–5 days, fever, abdominal cramping, and profuse bloody diarrhea begin. Myalgias, headache, and vomiting also commonly accompany infection. Symptoms typically last for a week or less, though prolonged infection can occur. *Campylobacter* infection has also been implicated as a causative agent of Guillain-Barré syndrome.

Yersinia

Yersinia enterocolitica is a gram-negative bacterium from the family Enterobacteriaceae that causes fever, abdominal pain, profuse watery or bloody diarrhea, and vomiting. Symptoms are due to direct invasion of the intestine, particularly the terminal ileum and the clinical syndrome it produces is commonly mistaken for acute appendicitis. Infection is spread from person to person via the fecal-oral route.

Escherichia coli

E. coli can cause diarrhea by several different mechanisms including toxin formation and direct invasion.

TABLE 71–1

Small Bowel and Colonic Pathogens

Pathogen	Small Bowel (noninflammatory)	Colon (inflammatory)
Bacteria	Salmonella[†] Escherichia coli* Clostridium perfringens Staphylococcus aureus Aeromonas hydrophila Bacillus cereus Vibrio cholerae	Campylobacter[†] Shigella Clostridium difficile Yersinia Vibrio parahaemolyticus Enteroinvasive E. coli Plesiomonas shigelloides
Virus	Rotovirus Norwalk agent	Cytomegalovirus[†] Adenovirus Herpes simplex virus
Protozoa	Cryptosporidium[†] Microsporidium[†] Isospora Cyclospora Giardia lamblia	Entamoeba histolytica

[†] Can involve both the small and large bowel, but are most likely to occur as listed.
*EPEC, EAggEC, EHEC, ETEC may all contribute; routine laboratories and cultures will not differentiate these from E. coli which are normal flora.

E. coli O157:H7 is the serotype responsible for enterohemorrhagic diarrhea. Most commonly acquired from eating undercooked beef, O157:H7 is most dangerous to children and the elderly. Hemolytic uremic syndrome and thrombotic thrombocytopenic purpura are two of the most feared complications of *E. coli* O157:H7 infection.

Viral

Rotavirus, the Norwalk virus, adenoviruses, and astroviruses all are known to cause epidemics of diarrhea, especially among children at schools and in daycare settings. Viral diarrhea may also pose a threat to immunocompromised adults (HIV infection).

Protozoa

Giardia lamblia is one of the principal agents of traveler's diarrhea and is spread by ingestion of contaminated water sources. Infection is common in the Rocky Mountain areas of the United States, in the states of the former Soviet Union, Latin America, and the Caribbean. Frequent, explosive, foul-smelling diarrhea commonly lasts 7–10 days, and reinfection is common unless antibiotic therapy is initiated.

Other protozoal causes of diarrhea include *Entamoeba histolytica*, *Cryptosporidium*, and *Isospora*. The latter two organisms are commonly implicated in the chronic diarrhea that occurs in patients with HIV infection.

PATHOPHYSIOLOGY

Diarrhea can be caused by a variety of pathophysiologic mechanisms. Secretory diarrhea results from increased secretion of water and electrolytes into the small intestine resulting in profuse watery stool. Osmotic diarrhea results when an increased osmotic load is delivered to the small intestine, preventing normal absorption of fluid from the gut lumen. Some pathologic processes cause severe inflammation of the gut mucosal lining resulting in altered absorption and diarrhea. Finally, some processes result in an increased transit time through the large and small intestine resulting in diarrhea simply from lack of adequate absorptive time. Infectious agents typically cause the secretory and inflammatory types of diarrhea.

causes. For example, *Staphylococcus aureus* and *Bacillus cereus* cause diarrhea via a preformed toxin that causes symptoms within 6 to 8 hours of ingestion. Viral agents and infection with enterohemorrhagic and enterotoxigenic *E. coli* typically cause symptoms 12 to 24 hours after exposure.

CLINICAL MANIFESTATIONS

Patients with infectious diarrhea typically present with loose stools, fever, abdominal cramping, and signs of dehydration. A careful food and travel history is helpful in determining the etiologic agent of the diarrhea (Table 71–2A and B). Additionally, the time from exposure to symptom onset can help narrow the likely infectious

DIFFERENTIAL DIAGNOSIS

- Mesenteric ischemia
- Gastrointestinal bleeding
- Inflammatory bowel disease
- Colon carcinoma
- Laxative abuse

TABLE 71–2A

Exposures Associated with Specific Intestinal Pathogens

Pathogen	Epidemiologic Clue(s) to Diagnosis
Bacteria	
Staphylococcus aureus	Beef, pork, poultry, eggs
Clostridium perfringens	Beef, pork, poultry, home-canned foods
Bacillus cereus	Beef, pork, fried rice (Chinese), vegetables
EHEC	Beef, pork, fast food restaurants (undercooked hamburger), apple cider, leaf lettuce, milk, cheese, extremes of age
EIEC	Milk, cheese
ETEC	Travelers to developing countries
Salmonella	Beef, pork, poultry, eggs (e.g., Caesar salad), raw milk, ice cream, vegetables (e.g., alfalfa sprouts), unpasteurized orange juice, pet ducklings, lizards, rattlesnake meat
Campylobacter	Poultry (undercooked at barbecues), raw milk and cheeses
Shigella	Daycare centers, vegetables (e.g., green onions)
Yersinia	Pork (not common), beef, milk, cheeses, hemochromatosis
Vibrio cholerae	Inadequately cooked seafood from South America, coconut milk from Thailand, airline outbreaks, shellfish
Vibrio parahaemolyticus	Ingestion of raw seafood, particularly in East Asia, shellfish, cirrhosis
Clostridium difficile	Hospitalization, inpatient or outpatient antibiotic(s) or chemotherapy within the last several weeks, daycare centers
Listeria	Beef, pork, poultry, milk, cheese, coleslaw, hot dogs, potato salad, pregnancy, neonates, "immunocompromised" patients

TABLE 71–2B

Exposures Associated with Specific Intestinal Pathogens

Pathogen	Epidemiologic Clue(s) to Diagnosis
Viruses	
Rotavirus	Daycare centers, nurseries, Australia
Norwalk-like viruses	Schools, nursing homes, cruise ships, camps, vegetables, waterborne, foodborne, and shellfish-associated outbreaks
Hepatitis A	Overcrowding, lack of clean water, patients and staff of institutions, daycare centers, homosexual men, IV drug users, travelers, military barracks, shellfish (clams, oysters, mussels)
Adenovirus	Infantile diarrhea, ?AIDS
Cytomegalovirus	HIV-infected homosexual men with AIDS, organ transplantation
Protozoa	
Giardia lamblia	Daycare centers, swimming pools, travel (e.g., St. Petersburg, mountainous areas with ingestion of stream water), fruit salad
Entamoeba histolytica	Travelers to endemic areas (e.g., Mexico) for more than one month, sexually active homosexual men, institutions
Cryptosporidium	Daycare centers, swimming pools, AIDS, farm animal exposure, city water supply contamination (e.g., Milwaukee)
Cyclospora	Raspberries (from Guatemala)
Isospora	Haiti, HIV infection
Microsporidium	AIDS (?travelers, ?fresh water)

- Malabsorption syndromes (celiac sprue, lactose intolerance)
- Thyrotoxicosis

DIAGNOSTIC EVALUATION

All patients with suspected infectious diarrhea should have stool sent for culture. Culture can identify infection with *Salmonella*, *Shigella*, *Campylobacter*, and *Yersinia* in a great majority of cases. Stool examination for ova and parasites can help identify infection with *Giardia*, *Entomoeba histolytica*, and *Cryptosporidium*. Abdominal radiography or computed tomography may be indicated to exclude other intra-abdominal processes as the cause of a patient's symptoms.

TREATMENT

Treatment of infectious diarrhea begins with measures to combat dehydration. The World Health Organization (WHO) has developed an oral rehydration solution (ORS) that is made up of a balanced mixture of water, salts, and sugar. This mixture has been instrumental in combating the significant mortality of infectious diarrhea in developing countries, though it is woefully underused in the United States where intravenous hydration and hospitalization remain the preferred method of treatment. The success of the WHO-ORS stems from the observation that in most diarrheal illnesses, the intestinal glucose-sodium transport mechanism remains intact. Thus, water can be effectively absorbed if the correct balance of salts and sugar are

TABLE 71–3A

Antimicrobial Therapy of Diarrhea: Bacterial Infections

Pathogen	First Choice	Second Choice	Comments
S. aureus B. cereus	Not required	Not required	Due to food poisoning and resolve with hydration only. TMP/SMX* can be used if susceptible; antibiotic therapy required only in severe cases (see text)
Salmonella	Usually not required (see text)	Oral quinolone[†] BID for 3 to 5 days	Same as above
Shigella	Oral quinolone[†] BID for 5 days	TMP/SMX* or ampicillin	Many strains now resistant to TMP/SMX* and ampicillin
Campylobacter	Oral quinolone[†] BID for 5 days	Macrolides[¶] or doxycycline	Antibiotics only in severe cases (see text). Quinolone resistance has been reported
Yersinia	Oral quinolone[†] BID for 7 to 10 days	TMP/SMX or doxycycline	Antibiotic therapy only in severe (systemic) cases
C. difficile	Metronidazole 250 mg PO QID	Vancomycin 125 mg PO QID	Duration of therapy 10 days; stop antibiotics, if possible; IV metronidazole if unable to tolerate oral therapy; IV metronidazole ± vancomycin fecal enemas for severe cases
ETEC	Oral quinolone[†] BID for 1 to 3 days	TMP/SMX,* doxycycline, furazolidone	
EIEC	Same as for shigellosis		
EHEC	Not recommended at this time	?oral quinolone[†]	
V. cholerae	Oral quinolone	Doxycycline	

*Trimethoprim/sulfamethoxazole 160/800 mg (DS tab) PO q 12 h.
[†]Norfloxacin 400 mg PO, ofloxacin 400 mg PO, ciprofloxacin 500 mg PO.
[¶]Erythromycin, clarithromycin, azithromycin.

provided to assist in transport across the gut mucosa. The ORS consists of:

- 1 liter of water
- 3.5 grams of sodium chloride
- 1.5 grams of potassium chloride
- 20 grams of glucose
- 2.5 grams of sodium bicarbonate

Initiation of antibiotic therapy should be considered for those patients who present with signs of bacterial infection (fever, bloody diarrhea, presence of fecal leukocytes), though rehydration remains the mainstay of therapy and most diarrheal illnesses are self-limited. Typical empiric regimens are listed in Table 71–3A and B.

Antimotility agents such as diphenoxylate or loperamide can be used for symptomatic relief. These agents are contraindicated in patients with enterohem-

TABLE 71–3B

Antimicrobial Therapy of Diarrhea: Nonbacterial Infections

Pathogen	First Choice	Second Choice	Comments
Amebiasis	Metronidazole 750 mg PO TID for 10 days	Dehydroemetine 1 to 1.5 mg/kg per day IM for five days	Both plus a luminal amebicide for invasive intestinal infection and hepatic abscesses (iodoquinol 650 mg PO TID for 20 days; paromomycin 500 mg PO TID for seven days); cyst passers without symptoms require luminicidal agent only
Giardiasis	Metronidazole 250 mg PO TID for 10 days	Tinidazole, quinacrine hydrochloride, furazolidone	Relapses may occur
Cryptosporidium	Paromomycin 500 mg PO BID	Azithromycin, hyperimmune bovine colostrum, nitozoxanide	Benefit and duration of any therapy unclear, spontaneous resolution without specific therapy in immunocompetent hosts, and in HIV-infected individuals with CD4 counts above 150 cells/mm^3
Microsporidium	Albendazole 200–400 mg PO BID for three months		Albendazole more effective for Encephalitozoon intestinalis than for Enterocytozoon bieneusi; available for compassionate use only
Isospora	TMP/SMX 1 DS PO QID for 10 days, then BID for three weeks	Pyrimethamine plus folinic acid	Maintainance therapy required in patients with AIDS
Cyclospora	TMP/SMX 1 DS PO BID for three to five days		

orrhagic *E. coli* infection as they may precipitate hemolytic-uremic syndrome.

◆ KEY POINTS ◆

1. Epidemiologic clues from the history of affected patients can help to identify the likely cause of diarrhea in many cases.

2. Shigella can cause infection after inoculation with as few as 10 organisms.

3. *Yersinia* infection can mimic acute appendicitis.

4. Rehydration is the key to the treatment of most infectious diarrheal illnesses.

72 Infectious Mononucleosis

Infectious mononucleosis (IM) is a disease characterized by fever, lymphadenopathy, and pharyngitis. It is a widespread disease caused by the Epstein-Barr virus (EBV).

EPIDEMIOLOGY

EBV, also known as human herpesvirus 4, is spread from person to person via contaminated saliva. Humans serve as the main reservoir of the virus. The majority of cases of IM occurs in adolescents and young adults, though infection can occur during any time in life. IM has a worldwide distribution, most infections are subclinical and almost 100% of adults show immunologic evidence of prior EBV exposure. Although not particularly contagious, IM cases tend to cluster among close contacts (dorm mates, family members) hence the moniker, "the kissing disease." Shedding of virus continues in the saliva for up to a year after clinical recovery, providing a mechanism for continued spread of the disease.

PATHOPHYSIOLOGY

EBV initially infects the epithelial cells of the oropharynx. The virus then replicates and spreads to B-lymphocytes throughout the lymphatic system. The incubation period for infection is between 1 and 2 months. Infection induces the proliferation of atypical lymphocytes and heterophile antibodies that are the immunologic hallmarks of the disease, and form the basis of the diagnosis of IM. The immune response to EBV infection is thought to be the cause of the symptoms of IM. EBV infection is also associated with African Burkitt's lymphoma.

CLINICAL MANIFESTATIONS

IM is characterized by high fever, severe exudative pharyngitis, and generalized lymphadenopathy. Malaise, severe fatigue, and headache may also be present. Physical examination may reveal splenomegaly and a diffuse maculopapular rash. For unclear reasons, the rash associated with EBV is more common following the administration of amoxicillin or ampicillin (many patients with EBV are mistakenly diagnosed with Group A streptococcal pharyngitis). Splenomegaly predisposes to acute traumatic or nontraumatic splenic rupture, a rare but potentially life-threatening complication of primary EBV infection. Neurologic manifestations, including Guillain-Barré syndrome, viral meningitis, and cranial nerve palsies, are rare. Symptoms typically last for 2–3 weeks, though the severe fatigue associated with infection often lasts longer. Recovery from infection confers long-lasting immunity.

DIFFERENTIAL DIAGNOSIS

- Pharyngitis
- Peritonsillar abscess

- Retropharyngeal abscess
- Cytomegalovirus infection
- Hepatitis
- Primary HIV infection

DIAGNOSTIC EVALUATION

IM should be considered in the differential diagnosis of all patients presenting with fever, sore throat, and lymphadenopathy. Routine laboratory evaluation may reveal a relative lymphocytosis with an elevated number of atypical lymphocytes on the peripheral smear. The "Monospot" is a latex agglutination test using horse red blood cells that detects the presence of heterophile antibodies in serum. Unlike the presence of atypical lymphocytes, the Monospot is specific for IM. Heterophile-negative mononucleosis occurs with cytomegalovirus, HIV, or toxoplasmosis infection. Specific testing for EBV virus is rarely needed due to the high sensitivity and specificity of heterophile antibody testing.

TREATMENT

Treatment of IM is entirely supportive. The pain from pharyngitis should be treated with analgesics, with corticosteroids—a controversial therapy—reserved for cases of impending upper airway obstruction. Patients should be counseled regarding the risk of transmission to others and the remote risks of splenic rupture.

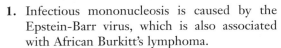

◆ KEY POINTS ◆

1. Infectious mononucleosis is caused by the Epstein-Barr virus, which is also associated with African Burkitt's lymphoma.
2. Clinically, IM is characterized by fever, sore throat, and lymphadenopathy.
3. The Monospot test, which detects the presence of heterophile antibodies in serum, is highly sensitive and specific for the diagnosis of IM.
4. Treatment is supportive.

73

Sexually Transmitted Diseases

EPIDEMIOLOGY

Although rarely the cause of acute life-threatening illness, sexually transmitted diseases (STDs) are responsible for significant morbidity and are a major cause of female infertility. More importantly, the practices that result in STD transmission also put patients at risk for infection with the human immunodeficiency virus.

GONORRHEA

Neisseria gonorrhoeae is a gram-negative intracellular diplococci that causes genital infection in both males and females. The incidence of gonococcal infection is rising, especially among adolescents and young adults.

Clinical Presentation

In males, gonococcal infection causes epididymitis, urethritis, or prostatitis. Dysuria and purulent penile discharge typically develop a week after infection. In females, asymptomatic infection is common (40%). In clinically evident infection, cervicitis and pelvic inflammatory disease are common presentations. Gonococcal cervicitis causes a mucopurulent discharge and an inflamed friable cervical mucosa (the so-called "strawberry cervix"). Disseminated gonococcal infection occurs in approximately 2% of patients and is characterized by widespread skin pustules, arthritis, fever, and in some cases meningitis or endocarditis. Monoarticu-

lar septic arthritis in a patient of reproductive age is a classic presentation of infection with *N. gonorrhea*.

Diagnostic Evaluation and Treatment

The diagnosis of gonorrhea is made by culture of cervical or penile discharge on chocolate agar, which has a sensitivity of 80–90%.

Ceftriaxone, cefixime, ofloxacin, or ciprofloxacin are all acceptable treatment regimens for gonorrhea (Table 73–1). Due to the high incidence of co-infection with *Chlamydia trachomatis*, single dose azithromycin or a 7-day course of doxycycline should be included. Treatment of all sexual partners is essential to prevent reinfection.

CHLAMYDIA

Chlamydia is caused by infection with the obligate intracellular organism *Chlamydia trachomatis*. It is a sexually transmitted disease that most commonly affects people in their teens and twenties and is a common cause of infertility in women of childbearing age. The Centers for Disease Control and Prevention (CDC) estimate that there are 4 million new *C. trachomatis* infections per year in the United States.

Clincal Presentation

Chlamydia causes a mucopurulent cervicitis in females characterized by purulent vaginal discharge and a

TABLE 73–1

Antibiotic and Antiviral Treatment of Sexually Transmitted Disease

Infection	First-Line Treatment	Alternative Treatment
Gonorrhea	Ceftriaxone 125 mg IM × 1	Cefixime 400 mg PO × 1
Chlamydia	Azithromycin 1 g PO × 1	Doxycycline 100 mg PO bid × 7 days
Syphilis	Benzathine penicillin G 2.4 million units IM × 1	Doxycycline 100 mg PO bid × 14 days
Genital herpes	Acyclovir 400 mg PO tid × 10 days	Valacyclovir 1 g PO bid × 10 days

friable, erythematous cervix. These symptoms are difficult to distinguish from gonoccocal cervicitis and many women are infected with both organisms. Asymptomatic infection is common in both sexes. Chlamydial infection in men typically causes urethritis or epididymitis.

Diagnostic Evaluation and Treatment

PCR of a voided urine specimen is both sensitive and specific for the diagnosis of chlamydia. Alternately, the diagnosis can be made by fluorescent antibody testing or traditional culture of cervical or urethral swabs. Single dose azithromycin and a 7-day course of doxycycline are both accepted treatment regimens for chlamydial infection (see Table 73–1). Seven-day courses of ofloxacin or erythromycin can also be used. Due to the high rate of co-infection with *Neisseria gonorrhoeae*, all patients with chlamydia should also be treated with ceftriaxone, cefixime, or ciprofloxacin and all sexual partners need to be treated to prevent reinfection.

SYPHILIS

Syphilis is a sexually transmitted disease caused by infection with the spirochete *Treponema pallidum*. Yaws is a tropical disease caused by a related spirochete, *Treponema pertenue*. Although a relatively rare disease, there has been a resurgence in new cases of syphilis over the last decade largely attributable to the acquired immunodeficiency syndrome (AIDS).

Clinical Manifestations

The clinical manifestations of syphilis can be divided into three stages. Primary syphilis is characterized by a painless chancre that develops at the site of inoculation.

Common sites are the shaft or tip of the penis or the vulva. The incubation period for primary syphilis averages 21 days. Secondary syphilis develops 3–6 days after the chancre resolves. Affected patients complain of sore throat, malaise, fever, and headache. A dull red, papular rash then develops on the palms, soles, and trunk. Tertiary syphilis presents years after initial infection and is characterized by multisystem involvement. Tabes dorsalis, leutic aortitis, paresis, and dementia may result from tertiary syphilis.

Diagnostic Evaluation and Treatment

The diagnosis of syphilis can be made in a variety of ways. Dark-field microscopy of material taken from a chancre or biopsy of the rash of secondary syphilis may reveal spirochetes. Several serologic tests are highly sensitive and specific for syphilis. Both the VDRL (Venereal Disease Research Laboratory) and RPR (rapid plasma reagin) can be performed on blood or cerebrospinal fluid. A positive test should be confirmed by specific antibody testing (fluorescent treponemal antibody absorbed).

Benzathine penicillin G is the treatment of choice for stage one and stage two syphilis (see Table 73–1). It is administered as a one-time dose of 2.4 million units intramuscularly. Tertiary syphilis is treated with 2.4 million units of benzathine penicillin G once a week for three weeks. Doxycycline or tetracycline can be substituted in penicillin-allergic patients.

GENITAL HERPES

Genital herpes is caused by infection with the herpes simplex virus type 1 (HSV 1). HSV 1 is one of the herpesvirus family of DNA viruses. Other members of the family are the Epstein-Barr virus (etiologic agent of infectious mononucleosis) and the cytomegalovirus.

Clinical Manifestations

Genital herpes manifests as painful vesicles that form 1 to 2 weeks after contact with an infected individual. Fever, headache, severe dysuria, and myalgias accompany the skin lesions. Generalized lymphadenopathy accompanies 80% of cases and viral meningitis has been reported. Untreated, the vesicular rash typically lasts 2 to 3 weeks and then resolves spontaneously. Recurrent infection occurs in 50–90% of cases and is brought on by stress, sunlight exposure, or even menses.

Diagnostic Evaluation and Treatment

The diagnosis of genital herpes is made primarily on clinical grounds. The diagnosis can be confirmed by Tzanck prep or PCR.

Acyclovir is the treatment of choice for primary herpes simplex infection (see Table 73–1). Valacyclovir or famciclovir are alternatives and all three drugs may be used for chronic suppressive therapy.

◆ KEY POINTS ◆

1. Gonorrhea is a common cause of pelvic inflammatory disease in women.

2. Patients with gonorrhea are commonly co-infected with *Chlamydia trachomatis*.

3. Primary syphilis is sensitive to benzathine penicillin G.

4. Genital herpes is a recurrent illness in 50–90% of affected individuals.

Part XII
Endocrine and
Metabolic
Emergencies

74

Acid-Base Disorders

The four primary acid-base disorders are respiratory acidosis, respiratory alkalosis, metabolic acidosis, and metabolic alkalosis. Acidosis (pH <7.38) results from the accumulation of acid (H^+) or elimination of base (HCO_3^-). Alkalosis (pH >7.42) results from the addition of base or elimination of acid. Metabolic disturbances occur when the primary disorder is due to a change in the concentration of bicarbonate (HCO_3^-). A respiratory disturbance occurs when the primary disorder is due to the concentration of carbon dioxide (CO_2) (Table 74–1).

ETIOLOGY AND PATHOPHYSIOLOGY

Table 74–2 identifies common causes of acid-base disturbances. Acids are continuously produced as a by-product of metabolism. A pH balance, however, is maintained between 7.35 and 7.45 largely by the bicarbonate-carbonic acid buffer ($CO_2 + H_2O \leftrightarrow H_2CO_3 \leftrightarrow HCO_3^- + H^+$). The primary organ systems that attempt to correct acid-base disturbances are the lungs and kidneys. The respiratory rate is adjusted to change the CO_2 level in order to correct a metabolic disturbance. The kidneys retain or secrete hydrogen ions or bicarbonate to correct a respiratory disturbance. Respiratory compensation is immediate while metabolic compensation usually takes 24–48 hours.

DIAGNOSTIC EVALUATION

Arterial blood gas and serum electrolytes can usually identify acid-base disorders. Other laboratory tests include urinalysis for glucose or ketones, serum osmolality for alcohol ingestions, toxicology screen, serum lactate, and serum ketones. Other considerations for diagnosis of acid-base disturbances are:

1. Determine whether the patient has a primary acidosis or alkalosis using pH, CO_2, and HCO_3 (see Table 74–1).

2. If the primary disorder is a metabolic acidosis then calculate the anion gap. $AG = Na - (Cl + HCO_3)$. If there is an anion gap check for ketonuria. If negative for ketonuria then check renal function, lactate, toxin screen, and osmolal gap.

3. If there is an anion gap, calculate the osmolal gap to determine if alcohol ingestion is the cause of the acidosis. Osmolal gap = Measured serum osmolality − (2 × Na + BUN/2.8 + glu/18).

DIFFERENTIAL

See Table 74–2 for the differential diagnosis of acid-base disorders.

TABLE 74–1

Respiratory versus Metabolic Disturbances

Type of Disturbance	Ph (7.35–7.45)	PCO_2 (40)	HCO_3 (24)
Respiratory acidosis	Decreased	**Increased:** COPD, airway obstruction	*Increased:* renal reabsorption
Respiratory alkalosis	Increased	**Decreased:** High altitude, hyperventilation	*Decreased:* renal secretion
Metabolic acidosis	Decreased	*Decreased:* hyperventilation	**Decreased:** diarrhea, DKA
Metabolic alkalosis	Increased	*Increased:* hypoventilation	**Increased:** vomiting

Bold indicates the primary disturbance and *italic* represents the compensatory response

TABLE 74–2

Causes of Acid-Base Disorders

Metabolic Acidosis

Metabolic acidosis can be divided into elevated and normal anion gap.

> **Elevated Anion Gap**
> ➤ Methanol
> ➤ Uremia-renal failure
> ➤ Lactic acidosis
> ➤ Ethylene glycol
> ➤ Paraldehyde
> ➤ Aspirin
> ➤ Ketoacidosis (e.g., diabetic, starvation, and alcoholic)

> **Normal Anion Gap:**
> ➤ Renal tubular acidosis
> ➤ Diarrhea
> ➤ Early renal failure
> ➤ Carbonic anhydrase inhibitor therapy (i.e., acetazolamide)

Metabolic Alkalosis
- Vomiting
- Nasogastric suction
- Volume depletion
- Diuretic therapy

- Mineralocorticoids—corticosteroid therapy, primary aldosteronism, Cushing's syndrome
- Alkali ingestion

Respiratory Acidosis (is caused by decrease in ventilation)
- Sedative therapy or overdose
- CNS lesions
- Neuropathies
- Myopathies
- Chest wall abnormalities—trauma or kyphosis
- Pleural disease
- Obstructive airway disease—COPD or asthma

Respiratory Alkalosis (is caused by an increase in ventilation)
- Anxiety
- Fever
- Hyperthyroidism
- Hypoxia-pulmonary embolism, pneumonia, pulmonary edema
- Stroke or brain tumor
- Liver disease
- Sympathomimetic therapy

TREATMENT

ABCs (airway, breathing, circulation) should be addressed first. Patients with respiratory acidosis or alkalosis may require supplemental oxygen or intubation. Hypovolemic patients require fluid resuscitation. Once stabilized, the primary goal of therapy is to correct the underlying problem. Most patients with acid-base disorders require admission to the hospital.

◆ KEY POINTS ◆

1. Acidosis (pH <7.35) results from the accumulation of acid (H^+) or elimination of base (HCO_3^-). Alkalosis (pH >7.45) results from the addition of base (HCO_3^-) or elimination of acid (H^+).

2. Metabolic disturbances occur when the primary disorder is due to a change in the concentration of bicarbonate (HCO_3^-).

3. Respiratory disturbances occur when the primary disorder is due to the concentration of carbon dioxide (CO_2).

4. The body responds to a primary metabolic disturbance by adjusting the respiratory rate (i.e., PCO_2) and responds to a primary respiratory disturbance by altering the excretion or retention of renal hydrogen ions (H^+/HCO_3).

5. Treatment of the underlying disorder will correct the acid-base abnormality.

75

Diabetic Ketoacidosis

Diabetic ketoacidosis (DKA) is a syndrome caused by insulin deficiency associated with hyperglycemia, ketonemia, and acidosis. It typically occurs in patients with insulin dependent diabetes mellitus (Type I).

ETIOLOGY

Predisposing factors for DKA include noncompliance with insulin, infectious process, stress, pregnancy, trauma, alcohol use, myocardial infarction, new onset diabetes, CVA, or GI bleeding.

PATHOPHYSIOLOGY

Insulin deficiency causes decreased peripheral use of glucose leading to hyperglycemia. In response to the stress of the precipitating illness, catecholamines, cortisol, and growth hormone are released, contributing to glucose production. Hepatic gluconeogenesis also contributes to hyperglycemia. Despite the abundance of glucose, the lack of insulin makes it unavailable for cellular metabolism. The liver begins to breakdown free fatty acids (i.e., lipolysis) as an alternative source of energy. Lipolysis produces ketoacids that are used by the brain and other tissues as substrates for energy, leading to ketonemia and metabolic acidosis. Intracellular potassium shifts to the extracellular space due to the acidosis. Hyperglycemia and ketoacidosis produce a hyperosmolar state and an osmotic diuresis that ultimately leads to volume depletion, electrolyte losses, and the sequela of DKA.

HISTORY

Symptoms of hyperglycemia include blurred vision, polyuria, polydipsia, or polyphagia. Symptoms of DKA include nausea, vomiting, abdominal pain, or a fruity, acetone odor. As DKA progresses, the osmotic diuresis causes signs of dehydration including dizziness and weakness. Patients may also present with altered mental status or shock.

PHYSICAL EXAMINATION

Look for signs of dehydration including hypotension, tachycardia, dry mucous membranes, and poor skin turgor. Patients may have abdominal tenderness due to gastric distention or stretching of the liver capsule. Patients may be tachypneic or have Kussmaul breathing as a compensatory response to the metabolic acidosis.

DIFFERENTIAL DIAGNOSIS

- Hyperosmolar/nonketotic coma (HHNC)
- Alcoholic ketoacidosis
- Sepsis

- Gastroenteritis
- Urinary tract infection
- Pancreatitis
- Appendicitis
- Alcohol or drug intoxication
- Uremia
- Methanol, ethylene glycol, or paraldehyde ingestion
- Starvation ketoacidosis
- Lactic acidosis

DIAGNOSTIC EVALUATION

The diagnosis of DKA is based on a glucose >250 mg/dl, HCO_3^- <15 meq/L, and pH <7.3 with ketonemia and ketonuria. Laboratory studies include urinalysis, electrolytes, BUN/Cr, serum glucose, CBC with differential, calcium, magnesium, and phosphate, serum ketones, beta HCG, and an ABG. The ABG should demonstrate metabolic acidosis with an anion gap. An electrocardiogram will evaluate for hyperkalemia or ischemia. A chest x-ray may help with the diagnosis of pneumonia as a precipitating cause.

TREATMENT

First evaluate ABCs (airway, breathing, circulation). Place the patient on a cardiac monitor, pulse oximeter, and give supplemental oxygen. Check bedside glucose and urine dipstick for ketones.

Fluid resuscitation should begin with 0.9% normal saline. Once the glucose is below 250, switch to glucose-containing solutions to avoid hypoglycemia. Begin an insulin drip to reverse ketogenesis and allow glucose to be utilized. Glucose should be monitored closely and insulin drip adjusted accordingly. The insulin drip can be tapered once plasma bicarbonate increases and the anion gap resolves. Electrolytes, especially potassium, should be monitored during treatment.

Complications of treatment include hypoglycemia, hypokalemia, hypophosphatemia, fluid overload, and cerebral edema. Most patients require admission to an ICU.

 KEY POINTS

1. Diabetic ketoacidosis (DKA) is a syndrome due to insulin deficiency associated with hyperglycemia, ketonemia, and anion gap acidosis.

2. Patients often present with vomiting, abdominal pain, fruity odor on the breath, and Kussmaul respirations.

3. Treatment includes IV fluids, insulin, and electrolyte repletion in addition to treating the precipitating event.

76 Hyperosmolar Hyperglycemic Nonketotic Coma

Hyperosmolar hyperglycemic nonketotic coma (HHNC) is a syndrome characterized by profound dehydration, hyperglycemia, hyperosmolarity, and decreased mental status functioning that can progress to coma. It is defined as a plasma glucose >600 mg/dl and a plasma osmolarity >350 mOsm/kg in the absence of ketoacidosis in patients with a decreased level of consciousness.

EPIDEMIOLOGY

Approximately 75% of patients who develop HHNC have no prior history of diabetes mellitus. However, upon recovery from HHNC most patients end up having a mild type II diabetes mellitus.

ETIOLOGY

HHNC most commonly occurs in Type II elderly diabetics with renal insufficiency who experience a stressful illness that precipitates worsening hyperglycemia and decreased renal function. HHNC may occur in patients who are not diabetic, especially after trauma, severe burns, dialysis, pancreatitis, or parenteral hyperalimentation. Certain medications including beta-blockers, phenytoin, corticosteroids, and thiazide diuretics have been implicated in the development of HHNC.

PATHOPHYSIOLOGY

HHNC usually results from a relative insulin deficiency in the undiagnosed or insufficiently treated diabetic. The insulin is sufficient to prevent ketoacidosis but not the hyperglycemia. The sustained hyperglycemia creates an osmotic diuresis, which leads to severe dehydration. It generally occurs under circumstances in which the patient is unable to drink sufficient fluids to offset the urinary losses. The average fluid deficit for patients with HHNC is between 9 and 12 liters.

HISTORY

Patients often present with altered mental status or coma. Patients may complain of polyuria, polydipsia and weight loss for days or weeks prior to presentation. Other symptoms include dizziness or weakness. HHNC can also present with a variety of neurologic findings including seizures, focal neurologic deficits, or aphasias.

PHYSICAL EXAMINATION

Vital signs often indicate dehydration (e.g., tachycardia and hypotension). In addition, patients may be orthostatic, have dry mucous membranes, and collapsed neck veins.

DIFFERENTIAL DIAGNOSIS

- DKA
- Hepatic failure
- Uremia
- Cerebrovascular accident
- Drug ingestion
- Hypoglycemia
- Sepsis

DIAGNOSTIC EVALUATION

Laboratory studies include serum glucose, electrolytes, BUN and Cr, CBC, urinalysis, serum osmolarity, and ABG. Liver function tests, amylase, lipase, coagulation studies, and cardiac enzymes may be helpful. An ECG and chest x-ray should be obtained to look for precipitating causes. A head CT is indicated if the patient is comatose or has a focal neurologic deficit. If the patient is febrile, urine and blood cultures should be sent.

MANAGEMENT

First assess ABCs (airway, breathing, circulation). Place patients on a cardiac monitor and a pulse oximeter, gain IV access, and give supplemental oxygen. A Foley catheter should also be placed to monitor urine output. Begin fluid resuscitation with normal saline. Replete electrolyte abnormalities as needed. Typically, insulin is reserved for patients who are acidemic, hyperkalemic, or in renal failure, since usually fluid alone resolves the hyperglycemia. Search for possible precipitants and treat accordingly. All patients with HHNC should be admitted to an intensive care unit for close monitoring.

◆ KEY POINTS ◆

1. Hyperosmolar hyperglycemic nonketotic coma (HHNC) is a syndrome characterized by profound dehydration, hyperglycemia, hyperosmolarity, and decreased mental status functioning that can progress to coma.

2. Most commonly occurs in mild Type II diabetics with a precipitating illness.

3. Patients may complain of polyuria, polydipsia, and weight loss for days or weeks prior to presentation.

4. Treatment includes aggressive fluid and electrolyte replacement and low dose insulin.

77 Potassium Disorders

Hypokalemia is defined as serum potassium level less than 3.5 mEq/L. Hyperkalemia is defined as serum potassium level greater than 5.0 mEq/L.

PATHOPHYSIOLOGY

Potassium is the major determinant of cellular membrane resting potential affecting the function of nerve and muscle cells. Potassium is primarily eliminated by renal excretion. However, multiple factors affect potassium homeostasis. Table 77–1 lists external factors that affect potassium balance.

HYPOKALEMIA

Etiology

Hypokalemia can be caused by decreased potassium intake, increased potassium excretion, and transcellular shifts. Table 77–2 outlines the etiologies of hypokalemia.

History

The manifestations of hypokalemia are generally mild but severe depletion can cause neuromuscular, cardiac, renal, and gastrointestinal symptoms. See Table 77–2 for signs and symptoms of hypokalemia.

Physical Examination

On physical exam, look for areflexia, paralysis, arrhythmias, orthostatic hypotension, and ileus (see Table 77–2).

Differential Diagnosis

- Lab error
- Intrinsic cardiac disease causing dysrhythmias
- Neuromuscular junction diseases including myasthenia gravis, organophosphate poisoning, and botulism
- Spinal cord disease
- Polyneuropathies
- Myopathies

Diagnostic Evaluation

Laboratory studies include electrolytes, magnesium, BUN, creatinine, urinalysis for myoglobin, and depending on clinical situation, an ABG for evaluation of acid-base status. An ECG will look for signs of hypokalemia including U waves, T-wave flattening or inversion, and ST segment depression.

Management

Patients with potassium between 2.5 and 3.5 mEq/L can usually be managed as outpatients with gradual oral potassium repletion. All patients who are sent home should have follow-up within 48 hours. Patients with severe hypokalemia (K <2.5 mEq/L) should be admitted to the hospital. These patients should be placed on a cardiac monitor and have IV access obtained. Typically, patients with severe hypokalemia require IV and oral potassium replacement. Hypovolemic patients require volume resuscitation in addition to potassium supplementation.

TABLE 77–1

Factors That Influence Potassium Balance

Factors that increase serum potassium concentrations (i.e., shift potassium out of cells)	• Acidemia • Insulin deficiency • Beta-blockers • Alpha-adrenergic agonists • Hyperosmolarity • Aldosterone deficiency
Factors that decrease serum potassium concentrations (i.e., shift potassium into cells)	• Alkalemia • Insulin • Beta-adrenergic agonists • Aldosterone

◆ KEY POINTS ◆

1. Hypokalemia is defined as K less than 3.5 mEq/L.
2. Alkalosis, insulin, and beta-adrenergic agonists cause potassium to shift into cells.
3. ECG findings associated with hypokalemia include U-waves, T-wave flattening or inversion, and ST segment depression.
4. Treatment includes oral and/or IV potassium replacement depending on severity of deficiency.

TABLE 77–2

Etiology and Symptoms of Hypokalemia

	Etiology	Signs and Symptoms	ECG Finding

Hypokalemia (K+ <3.5 mEq/L)	**Decreased Potassium Intake:**
	• Nutritional: inadequate dietary intake
	Increased Potassium Excretion:
	• Renal tubular disorders or damage
	• Primary or secondary Hyperaldosteronism
	• Magnesium deficiency
	• Drug induced
	  — Diuretics
	  — Aminoglycosides
	  — Amphotericin B
	• GI losses
	  — Vomiting
	  — Diarrhea
	  — Laxative abuse
	  — Villous adenoma
	Transcellular Shifts:
	• Alkalosis
	• Insulin excess
	• Adrenergic excess
	  — Beta-adrenergic agonists (i.e., albuterol, epinephrine)
	  — Stress (i.e., trauma, MI, sepsis)
	• Hypokalemic periodic paralysis
		Neuromuscular:
		• Weakness
		• Cramps
		• Paresthesias
		• Paralysis
		• Areflexia
		• Rhabdomyolysis
		Cardiovascular:
		• Palpitations
		• Postural hypotension
		• Dysrhythmias
		• Ectopy
		• Potentiation of digitalis toxicity
		Renal:
		• Polyuria
		• Polydipsia
		• Metabolic alkalosis
		GI:
		• Constipation
		• Nausea or vomiting
		• Abdominal distention
		• Ileus
			• U waves
			• T-wave flattening or inversion
			• ST-segment depression
			• Premature ventricular contractions (PVCs)
			• Wide QRS complex

TABLE 77–3

Etiology and Symptoms of Hyperkalemia

	Etiology	Signs and Symptoms	ECG Finding
Hyperkalemia (K+ >5.0 mEq/L)	**Pseudohyperkalemia:** • Hemolysis of sample • Leukocytosis or thrombocytosis • Laboratory error **Increased Potassium Load:** • Potassium supplements • Blood transfusions • Crush injuries • Burns • Rhabdomyolysis • Intravascular hemolysis • Potassium containing medications **Decreased Renal Excretion:** • Acute or chronic renal failure • Hypoaldosteronism • Drugs — NSAID — Heparin — ACE inhibitors — Potassium sparing diuretics (i.e., spironolactone) — Cyclosporin **Transcellular Shifts:** • Acidemia • Hyperkalemic periodic paralysis • Beta-blockers • Succinylcholine • Insulin deficiency • Digitalis toxicity • Hyperosmolarity — Mannitol — Hyperglycemia	**Cardiovascular:** • Palpitations • Dysrhythmias — Second and third degree heart block — Wide complex tachycardia — Ventricular fibrillation — Asystole **Neuromuscular:** • Weakness • Cramps • Paresthesias • Paralysis • Tetany • Focal neurologic deficits • Areflexia **Gastrointestinal:** • Nausea • Vomiting • Intestinal colic	**Early:** • Peaked T waves • Shortened QT interval **Late:** • Widened QRS complex • Increased PR interval • Low amplitude P waves • Elevation or depression of ST segment **Advanced:** • Absent P waves • Marked QRS widening • Sine wave pattern • Ventricular fibrillation • Asystole

HYPERKALEMIA

Etiology

Hyperkalemia can be caused by increased potassium load, impaired potassium excretion, or transcellular shifts. Table 77–3 gives the etiology and symptoms of hyperkalemia.

History

The primary manifestations of hyperkalemia include cardiovascular and neuromuscular dysfunction with cardiac manifestations being more common. Many patients present without any symptoms (see Table 77–3).

Physical Examination

Physical exam finding may include paralysis, areflexia, focal neurologic deficits, respiratory insufficiency, or cardiac arrest (see Table 77–3).

Differential Diagnosis

- Pseudohyperkalemia
- Primary cardiac disease causing dysrhythmias
- Tricyclic overdose

Diagnostic Evaluation

An ECG should be the first test obtained in patients with suspected hyperkalemia. As the potassium level rises, peaked T waves become present followed by PR prolongation, loss of P waves, and widening of the QRS complex. Figure 77–1 outlines the classic ECG findings of hyperkalemia (see also Table 77–3). Laboratory studies include electrolytes, glucose, BUN, creatinine, magnesium, and calcium.

Management

First access ABCs (airway, breathing, circulation). For patients who present in cardiac arrest with known or suspected hyperkalemia, follow the Advanced Cardiac Life Support guidelines and administer calcium chloride and sodium bicarbonate. All patients should be placed on a cardiac monitor, have IV access secured while obtaining an immediate ECG and repeating a potassium level. For symptomatic patients, begin treatment with calcium gluconate or calcium chloride for cardiac membrane stabilization. Next, give insulin and glucose to shift potassium into cells. In addition, albuterol nebulizer and sodium bicarbonate can also be used to

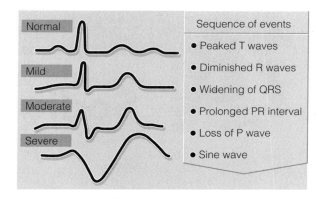

Figure 77–1 ECGs of increasingly severe hyperkalemia. An individual patient's response cannot be predicted from the plasma potassium level.

shift potassium into cells. Consider furosemide and Kayexalate to remove potassium from the body. For patients with renal failure or severe, refractory hyperkalemia, dialysis should be considered. Potassium levels should be monitored frequently during treatment. Ultimately, treat the underlying cause. For stable patients with mild elevations in potassium (<6.0 mEq/L) without ECG, changes can be discharged home with close follow-up within 48 hours.

◆ KEY POINTS ◆

1. Hyperkalemia is defined as K^+ greater than 5.0 mEq/L.

2. Classic ECG findings include peaked T waves, increased PR interval, loss of P waves, and widening of the QRS complex.

3. Stabilize the cardiac membrane with calcium chloride or calcium gluconate.

4. Shift potassium into cells with insulin plus glucose, sodium bicarbonate, and albuterol nebulizer.

5. Remove potassium from the body with Kayexalate or furosemide.

6. Consider dialysis for patients with renal failure or with severe refractory hyperkalemia.

78 Sodium Disorders

Thirst, antidiuretic hormone (ADH), and renal mechanisms closely maintain serum sodium concentration and serum osmolality. Hyponatremia is defined as a serum sodium concentration less than 135 mEq/L. Hypernatremia is defined as serum sodium greater than 146 mEq/L.

HYPONATREMIA

Etiology

Hyponatremia can be divided into three types (hypotonic, isotonic, and hypertonic) based on serum osmolality. Isotonic hyponatremia (i.e., pseudohyponatremia) is a falsely low serum sodium level due to hyperproteinemia or hyperlipidemia. Hypertonic hyponatremia (i.e., redistribute hyponatremia) is a low serum sodium level due to high levels of osmotically active substances (e.g., glucose), which cause water to move into the extracellular space diluting the serum sodium concentration. In both cases, treatment of the underlying problem will correct the apparent sodium imbalance. Hypotonic hyponatremia can be classified into three categories (hypovolemic, isovolemic, or hypervolemic) based on the patient's volume status. Table 78–1 lists the causes of hyponatremia.

History

The acutely hyponatremic patient (i.e., <48 hrs) is almost always symptomatic with serum sodium levels less than 120 mEq/L. Patients with chronic hyponatremia may tolerate much lower levels before becoming symptomatic. The primary symptoms of hyponatremia are related to central nervous system affects and include disorientation and confusion, agitation, ataxia, altered consciousness, seizures, and coma. Other nonspecific symptoms include headache, muscle cramps, anorexia, nausea and vomiting, and weakness.

Physical Examination

It is important to determine the volume status of patients with hypotonic hyponatremia in order to establish the cause. Signs of hypovolemia include tachycardia, poor skin turgor, dry mucous membranes, or oliguria. Signs of hypervolemia include pulmonary rales, elevated JVP, peripheral edema, or ascites.

Differential Diagnosis

- Hyperglycemia
- Hyperlipidemia
- Hyperproteinemia

Diagnostic Evaluation

Laboratory studies should include electrolytes, BUN, creatinine, and glucose. Obtain a urinalysis to determine urine sodium levels and osmolality. Calculate the serum osmolality as follows: $2NA + glucose/18 + BUN/2.8$ (normal, 290). This allows the separation into hypotonic, isotonic, and hypertonic.

TABLE 78–1

Etiology of Hyponatremia

Isotonic		• Hyperlipidemia • Hyperproteinemia
Hypertonic		• Hyperglycemia • Mannitol
Hypotonic	**Hypovolemic hyponatremia**	• GI losses: vomiting, diarrhea • Excessive sweating • Renal losses: salt wasting nephropathies, diuretics • Addison's disease • Cystic fibrosis • Third spacing: burns, peritonitis, pancreatitis
	Isovolemic hyponatremia	• Syndrome of inappropriate antidiuretic hormone (SIADH) • Psychogenic polydipsia • Water intoxication • Hypothyroidism • Cortisol deficiency
	Hypervolemic hyponatremia	• CHF • Cirrhosis • Nephrotic syndrome • Renal failure

Management

First evaluate ABCs (airway, breathing, circulation). The treatment of hyponatremia depends on the severity of symptoms, rate at which it developed, and underlying etiology. Patients with acute hyponatremia who present with severe central nervous system (CNS) symptoms (e.g., seizure or obtundation) should receive hypertonic (3%) saline. Once symptoms improve, typically when serum sodium is greater than 120 mEq/L,

further correction should be made with normal saline at a gradual rate. Too aggressive correction can lead to central pontine myelinolysis or cerebral edema. Patients should be admitted to an ICU.

For patients without severe manifestations, treatment should be directed at the underlying disorder. Correct hypovolemic hyponatremia with isotonic saline. Patients with isovolemic hyponatremia are treated with free water restriction. Patients with hypervolemic hypernatremia are treated with sodium and water restriction.

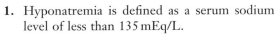

◆ **KEY POINTS** ◆

1. Hyponatremia is defined as a serum sodium level of less than 135 mEq/L.

2. Hypotonic hyponatremia is divided into three categories based on volume status: hypovolemic, isovolemic, and hypervolemic.

3. Treatment of acute symptomatic hyponatremia (e.g., seizure or coma) is with hypertonic saline (3%).

4. Too rapid correction of serum sodium can lead to development of central pontine myelinolysis or cerebral edema.

HYPERNATREMIA

Etiology

Hypernatremia results from free water deficit compared to sodium levels. Normally, small increases in the serum sodium concentration stimulate thirst and secretion of ADH causing renal water conservation. Hypernatremia can be divided into three categories based on volume status. Hypovolemic hypernatremia is the most common and is due to a loss of water and sodium, with water losses exceeding sodium losses. Isovolemic hypernatremia is due to water deficiency without sodium loss. Hypervolemic hypernatremia is due to accumulation of water and sodium, with sodium gain greater than water gain. Table 78–2 lists the etiologies of hypernatremia.

History

Signs and symptoms of hypernatremia are primarily related to central nervous system dehydration and include mental status changes, irritability, lethargy,

TABLE 78–2

Etiology of Hypernatremia

Hypovolemia hypernatremia	• Renal losses — Postobstructive, therapeutic or osmotic diuresis • Extrarenal causes — Excessive sweating — Lack of access to water: depressed mentation, intubated patient — Diarrhea/vomiting
Isovolemic hypernatremia	• Renal water losses — Diabetes insipidus: central or nephrogenic — Lithium treatment • Extrarenal water losses — Respiratory losses: hyperventilation — Defective thirst mechanism — Fever — Severe burns
Hypervolemic hypernatremia	• Iatrogenic-sodium bicarbonate, salt tablets, hypertonic saline, hypertonic renal dialysate • Sea water ingestion • Acute renal failure • Cushing's disease • Hyperaldosteronism • Adrenal hyperplasia • Exogenous corticosteroids

confusion, delirium, ataxia, seizures, and coma. Other symptoms include muscle spasticity, muscle weakness, and tremulousness.

Physical Examination

Signs of hypovolemic hypernatremia typically include tachycardia, orthostatics, dry mucous membranes, and poor skin turgor. Signs of hypervolemic hypernatremia typically include pulmonary edema, elevated JVP, and peripheral edema.

Differential Diagnosis

• Diabetic ketoacidosis
• Hyperosmolar coma
• Primary CNS lesions

Diagnostic Evaluation

Laboratory studies include electrolytes, BUN, creatinine, glucose, and urinalysis for sodium and osmolality.

Management

First evaluate ABCs (airway, breathing, circulation). As with hyponatremia, treatment of hypernatremia depends on the severity of symptoms, rate at which it developed, and underlying etiology. Treatment of symptomatic patients includes volume resuscitation the acute manifestations begin to improve. As with hyponatremia, rapid correction of hypernatremia can cause cerebral edema. Additional replacement should occur gradually.

Patients with hypovolemic hypernatremia and severe hypotension should be initially resuscitated with 0.9% normal saline to improve blood pressure and restore tissue perfusion. Once volume is restored change to D5W or hypotonic saline. Patients with isovolemic hypernatremia should have their water deficit replaced with D5W. Patients with central diabetes insipidus require administration of parenteral or intranasal vasopressin. Treatment of patients with hypervolemic hypernatremia consists of diuretics followed by infusion of hypotonic saline or D5W. Dialysis may be necessary for patients in renal failure.

◆ KEY POINTS ◆

1. Hypernatremia is clinically significant at sodium levels of 155 mEq/L.
2. Symptoms of hypernatremia are related to central nervous system dysfunction.
3. Acute hypovolemic hypernatremia should be corrected with normal saline.
4. Asymptomatic patients with hypernatremia should be corrected gradually to avoid rapid fluid shifts, cellular swelling, and cerebral edema.

79 Calcium Disorders

Hypocalcemia exists when total calcium [Ca] is less than 8.5 mg/dl or ionized calcium level [Ca+2] is less than 2.0 mEq/L. Hypercalcemia exists when total calcium is greater than 10.5 mg/dl or an ionized calcium level is greater than 2.7 mEq/L.

PATHOPHYSIOLOGY

Calcium participates in hundreds of enzymatic reactions including neurotransmission and skeletal and cardiac muscle contraction. Most calcium exists in bone or bound to proteins, but free ionized calcium is the physiologically active form. Calcium levels are regulated primarily by the interaction between parathyroid hormone (PTH) and vitamin D. Low serum calcium levels stimulates PTH release. PTH raises serum calcium levels by increasing bone resorption, renal tubular calcium reabsorption, and activation of vitamin D to 1,25 dihydroxycholecalciferol (1,25-DHCC). Activated vitamin D increases absorption of calcium from intestine and bone. High serum calcium levels suppress PTH release and stimulate the release of calcitonin, which enhances bone deposition, and renal excretion of calcium.

Systemic alkalosis increases calcium binding to serum proteins, lowering the free ionized calcium level without affecting the total plasma calcium level. Acidosis has the opposite effect. Total serum calcium levels may be falsely low in hypoalbuminemia because approximately 40% of serum calcium is bound to albumin.

Decreasing the serum albumin level by 1 g/dl lowers the total measured serum calcium by approximately 0.8 mg/dl.

HYPOCALCEMIA

Etiology and History

Table 79–1 lists the causes of hypocalcemia. Consider hypocalcemia in patients with history of renal failure, chronic malabsorption, and neck surgery or irradiation. Most of the clinical manifestations of hypocalcemia are due to the effects on neuromuscular function. Patients may complain of circumoral and distal extremity paresthesias, weakness, irritability, muscle cramps, tetany, and seizures. Severe hypocalcemia can also cause a decrease in myocardial contractility leading to hypotension and CHF (see Table 79–1).

Physical Examination

Physical examination findings can include:

- Trousseau's sign—carpal spasm in response to inflation of a blood pressure cuff to 20 mm Hg above systolic BP for 3 minutes.
- Chvostek's sign—twitching of the facial muscles after tapping over the facial nerve.
- Hyperreflexia
- Tetany

TABLE 79–1

Etiology and Symptoms of Hypocalcemia

	Etiology	Signs and Symptoms	ECG Finding
Hypocalcemia (total serum Ca+ <8.5 mg/dL)	• Hypoparathyroidism — Neck surgery — Neck irradiation • Renal failure • Vitamin D deficiency — Nutritional — Malabsorption — Rickets disease — Sepsis — Liver disease • Acute pancreatitis • Hyperphosphatemia • Hypoalbuminemia • Hypomagnesemia • Medications — Anticonvulsants — Chemotherapeutic agents — Cimetidine — Colchicine — Fluoride	**Neuromuscular:** • Weakness • Muscle cramps or spasm • Paresthesias • Hyperreflexia • Tetany • Seizures • Laryngeal stridor • Trousseau's sign • Chvostek's sign **Cardiovascular:** • Impaired contractility (CHF) • Hypotension • Arrhythmias **Psychiatric:** • Mental status changes • Depression • Irritability • Psychosis	• Prolongation of QT interval • Inverted T waves • Sinus bradycardia • Complete heart block • Ventricular dysrhythmias • Ventricular fibrillation

Differential Diagnosis

- Hypomagnesemia
- Severe alkalosis
- Strychnine poisoning
- Tetanus

Diagnostic Evaluation

Lab studies include electrolytes, BUN/creatine, glucose, serum albumin, calcium, magnesium, and phosphate. A serum-ionized calcium level confirms the diagnosis. A 12-lead ECG may show a prolonged QT interval.

Management

Symptomatic patients should be placed on a cardiac monitor and receive IV calcium. Calcium should be given cautiously to patients receiving digitalis because it can worsen digoxin toxicity or cause sudden death. Asymptomatic patients should receive oral calcium therapy. Patients with symptomatic hypocalcemia should be admitted. Patients who are asymptomatic may be discharged home with appropriate follow-up.

◆ KEY POINTS ◆

1. Hypocalcemia is defined as total serum calcium level less than 8.5 mg/dl or ionized calcium level less than 2.0 mEq/L.

2. Signs and symptoms of hypocalcemia are primarily related to neuromuscular effects, and may manifest by Trousseau's or Chvostek's sign.

3. QT prolongation may be present on ECG.

4. Treatment includes IV calcium for symptomatic patients and oral supplements for asymptomatic patients. The underlying disorder should be addressed.

TABLE 79–2

Etiology and Symptoms of Hypercalcemia

	Etiology	Signs and Symptoms	ECG Finding
Hypercalcemia (total Ca^{++} >10.5 mg/dL)	• **Endocrine disorders:** — Hyperparathyroidism — Hyperthyroidism — Adrenal insufficiency — Acromegaly — Pheochromocytoma — Zollinger-Ellison syndrome (MEN I) • **Malignancy:** — Breast — Lung (squamous cell) — Myeloma — Lymphoma • **Granulomatous disorders:** — Sarcoidosis — Tuberculosis — Histoplasmosis — Coccidioidomycosis • **Medications:** — Thiazides — Lithium — Vitamin A toxicity — Vitamin D toxicity — Calcium ingestion • **Miscellaneous:** — Prolonged immobility — Dehydration — Paget's disease — Milk alkali syndrome	**Neurologic:** • Weakness • Fatigue • Altered mental status • Coma • Hyporeflexia **GI:** • Nausea • Vomiting • Abdominal pain • Constipation • Ileus • Anorexia • Peptic ulcer disease **Renal:** • Renal calculi • Polyuria • Polydipsia • Dehydration • Oliguric renal failure **Cardiovascular:** • Hypotension or Hypertension • Arrhythmias • Asystole • Exacerbation of digoxin toxicity **Dermatologic:** • Pruritus	• Shortening of QT interval • Prolongation of PR interval • Widening of QRS complex • Sinus bradycardia • Bundle branch block • Ventricular dysrhythmias

HYPERCALCEMIA

Etiology

Primary hyperparathyroidism and malignancy are the two most common causes of hypercalcemia. Some tumors produce a PTH related protein that acts on the PTH receptor mimicking its action. Direct bone destruction by bony metastases and osteolytic tumors can also increase calcium levels. Other causes include enhanced intestinal absorption, increased renal absorption of calcium, and increased bone turnover (Table 79–2).

History

Patients may present with neurologic symptoms ranging from weakness, fatigue, and difficulty concentrating to confusion, obtundation, and coma. Gastrointestinal symptoms include anorexia, nausea, vomiting, abdominal pain, and constipation. Hypercalcemia also affects the concentrating ability of the kidney, leading to polyuria and dehydration. Patients with chronic hypercalcemia may give a history of recurrent nephrolithiasis or peptic ulcer disease (see Table 79–2).

Physical Examination

The physical exam is often unremarkable but may include dehydration, hypotension, decreased motor strength, hyporeflexia, fractures, ataxia, and altered mental status.

Differential Diagnosis

- Infection
- Primary CNS disorders
- GI system dysfunction
- Primary cardiac disorders

Diagnostic Evaluation

Elevated ionized or total calcium levels confirm the diagnosis. Other laboratory studies including albumin, PTH, vitamin D level, TSH, and phosphate may help determine the underlying etiology. A 12-lead ECG may show a short QT interval, prolonged PR interval, and widened QRS complex.

Management

Symptomatic hypercalcemia or a serum calcium level greater than 14 mg/dl should be treated emergently with IV fluids. Patients should be placed on a cardiac monitor and administered 1–2 liters of normal saline. Once intravascular volume is replete, IV furosemide is given to enhance urinary excretion of calcium. Calcitonin is given to those who respond poorly to saline diuresis or who cannot tolerate a saline load (e.g., patients with CHF). Hydrocortisone acts by inhibiting the action of vitamin D and is mainly effective in hypercalcemia due to hematologic malignancies, granulomatous disorders, and vitamin D toxicity. Dialysis should be considered when hypercalcemia is unresponsive to medical management or for patients with cardiac or renal disease.

Treatment of hypercalcemia is ultimately directed at the underlying cause. All patients with symptomatic hypercalcemia, calcium levels greater than 13 mg/dl or abnormal renal function should be admitted. Asymptomatic hypercalcemia or patients with calcium levels less than 13 mg/dl can be discharged home with close follow-up.

◆ KEY POINTS ◆

1. Hypercalcemia exists when [Ca] is greater than 10.5 mg/dl.
2. QT shortening, PR prolongation, and widened QRS may be seen on ECG.
3. Emergent treatment is required for symptomatic hypercalcemia or [Ca] greater than 14 mg/dl.
4. Treatment consists of IV hydration with isotonic saline followed by IV furosemide.

80 Thyroid Storm

Thyroid storm is a rare life-threatening complication of thyrotoxicosis (hyperthyroidism), characterized by fever, tachycardia, and dysfunction of the central nervous system, cardiovascular system, or gastrointestinal systems.

ETIOLOGY

A precipitating event causing adrenergic hyperactivity such as infection, surgery, or other stressors may trigger thyroid storm in a patient with:

- Graves' disease
- Toxic multinodular goiter
- Transient hyperthyroidism
  - Subacute thyroiditis
  - Postpartum thyroiditis
- Extra-thyroid source

Table 80–1 lists precipitating events in thyroid storm.

PATHOPHYSIOLOGY

Thyrotoxicosis is caused by excess thyroid hormone secretion, resulting in suppression of thyroid stimulating hormone (TSH).

HISTORY

The onset of thyroid storm is typically abrupt, but most patients have a history of Graves' disease or palpable goiter. Symptoms of thyrotoxicosis are usually present for at least six months prior to presentation (see Table 80–1).

PHYSICAL EXAMINATION

See Table 80–1 for a list of physical exam findings common in thyroid storm.

DIFFERENTIAL DIAGNOSIS

- Anxiety states
- Psychosis
- Cocaine toxicity
- Pheochromocytoma
- Heat stroke
- Malignant neuroleptic syndrome
- Diabetes mellitus
- Acute abdomen
- Cardiac disease
- Hypermetabolic states
  - Severe anemia, leukemia, polycythemia, cancer

TABLE 80-1

Signs and Symptoms of Hyperthyroidism and Thyroid Storm

Precipitating Events	Symptoms	Physical Exam Findings

• Infection
• Pulmonary embolism
• Surgery
• Burns
• Trauma
• Vascular accidents
• Hypoglycemia
• Diabetic ketoacidosis
• Hyperosmolar nonketotic coma
• Ingestion of thyroid hormone
• Premature withdrawal of antithyroid therapy
• Iodine therapy
	Systemic manifestation
	• Fever
	• Excessive sweating
	• Heat intolerance
	CNS dysfunction
	• Nervousness
	• Inability to sleep
	• Delirium
	• Tremor
	Cardiovascular
	• Chest pain
	• Palpitations
	Gastrointestinal
	• Weight loss
	• Frequent bowel movements
	• Diarrhea
	• Nausea and vomiting
	• Abdominal pain
		• Temperature >97.8
		• Diaphoresis
		• Proximal muscle weakness
		• Hyperreflexia
		• Tremor
		• Widen pulse pressure
		• Tachycardia
		• Congestive heart failure
		  — Pulmonary rales
		  — Elevated JVP
		• Palpable goiter with thrill or bruit
		• Ocular manifestations
		  — Proptosis and lid retraction
		  — Staring

DIAGNOSTIC EVALUATION

The diagnosis of thyroid storm is confirmed by elevated T4 and suppressed TSH level. An ECG may show sinus tachycardia.

MANAGEMENT

Patients should be placed on a cardiac monitor, have supplemental oxygen and IV access obtained. Initiation of cooling measures should begin with acetaminophen and cooling blankets. Congestive heart failure and dehydration should be managed accordingly.

Excessive thyroid hormone is controlled by:

1. Control thyroid hormone synthesis with propylthiouracil (PTU).
2. Inhibit thyroid hormone release with potassium iodine, Lugol's solution, or sodium iodine. (Iodide solutions should be given 1 hour after PTU to avoid synthesis of new hormone.)
3. Block peripheral effects of thyroid hormone with beta-blockers.
4. Prevent peripheral conversion of T4 to T3 with dexamethasone.

The underlying cause and precipitating event should be evaluated and treated. Patients with thyroid storm require admission to an intensive care unit.

◆ KEY POINTS ◆

1. Thyroid storm is a life-threatening complication of thyrotoxicosis.
2. Patients typically have a history of Graves' disease or palpable goiter.
3. Elevated T4 and suppressed TSH levels confirm the diagnosis of thyroid storm.
4. Treatment includes general supportive care, PTU, iodine solution, beta-blockade, and dexamethasone.

81 Hypothyroidism and Myxedema Coma

Patients with long-standing, untreated hypothyroidism may develop myxedema coma, a syndrome of hypothermia, altered mental status, respiratory insufficiency, and myxedema. Myxedema is a nonpitting, dry, waxy swelling of the skin caused by deposition of mucopolysaccharides in the dermis.

ETIOLOGY

Hypothyroid patients may develop myxedema following stressful events such as cold exposure, trauma, or infection. Causes of hypothyroidism are outlined in Table 81–1.

HISTORY AND PHYSICAL EXAMINATION

Patients may report a history of hypothyroidism, Graves' disease, or discontinuation of thyroid replacement hormone. Table 81–2 lists symptoms and physical findings of hypothyroidism and myxedema coma.

DIFFERENTIAL DIAGNOSIS

- Chronic renal failure
- Nephrotic syndrome
- Congestive heart failure
- Hypoalbuminemia
- Sepsis
- Depression
- Other causes of coma

DIAGNOSTIC EVALUATION

An elevated TSH with suppressed T3 and T4 levels confirm the diagnosis of hypothyroidism. Other laboratory tests serve mainly to exclude alternative diagnoses. Common lab findings include hyponatremia, hypochloremia, and hypoglycemia. Chest x-ray may show pulmonary edema or enlarged cardiac silhouette, and ECG may show bradycardia, prolonged PR interval, low voltage, and inversion of T waves.

MANAGEMENT

Treatment includes cardiac monitor, IV fluids, and rewarming as indicated. Hypotension is treated with IV fluids and pressors as required. Hyponatremia and hypoglycemia are treated accordingly. Hydrocortisone is administered for presumptive adrenal insufficiency. The cornerstone of treatment for myxedema coma is thyroid hormone replacement with intravenous L-thyroxine. Precipitating events should be addressed and the patient should be admitted to the hospital.

TABLE 81–1

Causes of Hypothyroidism

- Congenital
- Idiopathic
- Iatrogenic
  — Surgical or medical ablation
  — Antithyroid drugs (e.g., lithium)
- Autoimmune
  — Hashimoto's thyroiditis
  — Hypothyroidism
- Iodine deficiency
- Secondary hypothyroidism
  — Pituitary tumors
  — Infiltrative disorders
  — Postpartum hemorrhage

◆ KEY POINTS ◆

- Myxedema coma is a life-threatening form of hypothyroidism.
- Treatment includes supportive care, levothyroxine, and hydrocortisone.

TABLE 81–2

Signs and Symptoms of Hypothyroidism and Myxedema Coma

Precipitating Events	Symptoms	Physical Exam Findings
• Cold environment	• Weakness/fatigue	• Temperature <37°C
• Infection	• Cold intolerance	• Scant body hair
— Pulmonary	• Weight gain despite decreased appetite	• Thinning of lateral 1/3 of eyebrows
• Hemorrhage	• Constipation	• Prolonged deep tendon reflexes
— Gastrointestinal	• Abdominal distention	• Periorbital puffiness
• Trauma	• Urinary retention	• Large tongue
• Cerebrovascular accident	• Menstrual irregularities	• Myxedema—dry, waxy swelling of skin
• Congestive heart failure	• Muscle cramps	• Pale, cool, rough skin
• Drugs	• Deepened or hoarse voice	• Goiter
— Sedative hypnotics	• Dry skin and hair	• Bradycardia
• Hypoxia	• Paresthesias	• Hypotension
• Hypercapnia		• Hypoventilation
• Hyponatremia		• Hypoxia
• Hypoglycemia		• Coma/altered mental status

82

Adrenal Insufficiency and Adrenal Crisis

Adrenal crisis is a medical emergency that occurs when patients with adrenal insufficiency experience a stressful event such as infection, trauma, burns, pregnancy, or surgery.

ETIOLOGY

Patients with chronic adrenal insufficiency, acute adrenal hemorrhage, rapid steroid withdrawal, and steroid dependence are at risk of developing adrenal crisis. Table 82–1 lists causes of both primary and secondary adrenal failure.

PATHOPHYSIOLOGY

Adrenal crisis occurs when glucocorticoids are unable to meet the body's metabolic requirements. Primary adrenal insufficiency (Addison's disease) is due to disease or destruction of adrenal cortex. It causes lack of both cortisol and aldosterone, providing no feedback inhibition to the pituitary gland and thus high levels of adrenocorticotropic hormone (ACTH). Secondary adrenal insufficiency is due to disease or destruction of the pituitary gland resulting in lack of ACTH secretion and thus a lack of cortisol production.

HISTORY

Patients may present with vague symptoms including weakness, fatigue, nausea, vomiting, diarrhea, abdomi-

nal pain, and weight loss. Patients with secondary adrenal insufficiency may also have symptoms related to pituitary disease including headache, visual changes, menstrual irregularities, loss of sexual performance, or galactorrhea.

PHYSICAL EXAMINATION

Findings may include orthostatic hypotension, tachycardia, mental status changes, fever, or shock. Patients with primary adrenal insufficiency often have hyperpigmented skin.

DIFFERENTIAL DIAGNOSIS

- Myocardial infarction
- Congestive heart failure
- Hypovolemia
- Sepsis
- Pulmonary embolus
- Thyrotoxicosis
- Occult malignancy
- Anorexia nervosa
- Hemochromatosis
- Panhypopituitarism

TABLE 82–1

Etiology of Primary and Secondary Adrenal Insufficiency

Primary Adrenal Insufficiency	Secondary Adrenal Insufficiency
• Idiopathic — Autoimmune • Infectious — Granulomatous (TB) — Bacterial (meningococcemia) — Fungal (histoplasmosis) — Viral (CMV) • Infiltrative — Sarcoidosis — Amyloidosis — Hemochromatosis • Hemorrhage — Sepsis — Pregnancy — Anticoagulants — Abdominal trauma • Congenital-adrenal hyperplasia • Postadrenalectomy • Adrenal infarction — Waterhouse-Friderichsen syndrome	• Iatrogenic (glucocorticoids) • Pituitary tumors • Head trauma • Pituitary hemorrhage • Infection • Isolated ACTH deficiency • Infiltrative — Sarcoidosis — Amyloidosis — Hemochromatosis • Infarction — Sheehan's syndrome

DIAGNOSTIC EVALUATION

Lab studies include electrolytes, glucose, BUN, creatine, CBC, ACTH, and cortisol. Patients with primary adrenal insufficiency classically have hyponatremia, hyperkalemia, and hypoglycemia. Since ACTH levels to confirm adrenal insufficiency are not available to the emergency physician, treatment should begin based on clinical suspicion.

MANAGEMENT

Treatment of adrenal crisis should begin with rapid infusion with 5% dextrose and isotonic saline. Continue to treat hypotension with IV fluids and pressors as needed. Treat hyperkalemia as indicated. Glucocorticoid and mineralocorticoid replacement with hydrocortisone is the mainstay of treatment. In addition, identify and treat the underlying precipitant. All patients with adrenal crisis should be admitted to an intensive care unit.

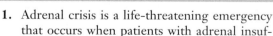

♦ **KEY POINTS** ♦

1. Adrenal crisis is a life-threatening emergency that occurs when patients with adrenal insufficiency experience a stressful event.

2. Primary adrenal insufficiency causes lack of both cortisol and aldosterone.

3. Lab abnormalities seen in primary adrenal insufficiency include hyponatremia, hyperkalemia, and hypoglycemia.

4. Treatment of adrenal crisis includes IV glucose, saline, and hydrocortisone.

Part XIII
Hematologic and Immunologic Emergencies

83

Anaphylaxis and Allergic Reactions

Anaphylaxis is an acute life-threatening condition due to massive release of chemical mediators from mast cells and basophils throughout the body.

ETIOLOGY AND PATHOPHYSIOLOGY

Table 83–1 outlines the common causes of anaphylaxis and allergic reactions. Anaphylaxis is a type I hypersensitivity reaction that occurs in previously sensitized individuals. On re-exposure, the antigen combines with an antibody (IgE) bound to mast cells or basophils causing release of chemical mediators. The chemical mediators released include histamine, prostaglandins, platelet-activating factor, leukotrienes, and kallikrein, causing the symptoms of anaphylaxis. These mediators produce vasodilation, increased vascular permeability, and smooth muscle spasm resulting in hypotension, urticaria, bronchospasm, and angioedema of the skin, upper airway, and GI tract.

HISTORY

Patients often have a history of exposure to a bee sting, food substance, or drug. Anaphylaxis can include any combination of symptoms related to allergic reactions in addition to hypotension or airway compromise. Symptoms can begin seconds to minutes after contact with the offending antigen (Table 83–2).

PHYSICAL EXAMINATION

See Table 83–2 for physical examination findings in allergic reaction and anaphylaxis.

DIFFERENTIAL DIAGNOSIS

- Carcinoid syndrome
- Hereditary angioedema
- Vasovagal reaction
- Epiglottitis
- Status asthmaticus
- Foreign-body airway obstruction
- Mastocytosis
- Drug reaction
- Pulmonary embolus
- Myocardial infarction

DIAGNOSTIC EVALUATION

The diagnosis of anaphylaxis is based on history and physical exam.

MANAGEMENT

Patients who present with profound hypotension or imminent airway obstruction require IV epinephrine, IV

TABLE 83–1

Etiology of Allergic Reaction and Anaphylaxis

Foods	• Peanuts
	• Nuts
	• Shellfish
	• Milk
	• Eggs
	• Strawberries
Drugs	• Penicillin and related antibiotics
	• Sulfonamides
	• Nonsteroidal anti-inflammatory drugs
	— Aspirin
	— Ibuprofen
Venoms	• Hymenopteran stings
	— Yellow jacket
	• Fire ant
	• Rattlesnake
	• Jellyfish
Other	• Molds
	• Pollens
	• Danders
	• Radiographic contrast material

fluids, and pressors as required. Patients who present with hoarseness, stridor, dysphagia, or a lump in their throat should receive subcutaneous epinephrine. All patients should receive corticosteroids to prevent late phase reactions. Patients should also receive antihistamines—both H1 and H2 blockers—including diphenhydramine and ranitidine. Patients with persistent bronchospasm can be treated with beta-agonists (e.g., albuterol).

Patients who respond quickly and completely can be monitored for several hours and safely discharged home. These patients should be discharged on oral steroids, H1 and H2 blockers. Patients should also follow up with an allergist.

◆ KEY POINTS ◆

1. Anaphylaxis is a life-threatening condition due to massive release of bioactive substances from mast cells or basophils in response to an offending antigen.

2. Patients present with pruritus, cutaneous flushing, urticaria followed by a sense of fullness in the throat, shortness of breath, lightheadedness, and finally loss of consciousness minutes after exposure to an offending antigen.

3. Treatment includes epinephrine, corticosteroids, and antihistamines.

TABLE 83–2

Signs and Symptoms of Allergic Reaction and Anaphylaxis

Reaction	Sign	Symptom
Urticaria	Itching	Raised wheal
Rhinitis	Nasal congestion and runny nose	Mucosal edema
Conjunctivitis	Tearing and itchy eyes	Lid edema, injected sclera, and chemosis
Bronchospasm	Cough, chest tightness, dyspnea	Wheezing, tachypnea, retractions
Angioedema	Tingling of affected area	Swelling of lips, tongue, eyes, uvula, hands
Laryngeal edema	Hoarseness, dysphagia, lump in throat, airway obstruction,	Inspiratory stridor, intercostal and clavicular retractions, cyanosis
Hypotension	Dizziness, syncope, confusion	Hypotension, tachycardia
Gastrointestinal	Nausea, vomiting, abdominal pain, diarrhea	

ANGIOEDEMA

Angioedema of the tongue, lips, and face can occur in patients taking angiotensin-converting enzyme (ACE) inhibitors. Most cases of angioedema are mild and short lived. However, the airway can become rapidly occluded and needs to be monitored carefully. Symptoms may develop months after institution of therapy.

PATHOPHYSIOLOGY

Angiotensin-converting enzyme converts angiotensin I to angiotensin II, a potent vasoconstrictor and inactivates the potent vasodilator, bradykinin. ACE inhibitors block this reaction and thus cause the accumulation of bradykinin and angiotensin I leading to vasodilation, hypotension, and angioedema. In addition, it is not associated with an elevation in IgE. For these reasons angioedema is typically refractory to the standard medical treatment (e.g., epinephrine, antihistamines, and steroids) of allergic reactions.

MANAGEMENT

Management of angioedema is supportive, paying particular attention to the airway, which can rapidly become occluded.

Although epinephrine, antihistamines, and steroids are not proven to be beneficial, they are still used. Patients with moderate to severe swelling, dysphagia, or respiratory compromise need to be admitted and monitored closely. Patients with mild swelling and without airway compromise can be observed in the emergency department for several hours and then discharged home if the swelling resolves. Rebound or recurrent symptoms will not occur unless the patient is re-exposed to ACE inhibitors. Therefor, ACE inhibitors need to be immediately stopped and another antihypertensive agent should be prescribed.

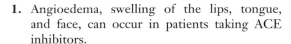

◆ KEY POINTS ◆

1. Angioedema, swelling of the lips, tongue, and face, can occur in patients taking ACE inhibitors.

2. Management is primarily supportive care, paying particular attention to airway compromise.

84

Transfusion Reactions

Transfusion reactions consist of any adverse effects caused by receiving blood products. Table 84–1 lists types of transfusion reactions.

PATHOPHYSIOLOGY

The most significant reaction is the hemolytic transfusion reaction (HTR), which occurs when incompatible red blood cells are attacked by circulating antibodies, activating the complement cascade and causing lysis to the red cells. During HTR, intravascular hemolysis causes activation of the coagulation system leading to inflammation, shock, and disseminated intravascular coagulation (DIC). Febrile reaction, the most common complication, is due to antigen-antibody reaction to transfused blood components, primarily leukocytes, platelets, and plasma. See Table 84–1 for other mechanisms of transfusion reactions.

HISTORY

Typically, patients are receiving blood when the acute transfusion reaction starts. Delayed reactions may occur hours to years later.

PHYSICAL EXAMINATION

See Table 84–1 for signs of transfusion complications.

DIFFERENTIAL DIAGNOSIS

- Allergic reaction or anaphylaxis due to medication
- Sepsis

DIAGNOSTIC EVALUATION

Lab studies include repeat type and crossmatch, CBC, electrolytes, creatinine, PT and PTT, haptoglobin, bilirubin, direct and indirect Coombs test, plasma free hemoglobin, LDH, and urinalysis for hemoglobin.

MANAGEMENT

If HTR is suspected, stop the infusion immediately and recheck blood identification information. Redraw blood sample for repeat ABO and Rh typing and direct antiglobulin testing. Aggressively hydrate in order to maintain a brisk diuresis for at least 24 hours. Furosemide may be required to maintain brisk diuresis. Treat hypotension with IV fluids and pressors as needed.

Treat febrile reactions with acetaminophen and meperidine as required. Treat allergic reactions with antihistamines, epinephrine, and steroids as indicated. Treat circulatory overload by slowing transfusion rate and diuretics as needed.

Patients with acute HTR, pulmonary complications, anaphylaxis, and sepsis will need to be admitted to an intensive care unit. Patients who have febrile reactions or

TABLE 84–1

Types of Transfusions Reactions

Complication	Etiology	Signs and Symptoms
Acute		

Hemolytic transfusion reaction (HTR)	• Circulating antibodies
	  — ABO incompatibility
	  — RH, or minor groups incompatibility
	• Blood type identification error
	• Mechanical damage
	  — Dilution of erythrocytes with hypotonic solutions
	  — Overheating or freezing transfusion
	  — Transfusion through small-bore needle
		• Fever
		• Chills
		• Heat or pain at infusion site
		• Low back pain
		• Flushing
		• Dyspnea
		• Tachycardia
		• Shock
		• Hemoglobinuria
		• Oliguria or anuria

Febrile (nonhemolytic) reaction	• Antigen-antibody reaction involving plasma, platelets, or WBC that are passively transfused with RBC • Most common in multiparous women or patients who have had multiple transfusions • Bacterial, viral, parasitic contamination	• Fever • Chills
Allergic reaction	• Passive transfer of allergens in plasma proteins • Most common in IgA-deficient patients • Platelet and leukocyte antibodies	• Skin erythema • Urticaria • Pruritus • Bronchospasm • Hypotension • Tachycardia • Shock
Circulatory overload	• Volume overload	• Dyspnea • Tachycardia • Hypertension • JVD • Pulmonary edema • Hypoxia
Delayed		
Delayed extravascular hemolytic reaction	• Antigen-antibody reaction	• 7–10 days • Asymptomatic
Infection	• Hepatitis B or C • HIV • HTLV-1	

TABLE 84–2

Treatment and Diagnosis of Transfusion Reactions

Complication	Diagnosis	Treatment
Acute		
Hemolytic transfusion reaction (HTR)	• Elevated plasma free hemoglobin • Elevated haptoglobin • Elevated bilirubin • Hemoglobinuria • Coombs test positive	• Stop transfusion • Treat hypotension — IV fluids — Dopamine • Aggressive hydration to maintain brisk diuresis • Furosemide or mannitol if oliguric
Febrile reaction	• Temperature >1°C, with chills	• Stop transfusion • Rule out HTR • Antipyretics — Acetaminophen — NSAIDs • Treat chills with meperidine
Allergic reaction	• Mild — Urticaria — Pruritus • Severe — Dyspnea — Bronchospasm — Hypotension — Tachycardia — Shock	• Discontinue transfusion while patient is evaluated and treated • Transfusion can be restarted if mild reaction and patient improves after treatment • Antihistamines — Diphenhydramine • Epinephrine for respiratory symptoms • Steroids — Solu-Medrol
Circulatory overload	• Dyspnea • Tachycardia • Hypertension • JVD • Pulmonary rales • Hypoxia	• Stop transfusion or slow down rate • Diuresis — Furosemide
Massive transfusion	• Bleeding — DIC — Platelet dysfunction — Coagulopathy • Hypothermia	• Treatment should be guided by clinical situation

allergic reactions can be safely discharged home once stabilized. Table 84–2 outlines the treatment of transfusion reactions.

◆ KEY POINTS ◆

1. Hemolytic transfusion reaction (HTR) is the most significant life-threatening complication of blood transfusions.

2. Symptoms of HTR include fever, chills, low back pain, flushing, dyspnea, tachycardia, shock, and hemoglobinuria.

3. Treatment includes immediately stopping the transfusion, IV hydration to maintain diuresis, and cardiorespiratory support as indicated.

Part XIV
Toxicologic Emergencies

85 General Approach to Overdose

Curious children and adults with psychiatric illness commonly present to the emergency department after toxic ingestions. In all cases, management of the airway, breathing, and circulation should take priority over further attempts at diagnosis. In the unconscious patient, hypoxia, hypoglycemia, and opiate overdose can be rapidly and safely treated by the empiric administration of oxygen, glucose, and naloxone. History is the key aspect of the evaluation of a toxic ingestion. Patients, family members, hospital records, pharmacies, and prehospital personnel may provide information about possible ingested substances.

The vital signs are the most important portion of the physical exam and a complete set, including oxygen saturation and rectal temperature, should be obtained in all patients. A careful physical examination should be conducted on all patients to rule out nontoxicologic causes of the patient's condition such as trauma. A 12-lead EKG and rhythm strip should be obtained on all patients to evaluate for arrhythmia. Finally, blood should be sent for chemistries, complete blood count, and serum and urine toxicology screens.

TOXIDROMES

Many overdose cases can be classified into one of four common "toxidromes." The sedative-hypnotic toxidrome is characterized by decreased level of consciousness, bradypnea, respiratory depression, hypotension, and miosis. Opiates, ethanol, benzodiazepines, and barbiturates are the most common causes of the sedative-hypnotic toxidrome.

The anticholinergic toxidrome is commonly caused by overdose of over-the-counter medicines such as benadryl or plants such as *Atropa belladonna*. Clinically, patients present with tachycardia, pyrexia, dry mouth, dilated pupils, and flushed skin.

The cholinergic toxidrome is characterized by salivation, lacrimation, urination, diarrhea, gastrointestinal distress, and emesis (mnemonic S-L-U-D-G-E). Agricultural exposure to organophosphate-based pesticides and industrial accidents are the primary means of exposure.

Cocaine, methamphetamine, ephedrine, and ecstasy (3,4-methylenedioxymethamphetamine) all can give rise to the sympathomimetic toxidrome. Hypertension, tachycardia, dilated pupils, and arrhythmias are to be expected.

MANAGEMENT

Activated charcoal has replaced ipecac-induced vomiting or oral-gastric lavage as the gastrointestinal decontamination method of choice. Ethanol, hydrocarbons, lithium, bromides, and alkalis do not adsorb to activated charcoal. Gastric lavage with a large-bore orogastric tube may still play a role in acute (within 1 hour of ingestion) life-threatening overdoses. Further management beyond activated charcoal and supportive measures should be based on the specific agent ingested.

◆ KEY POINTS ◆

1. The ABCs (airway, breathing, and circulation) are priorities in management of ingestions.

2. The sedative-hypnotic toxidrome is the most common and is characterized by a depressed level of consciousness.

3. The cholinergic toxidrome is characterized by salivation, lacrimation, urination, diarrhea, gastrointestinal distress, and emesis.

4. Activated charcoal has replaced gastric lavage as the gastrointestinal decontamination procedure of choice.

86 Acetaminophen

Due to the widespread use and availability of acetaminophen (APAP), it is an extremely common drug overdose.

PATHOPHYSIOLOGY

The majority of ingested APAP is metabolized in the liver and excreted in the urine. Of the remaining APAP, some is excreted unchanged in the urine and a similar amount is metabolized into a highly reactive intermediate by the hepatic P450 system. During therapeutic doses, this intermediate is conjugated to glutathione and excreted as an inactive substance. During overdose, hepatotoxicity occurs due to glutathione depletion, allowing the toxic intermediate to affect the liver.

HISTORY AND PHYSICAL EXAMINATION

The clinical presentation of APAP poisoning can be divided into four phases (Table 86–1).

DIFFERENTIAL DIAGNOSIS

- Reye's syndrome
- Infectious hepatitis
- Gastroenteritis
- Iron toxicity
- Mushroom toxicity
- Pancreatitis
- Renal failure
- Sepsis

DIAGNOSTIC EVALUATION

The diagnosis depends on a serum acetaminophen level. The measured acetaminophen level is then plotted on the Rumack-Matthew nomogram, which assesses the degree of toxicity. Treatment is required when the level is 150 μg/ml at 4 hours post ingestion. Other lab studies include liver enzymes, PT, bilirubin, electrolytes, BUN, creatine, and glucose.

MANAGEMENT

Address ABCs (airway, breathing, circulation). Gastric decontamination begins with the administration of activated charcoal. The mainstay of treatment for acetaminophen poisoning is the administration of the antidote *N*-acetylcysteine (NAC). NAC, a glutathione precursor, works by replenishing glutathione stores and inhibiting the binding of toxic metabolites to hepatic proteins. NAC should be administered within 8 hours of ingestion.

TABLE 86-1

Phases of Acetaminophen Poisoning

Stage	Time After Ingestion	Signs and Symptoms	Stage	Time After Ingestion	Signs and Symptoms

Phase 1	0.5–24 hours	• Anorexia
		• Nausea
		• Vomiting
		• Malaise
		• Pallor
		• Diaphoresis
			Phase 3	3–5 days	• Anorexia, nausea, vomiting, malaise may reappear
					• Progressive evidence of hepatic failure
					  — Jaundice
					  — Encephalopathy
					  — Coagulopathy
					• Renal failure
					• Coma
					• Death

Phase 2	24–72 hours	• Decreased GI symptoms • Right upper quadrant pain and tenderness • Increases in liver enzymes, PT, and bilirubin • Oliguria	Phase 4	4–10 days	• Resolution of hepatic dysfunction in survivors • Progression fulminant hepatic failure
Phase 3	3–5 days	• Peak liver function abnormalities			

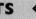

◆ KEY POINTS ◆

1. Acetaminophen causes hepatotoxicity through an intermediate metabolite when glutathione stores are depleted.

2. The Rumack-Matthew nomogram assesses the degree of toxicity.

3. Treatment of acetaminophen poisoning consists of GI decontamination, *N*-acetylcysteine (NAC), and supportive care.

87

Sedative-Hypnotics

Barbiturates and benzodiazepines are widely used for anxiety, insomnia, and pain disorders and as muscle relaxants, anticonvulsants, and hypnotics. In overdose, barbiturates cause respiratory depression and death. In contrast, benzodiazepines have a wide therapeutic index and seldom cause serious toxicity and death unless combined with other central nervous system (CNS) depressants (e.g., alcohol).

PATHOPHYSIOLOGY

Barbiturates and benzodiazepines enhance the function of γ-aminobutyric acid (GABA) especially in the CNS. GABA, an inhibitory neurotransmitter, causes depression of excitable tissues by opening chloride channels and inhibiting depolarization. Benzodiazepines bind to a specific site associated with the GABA receptor.

Barbiturates do not bind to any specific site, but appear to interact with other sites on the chloride channel. They suppress respiration by inhibiting the hypoxic and CO_2 response of chemoreceptors. Barbiturates also cause direct myocardial depression and inhibition of vascular smooth muscle.

HISTORY

History should include name, time, and amount of drugs ingested; known medical and psychiatric illnesses; and current drug therapy.

PHYSICAL EXAMINATION

Common findings on physical exam for both benzodiazepines and barbiturates include miosis, drowsiness, altered mental status, ataxia, hypotonia, and respiratory depression. In barbiturate toxicity, hypothermia, decreased GI motility, bradycardia, hypotension, and "barbiturate burns" (hemorrhagic bullous lesions over pressure points in deeply comatose patients) may also be seen.

DIFFERENTIAL DIAGNOSIS

- Overdose of other drugs (e.g., antidepressants-antipsychotics, ethanol, narcotics)
- Uremia and renal failure
- Post ictal state
- Liver failure
- Carbon monoxide poisoning
- Hypoglycemia
- Head trauma
- CVA
- CNS infections
- Hypothyroidism

DIAGNOSTIC EVALUATION

Lab studies include a CBC, electrolytes, BUN, creatine, glucose, creatine kinase, toxicology screen, beta HCG, and urinalysis. Patients down for a long time may have elevated potassium, creatine kinase, and rhabdomyolysis from muscle breakdown. Stuporous and comatose patients should have a chest x-ray to rule out aspiration, ECG, and a head CT scan. Patients with fever may require a lumbar puncture to rule out meningitis.

MANAGEMENT

Assess ABCs (airway, breathing, and circulation). The treatment of acute barbiturate and benzodiazepine poisoning is mainly supportive. Patients with CNS depression should be given naloxone, thiamine, and glucose (or check finger stick). Hypotension is treated with IV fluids and pressors as required. Rewarm patients with hypothermia. Gastrointestinal decontamination should begin with activated charcoal. Treat electrolyte abnormalities accordingly. For barbiturate toxicity, consider hemodialysis for patients with renal failure or who fail to respond to supportive measures. For pure acute benzodiazepine toxicity, flumazenil may be used with caution in patients with altered mental status and respiratory depression, but not in patients with the possibility of long-term benzodiazepine use or seizure

disorders. Patients who present with mild benzodiazepine or barbiturate toxicity can be observed in the emergency department until they recover. Psychiatric evaluation should occur as needed.

◆ KEY POINTS ◆

1. Barbiturates and benzodiazepines act by enhancing the inhibitory effect of GABA on the central nervous system.

2. Barbiturates produce sedation, hypnosis, coma, and death.

3. Benzodiazepines rarely cause death when ingested alone.

4. Treatment of both barbiturates and benzodiazepines includes supportive measures and GI decontamination.

5. Hemodialysis may be indicated for severe barbiturate toxicity.

6. Flumazenil is sometimes used cautiously to reverse benzodiazepine overdose.

88

Tricyclic Antidepressants

Tricyclic antidepressants (TCA) are used primarily for the treatment of major depression. In overdose, these drugs can produce life-threatening cardiac dysrhythmias, seizures, and coma.

PATHOPHYSIOLOGY

TCAs block norepinephrine and serotonin reuptake. In addition, they have anticholinergic, alpha blockade, and antihistaminic effects, which account for their major side effects. Cardiovascular toxicity results from TCA-induced sodium channel blockade, causing depolarization and conduction abnormalities.

HISTORY

Presentation of TCA overdose may range from asymptomatic to full cardiac arrest. Symptoms may include dry mouth, constipation, blurry vision, slurred speech, confusion, and drowsiness. History should include time, amount, and name of all agents ingested.

PHYSICAL EXAMINATION

Patients may present initially with tachycardia and hypertension due to norepinephrine reuptake blockade and anticholinergic effects. As norepinephrine is metab- olized, patients develop a catecholamine depletion state, which causes hypotension, bradycardia, and cardiogenic shock. Other signs include absent bowel sounds, urinary retention, dilated pupils, flushed hot skin, agitation, and dry mucous membranes.

DIFFERENTIAL DIAGNOSIS

- Hyperkalemia
- Neurologic disease
- Toxicity from other drugs
- Alcohol withdrawal
- Cardiac disease

DIAGNOSTIC EVALUATION

Lab studies include electrolytes, glucose, and toxicology screen. ECG often exhibits sinus tachycardia, right-axis deviation (RAD), and prolongation of PR, QRS, and QT intervals. A chest x-ray should be obtained to rule out aspiration pneumonia.

MANAGEMENT

Initial stabilization with standard advance cardiac life support (ACLS) protocols should be started. Patients require IV access, continuous cardiac monitoring and an ECG. Hypotension should be treated with IV fluids and pressors as needed. Seizures should be treated with diazepam or lorazepam. Sodium bicarbonate should be used for patients with ventricular dysrhythmias, with hypotension, who are unresponsive to fluids, or who have QRS widening greater than 100 ms. In addition, patients should receive activated charcoal for gastric decontamination.

◆ KEY POINTS ◆

1. Tricyclic antidepressant toxicity can cause life-threatening cardiac dysrhythmias.

2. Classic ECG findings include sinus tachycardia, prolongation of PR, QRS, and QT intervals.

3. Treatment includes general supportive care, sodium bicarbonate, and benzodiazepines for seizures.

89 Drugs of Abuse

HEROIN

Heroin is a commonly abused substance. It can be injected, smoked, or snorted and overdoses are characterized clinically by miosis (pinpoint pupils) and respiratory depression. Complications of heroin use include endocarditis, cellulitis, and cutaneous abscesses from skin injection. Endocarditis is typically "right-sided" (affecting the pulmonic and tricuspid valves) due to seeding of the bloodstream with non-sterile drug material. Tetanus and non-cardiogenic pulmonary edema are other serious complications of heroin use.

Treatment of heroin overdose is symptomatic and involves support of oxygenation and ventilation as well as administration of naloxone. Naloxone is an opiate receptor antagonist that works immediately to reverse the respiratory depression caused by heroin.

COCAINE

Cocaine is a compound synthesized from the South American plant *Erythroxylon coca*. It can be absorbed across mucosal surfaces such as the nasal epithelium and can also be snorted or smoked. Cocaine acts locally as an anesthetic and systemically as a stimulant through activation of the sympathetic nervous system and blockade of the reuptake of dopamine, serotonin, and norepinephrine. Clinically, cocaine affects multiple organ systems. Cocaine's cardiovascular effects include tachycardia, arrhythmias, hypertension, ischemia, and infarction. The spectrum of central nervous system effects range from simple euphoria to seizures and intracranial hemorrhages. Pulmonary effects include asthma, pulmonary hemorrhage, and noncardiogenic edema. The gastrointestinal effects of cocaine are most often the result of "body packers." Packers are people who ingest large quantities of cocaine packaged in bags in order to transport drugs.

Treatment of the cardiac effects of cocaine is identical to the treatment of atherosclerotic ischemic heart disease with the exception of the use of beta-blockade. Beta-blockers are contraindicated in cases of cocaine chest pain because their use leads to unopposed alpha-adrenergic stimulation and worsened vasoconstriction.

AMPHETAMINES

Methamphetamine (ice and crank), ecstasy, and ephedrine are all examples of amphetamines. Amphetamines refer to a class of compounds that cause a "hyper-adrenergic" state resulting from a decreased uptake and inhibition of the breakdown of endogenous catecholamines. This is manifested clinically by pupillary dilation, tachycardia, hypertension, insomnia, anorexia, and psychosis.

Treatment of amphetamine overdose is largely supportive. Activated charcoal is indicated in cases of suspected polysubstance overdose. Benzodiazepines can be used for treatment of seizures and agitation.

HALLUCINOGENS

Marijuana, phencyclidine (PCP), mushrooms, and lysergic acid diethylamide (LSD) are all commonly abused hallucinogenic drugs. They cause alterations in consciousness that allow persons who use them to escape from reality. The biggest danger in cases of hallucinogen overdose is injury to the patient while he or she is intoxicated. Treatment is supportive with benzodiazepines being the drug of choice to control acute psychomotor agitation. The effects of hallucinogens are temporary, with most patients returning to a normal mental status in 6–12 hours.

 KEY POINTS

1. Respiratory depression is the hallmark of heroin overdose.

2. Treatment of cocaine chest pain does not include beta-blocker use.

3. Ecstasy is a commonly misused designer amphetamine.

90 Toxic Alcohols

ISOPROPYL ALCOHOL

Isopropyl (rubbing) alcohol is commonly ingested as a substitute for ethanol or by curious children. It is rapidly absorbed through the gastrointestinal (GI) mucosa, though significant toxicity can result from transdermal absorption. Up to 50% is excreted unchanged by the kidneys while the remainder is metabolized in the liver to acetone. A potent central nervous system (CNS) depressant, ingestions of more than 200 mL are potentially lethal in adults.

Clinical Manifestations

Isopropyl alcohol predominantly affects the CNS and GI systems. Mild intoxication is characterized by headache, ataxia, confusion, and difficulty with fine motor control and may be difficult to differentiate from acute ethanol intoxication. Typical GI complaints include nausea, vomiting, and abdominal pain. These manifestations are due to the direct irritant effect of isopropyl alcohol on the GI tract. Coma, hypotension, renal failure (from rhabdomyolysis), and respiratory failure herald severe ingestions.

Diagnostic Evaluation

The clinical presentation of isopropyl alcohol ingestion mimics that of a myriad of other conditions including stroke, diabetic ketoacidosis (DKA), alcohol intoxication, and ethylene glycol and methanol poisoning. Blood should be obtained for toxicology, complete blood count, serum osmolality, serum, ketones, electrolytes, BUN, creatinine, and serum glucose. A urinalysis should be obtained. Isopropyl alcohol ingestion commonly causes an osmolal gap and ketosis without acidosis (as opposed to DKA, ethylene glycol, and methanol).

Treatment

Treatment of isopropyl alcohol ingestions is largely supportive. Activated charcoal does not absorb alcohols, but should be administered in suspected multi-agent overdoses. Hypotension and coma should be aggressively treated with fluids and vasopressors. Dialysis is indicated for refractory hypotension or isopropyl levels greater than 400 mg/dL.

METHANOL

Methanol is a clear, sweet fluid produced in the wood distilling process that is a component in a variety of commercial applications including glass cleaners, de-icing products, and antifreeze. Methanol is rapidly absorbed from the GI tract and converted to formaldehyde by alcohol dehydrogenase. Formaldehyde is then converted by aldehyde dehydrogenase to formic acid. Formic acid is responsible for much of the clinical toxicity in cases of methanol ingestions. Approximately 0.4 mL/kg of 40% methanol is considered a potentially lethal dose.

Clinical Manifestations

The CNS, eyes, and GI tract are the organs primarily affected in cases of methanol ingestions. Typical CNS findings include vertigo, headache, and extremity paresthesias, while the ocular manifestations have been likened to driving at night in a snowstorm. Nausea, vomiting, and abdominal pain are typical GI symptoms. Death occurs from respiratory arrest and may occur precipitously.

Diagnostic Evaluation

Blood should be obtained for toxicology, complete blood count, serum osmolality, serum, ketones, electrolytes, BUN, creatinine, and serum glucose. A urinalysis should be obtained as well. Methanol causes a severe anion gap metabolic acidosis due to the accumulation of formic and lactic acid. An osmolal gap is also present. Diabetic ketoacidosis, isopropyl alcohol or ethylene glycol poisoning, stroke, intracranial hemorrhage, hypoglycemia, seizures, and CNS infections should all be considered in the differential of methanol ingestions.

Treatment

Initial treatment of any overdose requires rapid assessment of the ABCs (airway, breathing, and circulation). If the patient presents within 1 to 2 hours of ingestion, gastric lavage may remove residual toxin. Activated charcoal is indicated if other substances were ingested. Administration of ethanol or 4-methylpyrazole effectively blocks the conversion of methanol (and ethylene glycol) to the toxic metabolites responsible for the clinical sequelae of ingestions. Dialysis is indicated for patients with severe metabolic acidosis, renal failure, or methanol levels greater than 25 mg/dL.

ETHYLENE GLYCOL

Ethylene glycol is a colorless, sweet tasting compound used in antifreeze, industrial, and automotive coolants and as a de-icer. Due to its appealing taste and the propensity for parents to store the substance in 2-L soda bottles, children are often the victims of accidental ingestions. Ethylene glycol is converted to glycoaldehyde by alcohol dehydrogenase. Glycoaldehyde is further degraded to oxalic acid, which is responsible for the clinical manifestations of ethylene glycol ingestions.

Clinical Manifestations

Clinically, ingestions of ethylene glycol are characterized by profound anion gap metabolic acidosis. Initially, ataxia, hallucinations, and CNS depression predominate. Progressive renal dysfunction (from the precipitation of calcium oxalate crystals in the renal parenchyma) develops 1–2 days after ingestion. SIRS may develop in severe ingestions.

Diagnostic Evaluation

Blood should be sent for chemistries, complete blood count, arterial blood gases, osmolality, and urinalysis (to look for crystalluria). In cases of ethylene glycol poisoning from ingestion of antifreeze, a Wood's lamp applied to a fresh sample of urine may cause a diagnostic fluorescence due to the additive fluorescein.

Treatment

Treatment of ethylene glycol is similar to that of methanol and revolves around the antagonism of alcohol dehydrogenase to prevent the formation of toxic metabolites.

◆   KEY POINTS   ◆

1. Isopropyl alcohol is frequently ingested as an ethanol substitute.

2. Treatment of isopropyl alcohol ingestion is largely supportive.

3. Methanol is broken down into formic acid, which may cause blindness.

4. Ethylene glycol causes a profound metabolic acidosis and renal dysfunction due to the formation of calcium oxalate crystals.

5. Treatment of both methanol and ethylene glycol ingestions is accomplished by competitive inhibition of alcohol dehydrogenase with either ethanol or 4-methylpyrazole and by dialysis.

91 Salicylates

Aspirin (acetylsalicylic acid or ASA) is a common analgesic found in prescription and over-the-counter preparations, making toxicity a common occurrence.

PATHOPHYSIOLOGY

Aspirin is absorbed in the stomach and small intestine where it is converted by plasma esterases to its active metabolite salicylic acid. At physiologic pH (7.4) almost all salicylate molecules are ionized. If pH decreases, more of the molecules become un-ionized and will freely cross cellular membranes.

Salicylate toxicity causes a metabolic acidosis by inhibiting the Krebs cycle leading to production of lactic acid. Salicylates also produce a respiratory alkalosis by directly stimulating the respiratory center causing hyperventilation.

HISTORY

Acute salicylate intoxication is usually intentional and patients frequently have psychiatric or prior overdose history. The history should include time and amount of ingestion. Typical symptoms include:

- Nausea and vomiting
- Tinnitus
- Epigastric pain
- Diaphoresis
- Hematemesis
- Mental status abnormalities: hallucinations, seizures, and coma

PHYSICAL EXAMINATION

Signs of acute salicylate toxicity include tachypnea, hyperpnea, tachycardia, hyperthermia, diaphoresis, pulmonary edema, and ataxia.

DIFFERENTIAL DIAGNOSIS

- Other intoxications: methanol or ethylene glycol
- Sepsis
- Pneumonia
- Gastritis
- Alcohol withdrawal

DIAGNOSTIC EVALUATION

A serum salicylate level should be obtained at presentation and every 2 hours until the level begins to decline. Toxicity occurs at greater than 25 mg/dL. However, management should be based on clinical findings and not the level alone.

Other lab studies include a toxicologic screen to rule out co-ingestion, ABG, electrolytes, glucose, BUN, creatine, urinalysis with urine pH, CBC, liver function tests, and PT and PTT. Patients should also have an ECG and CXR.

MANAGEMENT

First assess ABCs (airway, breathing, and circulation). Fluid and electrolyte disturbances should be treated accordingly. Hypotension should be treated with IV crystalloid. All patients should receive activated charcoal, since it reduces the absorption of salicylates. Whole bowel irrigation may be beneficial especially for patients who ingested sustained-release or enteric-coated preparations. Urinary alkalinization with sodium bicarbonate promotes renal elimination of salicylates.

Hemodialysis is the treatment of choice for severe toxicity because it can normalize acid-base and electrolyte abnormalities in addition to removing salicylates. Hemodialysis should be considered in patients with ARDS, altered mental status, severe acid-base disorders, renal failure, and clinical deterioration despite therapy.

 KEY POINTS

1. Salicylate toxicity causes a metabolic acidosis and respiratory alkalosis.

2. The main goals of treatment include correction of volume depletion and metabolic derangements, GI decontamination, and urinary alkalinization with sodium bicarbonate.

3. Hemodialysis is the treatment of choice for severe toxicity.

92 Anticholinergic Intoxication

Many classes of drugs possess anticholinergic activity including antihistamines, antipsychotics, antispasmodics, skeletal muscle relaxants, and tricyclic antidepressants. Common systemic anticholinergic drugs include atropine, benzotropine, dicyclomine, oxybutyrin, scopolamine, and glycopyrrolate. Many over-the-counter cold and allergy formulations have relatively strong anticholinergic properties. Certain plants (e.g., jimsonweed) and mushrooms (e.g., *Aminata muscaria*) also contain alkaloids with anticholinergic activity. Severe anticholinergic poisoning may result in death.

PATHOPHYSIOLOGY

Anticholinergic agents act as competitive inhibitors to acetylcholine at peripheral muscarinic acetylcholine receptors as well as central receptors. Muscarinic acetylcholine receptors are typically located at the site of parasympathetic nerve innervation. Sweat glands, salivary glands, and smooth muscle cells are usually the most affected structures. Absorption of orally ingested anticholinergic agents may be delayed since they cause gastric motility slowing.

HISTORY

Patients with anticholinergic poisoning are typically brought to the emergency department for the evaluation of an abnormal mental status. Details should be elicited regarding the time of onset of the abnormal mental state, how it progressed over time, currently used medications (including over-the-counter formulations), recent illnesses or fever, recent head trauma, the possibility of intentional or unintentional illicit drug exposure, and the use of herbal remedies.

PHYSICAL EXAMINATION

Individuals are often agitated, tachycardic, and hypertensive. They also typically present with delirium, warm dry flushed skin, a dry mouth, mydriasis (dilated pupils), jerky movements or choreoathetosis, and urinary retention. More significant toxicity may result in hyperthermia, respiratory arrest, coma, and death. Seizures are rare. A thorough physical examination is critical since the differential diagnosis includes many serious entities such as hypo- or hyperglycemia, hypoxia, meningitis, encephalitis, cerebral contusion, and intracranial hemorrhage. Blood analysis typically includes electrolytes, glucose, a complete blood count with differential, and toxicology screen. An electrocardiogram should also be performed and may reveal findings indicative of a tricyclic antidepressant overdose. Unless the history is undoubtedly consistent with anticholinergic intoxication, patients may also undergo CT imaging of the brain, as well as a lumbar puncture for analysis of their cerebral spinal fluid. The diagnosis of anticholinergic intoxication is primarily based on the history and the presence of typical features such as dilated pupils and flushed skin.

TREATMENT

Individuals suspected of an unknown oral poisoning usually warrant the administration of activated charcoal. Complications of anticholinergic intoxication should generally be treated with supportive care (e.g., the treatment of hyperthermia or seizures if present). Physostigmine will reverse the complications of anticholinergic intoxication by its action as a cholinesterase inhibitor, which ultimately increases the amount of available acetylcholine. Physostigmine may be used both diagnostically and therapeutically (0.5–1 mg IV) in an adult suspected of pure anticholinergic intoxication. However, since physostigmine is capable of causing hypersalivation, atrioventricular block, asystole, and seizures (especially among those with a tricyclic antidepressant overdose), its use is usually limited to severely ill patients whose diagnosis of anticholinergic intoxication is certain.

 KEY POINTS

1. Many classes of drugs possess anticholinergic activity including antihistamines, antipsychotics, antispasmodics, skeletal muscle relaxants, and tricyclic antidepressants.

2. Anticholinergic agents act as competitive inhibitors to acetylcholine at peripheral muscarinic acetylcholine receptors as well as central receptors.

3. The diagnosis of anticholinergic intoxication is primarily based on the history and the presence of typical features such as dilated pupils and flushed skin.

4. Since physostigmine is capable of causing hypersalivation, atrioventricular block, asystole, and seizures, its use is limited to severely ill patients whose diagnosis of anticholinergic intoxication is certain.

93 Carbon Monoxide Poisoning

Carbon monoxide (CO) is a clear, colorless, odorless, toxic gas that is slightly heavier than air, and is generated by the incomplete combustion of carbon-based compounds. Carbon monoxide poisoning (COP) is the most common cause of lethal poisoning in the United States resulting in at least 3,800 deaths per year. Accidental poisonings have been reported to result from many sources including house fires, fireplaces, home heating units, automobiles, boats, charcoal grills, and propane-powered machinery. As many as one-third of accidental carbon monoxide poisonings may go unrecognized.

PATHOPHYSIOLOGY

Carbon monoxide readily crosses the alveolar-capillary membrane in the lungs and binds to hemoglobin with a 200-fold greater affinity than oxygen to form carboxyhemoglobin (COHb). The affinity of CO for fetal hemoglobin is even greater. The half-life of COHb is believed to be approximately 4 to 6 hours on room air at sea level (1 atm), 90 minutes on 100% oxygen at 1 atm, and 20 minutes on 100% oxygen at 3 atm. In the presence of COHb, oxygen availability to the tissues is reduced by the lowered oxygen-carrying capacity of the blood as well as by a leftward shift in the oxyhemoglobin dissociation curve. The cellular utilization of oxygen may also be impaired. Renal dysfunction may result from rhabdomyolysis. Neurologic toxicity from CO pri-

marily results in white matter demyelination and hallmark grey matter necrosis within the globus pallidus.

HISTORY

The high incidence of unrecognized carbon monoxide poisoning is likely due to the difficulty in detecting the poisonous gas as well as the nonspecific, viral-like symptoms that it creates. A thorough history is critical and may be the only means of diagnosis in many cases. Symptoms of patients with COP may include the following: headache, general malaise, lethargy, fatigue, dyspnea, nausea, confusion, angina, seizures, and coma. Additional clues to the diagnosis of carbon monoxide poisoning may include multiple individuals presenting from the same location with similar symptoms, known exposure to carbon monoxide producing equipment, and the beginning of cooler weather that may prompt the re-ignition of fireplaces and dormant heating units.

PHYSICAL EXAMINATION

Similar to symptoms, the findings on physical examination of patients with COP are usually nonspecific. Patients may exhibit hemodynamic abnormalities that result from the cardiovascular effects. Tachypnea may be present. The "cherry red" skin discoloration often ascribed to COP is exceedingly rare and may only exist as the COHb level approaches 80%. Patients may exhibit alterations in mental status as well as focal neurologic findings and seizure.

DIAGNOSIS

The partial pressure of oxygen in the arteries (PaO_2) may be normal or low. Transcutaneous blood oxygen saturation monitors are typically unable to distinguish oxyhemoglobin from carboxyhemoglobin, and thus often report a falsely high measurement. Similarly, the oxyhemoglobin saturation as determined indirectly by mathematical calculation in blood gas analysis typically generates falsely elevated measurements. Normal COHb levels are usually zero among nonsmoking rural-living individuals, and 2–10% in smokers and urban dwellers. A COHb level elevated over 10% is usually indicative of an abnormally high CO exposure. An electrocardiogram should be performed on all patients, and a pregnancy test on all women suspected of COP. Hemodynamically unstable individuals and those of concern for an acute coronary syndrome should receive continuous cardiac monitoring for dysrhythmia detection as well as blood cardiac enzyme evaluation. Patients with altered levels of consciousness typically require CT imaging of the brain to rule out other etiologies.

TREATMENT

Victims of COP require general supportive care and the delivery of supplemental oxygen. Patients should be placed on high-flow oxygen by non-rebreather face mask to hasten the dissociation of COHb. Controversy exists over the use of hyperbaric oxygen (HBO) for the treatment of COP. Although HBO therapy has numerous physiologic effects, it is believed to benefit patients with COP primarily by increasing the atmospheric pressure around the patient (e.g., 3 atm) and enabling the delivery of supranormal quantities of supplemental oxygen. There appear to be short-term neurobehavioral and cognitive benefits from HBO, compared to oxygen, delivered at sea level for patients with COP. However, the extent and duration of the benefits are still unclear. In general, patients considered for HBO therapy include those with neurologic deficits, cardiac abnormalities, and women who are pregnant.

◆ KEY POINTS ◆

1. Carbon monoxide is a clear, colorless, odorless, toxic gas generated by the incomplete combustion of carbon-based compounds.

2. Symptoms of COP are nonspecific.

3. Consider CO poisoning in patients with headache and vague complaints during the winter months.

4. Clues to the diagnosis of carbon monoxide poisoning may include multiple individuals presenting from the same location with similar symptoms, known exposure to carbon monoxide producing equipment, and the beginning of cooler weather that may prompt the re-ignition of fireplaces and dormant heating units.

5. Victims of COP require general supportive care and the delivery of supplemental oxygen.

6. Treatment with hyperbaric oxygen should be considered.

94 Digoxin Toxicity

Digitalis is a plant-derived cardiac glycoside that is currently used in the treatment of congestive heart failure and atrial fibrillation. Glycoside-containing plants include foxglove, oleander, lily of the valley, red squill, and rhododendron. Digoxin is the most common preparation of digitalis in the United States, whereas digitoxin is more popular in Europe, Canada, and Latin America. Digoxin toxicity may result from acute or chronic ingestions. Older age and chronic digoxin toxicity are associated with a higher mortality. As little as 1 mg of digoxin in children and 3 mg in adults may be toxic. Just a few leaves from the foxglove or oleander plants may contain even larger doses of the active drug.

PATHOPHYSIOLOGY

Digoxin causes increased mycocardial contractility as well as the slowing of electrical conduction at the atrioventricular (AV) node. Additionally, vagal tone is potentiated and automaticity in the Purkinje fibers is increased. Digoxin acts as an inhibitor of the membrane-bound sodium potassium-ATPase ion exchanger. This ion exchanger normally works to pump sodium and potassium back against their concentration gradients (to the extracellular and intracellular spaces, respectively) following cellular depolarization (Fig. 94–1A). When this ion exchanger is inhibited, intracellular concentrations of sodium and calcium rise, as does the extracelluar concentration of potassium (Fig. 94–1B). Improved cardiac contractility is believed to result from the increased intracellular concentration of calcium. At therapeutic levels of digoxin, these electrolyte changes are minimal; however, in the presence of digoxin toxicity, extracellular concentrations of potassium and intracellular concentrations of sodium and calcium may rise markedly. Hypomagnesemia, hypokalemia, and hypercalcemia make individuals more susceptible to digoxin toxicity. Following an acute ingestion, peak digoxin levels are usually achieved within 1.5 to 2 hours, and steady-state concentrations within 6 to 8 hours. Falsely elevated digoxin levels may result if the blood is drawn too soon after oral ingestion. The serum half-life of digoxin (large volume of distribution, renally excreted) is 40 hours, and digitoxin (small volume of distribution, hepatically metabolized) is 7 days.

HISTORY

A complete history should include details about the time of ingestion, dose of pills taken, number of pills ingested, recent illness or dehydration, past medical history, and current medications. Symptoms associated with digoxin toxicitiy include malaise, fatigue, headache, weakness, nausea, vomiting, diarrhea, visual abnormalities such as blurring or color aberrations, palpitations, confusion, and seizures.

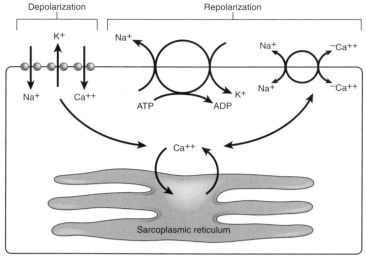

A   **Cardiac Muscle Cell**

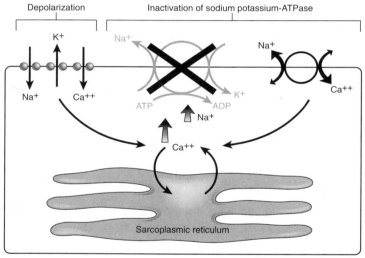

B   **Cardiac Muscle Cell Exposed to Digoxin**   **Figure 94–1**

PHYSICAL EXAMINATION

Digoxin toxicity is usually associated with bradycardia, which may also be accompanied by hypotension. There are no signs on the physical examination specific only to digoxin toxicity.

DIAGNOSTIC EVALUATION

The most common electrocardiographic abnormality associated with digoxin toxicity is premature ventricular contractions. Cardiac rhythm disturbances may include bradycardia, sinoatrial arrest, junctional escape, second- or third-degree AV block, tachydysryhthmias (e.g., accelerated junctional, atrial tachycardia, ventricular tachycardia), torsades de pointes, and ventricular fibrillation.

Laboratory blood work should include a digoxin level and an electrolyte panel (including potassium, magnesium, and calcium). A complete blood count and cardiac enzymes may also be indicated. A normal digoxin level is 0.5–2 ng/mL, and that for digitoxin is 10–30 ng/mL. It is important to note that although medication levels are neither sensitive nor specific in the diagnosis of digoxin toxicity (i.e., toxic individuals may have a level within the normal range, and therapeutic individuals may have a level slightly above the normal range), very high levels (especially in the setting of chronic ingestion) likely represent toxicity. The diagnosis of digoxin toxicity is made clinically and typically relies on a history of overdose associated with characteristic dysrhythmias. Serum potassium levels greater than 5.5 meq/L in the setting of a digoxin overdose are indicative of severe poisoning.

TREATMENT

Patients suspected of digoxin toxicity should receive continuous cardiac monitoring. Following an oral digoxin overdose, patients should be treated with activated charcoal. Repeated doses of charcoal may be more helpful in cases of digitoxin toxicity due to the much larger enterohepatic circulation of the drug compared to digoxin. Patients with hypokalemia (usually seen in chronic toxicity) should generally not receive supplemental potassium unless their potassium level is lower than approximately 3.3 meq/L. Hypomagnesemia may be corrected slowly as well. Hyperkalemia greater than 5.5 meq/L should be treated with sodium bicarbonate (1 meq/kg IV), glucose (0.5 meq/kg IV), regular insulin (0.1 u/kg IV), and polystyrene sulfonate (i.e., Kayexalate 0.5 g/kg PO). Calcium is generally contraindicated for hyperkalemic patients due to the concern of creating cardiac tetany among cells that already contain higher-than-normal concentrations of calcium, and worsening dysrhythmias. Indications for digitalis antibody therapy typically include significant dysrhythmia or a serum potassium greater than 5 meq/L. Digibind consists of the Fab fragments of digoxin-specific antibodies, and acts to bind digoxin (and other digitalis preparations to a lesser extent) thus forming an inactive complex that is highly excretable in the urine. The administration of Digibind may lead to a lowering of the serum potassium level due to the intracellular shift of potassium as the sodium potassium-ATPase is reactivated. The number of Digibind vials necessary is variable and depends on digoxin level and body weight. Bradycardia or heart block may be responsive to atropine (0.5–3 mg IV), but may also require the placement of a temporary pacemaker. Phenytoin and lidocaine are the antiarrhythmics of choice for treating ventricular dysrhythmias.

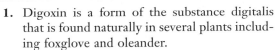

◆ KEY POINTS ◆

1. Digoxin is a form of the substance digitalis that is found naturally in several plants including foxglove and oleander.

2. Digoxin inhibits the membrane-bound sodium potassium-ATPase ion exchanger.

3. The diagnosis of digoxin toxicity is made clinically and typically relies on a history of overdose associated with characteristic dysrhythmias.

4. Hyperkalemia greater than 5 meq/L and significant dysrhythmias in the setting of digoxin toxicity typically warrant Digibind (Fab fragments of digoxin-specific antibodies).

5. Digibind combines with digoxin to form a complex that is highly excretable in the urine.

Part XV
Environmental Emergencies

Hypothermia

Hypothermia is defined as a core body temperature that is less than 35°C (95°F). As the temperature drops below this level, the body is unable to generate enough heat to perform functions efficiently. "Mild hypothermia" is defined as a core body temperature of 32 to 35°C (90 to 95°F). A core body temperature of 30 to 32°C (86 to 90°F) constitutes "moderate hypothermia," and temperatures less than 30°C (86°F) indicate "severe hypothermia." Hypothermia not only occurs in extreme environments, but also occurs in moderate climates including air-conditioned indoors. Factors associated with an increased susceptibility to hypothermia include extremes of age, significant skin barrier disruption, metabolic diseases (e.g., hypothyroidism, hypoadrenalism, hypoglycemia, and hypopituitarism), sepsis, medications that alter the body's ability to generate heat (e.g., beta-blockers), and an altered sensorium (e.g., alcohol intoxication) that may prevent appropriate behavioral changes such as adding clothes and moving to warmer environments.

PHYSIOLOGY

The body normally loses heat via conduction (i.e., heat transfer from a warmer object to a cooler one during direct contact), convection (i.e., heat loss due to movement and the disruption of the warm air layer surrounding the body), radiation (i.e., heat transfer into a cooler environment via electromagnetic waves), and evaporation (i.e., the change in state of liquid water to gaseous vapor). The body generates heat by increasing the metabolic rate, shunting blood centrally from the periphery, shivering, and behavioral responses. The initial response to hypothermia includes tachycardia, tachypnea, and increased cardiac output. As hypothermia worsens, complications may include tissue hypoxia, a leftward shift of the oxyhemoglobin dissociation curve, impaired renal concentrating ability with subsequent "cold diuresis," third spacing of intravascular plasma, bradycardia, hypotension, and hypoventilation. Later, depressed consciousness, disseminated intravascular coagulation, life-threatening cardiac dysrhythmias, coma, and death may ensue. The risk of cardiac dysrhythmia does not typically occur until severe hypothermia ensues. The Osborn (i.e., "J") wave (Fig. 95–1) on the electrocardiogram is a slow, positive deflection at the end of the QRS complex that is characteristic of hypothermia, but not specific to the diagnosis.

HISTORY

A detailed and complete history should be elicited to identify the potentially reversible metabolic, medication-related, and environmental causes of the hypothermia.

PHYSICAL EXAMINATION

Since most clinical thermometers only measure as low as 34.4°C (94°F), a specialized low-reading thermome-

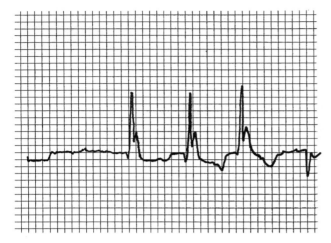

Figure 95–1   Osborne wave.

ter may be necessary for accurate temperature measurement. Rectal temperature measurement is the most accurate, readily available, noninvasive measure of body temperature. Vital signs and the electrocardiogram should be monitored continuously. Physical examination may reveal signs of reversible metabolic disease, or evidence of trauma that may have predisposed the patient to increased heat losses and subsequent hypothermia. Care should be taken not to move patients with severe hypothermia vigorously due to increased cardiac irritability. Patients with significant hypothermia typically require laboratory blood evaluation including glucose, electrolytes, BUN, creatinine, complete blood count, and coagulation studies. Further studies that may be indicated include an arterial blood gas, a toxicologic screen, and thyroid as well as liver function tests. Chest and abdominal x-rays may be indicated. If trauma is suspected appropriate radiographic imaging should be obtained.

TREATMENT

The treatment of hypothermia includes supportive care and rewarming. Airway and hemodynamic stabilization takes precedence over rewarming. Patients typically require the placement of two large-bore intravenous catheters. The administration of antibiotics, stress dose steroids, and thyroid hormone should be individualized. Rewarming techniques are classified as passive (e.g., insulation), active external (e.g., warm water immersion, heated blankets, radiant heat), and active internal (e.g., warm gas inhalation, heated intravenous fluids, peritoneal lavage, pleural lavage, mediastinal lavage, and cardiopulmonary bypass). Although the best rewarming strategy for hemodynamically stable patients remains controversial, hemodynamically unstable patients should be rewarmed rapidly.

Cardiopulmonary bypass and water immersion are the fastest means of rewarming. Due to metabolism slowing, hypothermic patients may tolerate longer than usual periods of hypoperfusion and anoxia. For this reason, death should generally not be pronounced in a hypothermic patient until they have been rewarmed.

◆ KEY POINTS ◆

1. Hypothermia is defined as a core body temperature that is less than 35°C (95°F).

2. Hypothermia not only occurs in extreme environments, but also occurs in moderate climates including air-conditioned indoors.

3. The risk of cardiac dysrhythmia does not typically occur until severe hypothermia (i.e., core temperature less than 30°C [86°F]) ensues.

4. Care should be taken not to move patients with severe hypothermia vigorously as their increased cardiac irritability coupled with the harsh movement may induce a lethal dysrhythmia.

5. Rewarming techniques are classified as passive, active external, and active internal.

6. Death should generally not be pronounced in hypothermic patients until they have been rewarmed.

96 Heat Illness

The possible manifestations of heat illness are on a continuum and include (more benign to severe): heat edema, heat rash, heat cramps, heat syncope, heat exhaustion, and heat stroke. Heat stroke accounts for more than 4,000 deaths annually in the United States, and is the second leading cause of death in young athletes. The body's regulation of temperature within a specific range is complex but critical for proper physiologic function. Individuals at increased risk for developing heat illness include those who are dehydrated, at extremes of age, obese, alcoholics, have cardiovascular disease, or take medications such as antipsychotics, anticholinergics, or cardiovascular medications that may interfere with the body's temperature regulating mechanisms.

PATHOPHYSIOLOGY

Body temperature is the final result of the total heat loss and heat gained. Heat transfer occurs when a gradient exists between the temperatures of two objects. The transfer of heat occurs via conduction (i.e., during direct contact), convection (i.e., disruption of the warm air layer surrounding an object), radiation (i.e., electromagnetic waves), and evaporation (i.e., the change in state of liquid water to gaseous vapor). Fever, as seen with infections, differs from hyperthermia in that it results from a resetting of the temperature set point in the hypothalamus, thereby enabling medications that readjust the set point (e.g., acetaminophen or aspirin) to be effective.

HISTORY

A thorough history including a description of recent activity, location, preexisting medical conditions, current medications, drug allergies, recreational drug use, and the living environment may provide insight into the cause of the heat illness.

PHYSICAL EXAMINATION

Rectal temperature measurement is the most accurate, readily available, noninvasive measure of body temperature. Milder forms of heat illness may not present with significantly elevated body temperatures. A complete physical examination should be performed and include an accurate neurologic evaluation. Ancillary tests such as blood analysis and imaging studies are not always necessary and should be individualized to the patient.

TREATMENT

Heat edema is typically benign and presents as swollen feet and ankles. Those with cardiovascular disease and the elderly are believed to be more susceptible. Heat edema is usually minimal and primarily results from vasodilation with vascular leak. The edema is treated by extremity elevation and usually resolves after a couple of weeks (i.e., after climate acclimatization) or a return to a cooler environment. Heat rash (i.e., prickly heat) is a relatively minor illness that results from the blockage of sweat gland pores and is frequently accompanied by staphylococcal infection. Heat rash typically presents with pruritic vesicles on an erythematous base on clothed areas of skin and may take weeks to completely resolve. The treatment of heat rash typically includes topical chlorhexidine antibacterial cream, 1% salicylic acid for small areas, and oral antibiotics for more severe manifestations.

Heat cramps are severe muscle cramps resulting from overexertion in hot environments. They typically occur just after the cessation of activity. Salt deficiency is believed to play a major role in this relatively benign illness. Milder cases of heat cramps may be treated with an oral salt solution, while more severe cases typically require intravenous normal saline or small amounts of hypertonic saline. Heat syncope (i.e., temporary loss of consciousness) is caused by brain hypoperfusion and results from the relative hypotension created by peripheral vasodilation and vascular leak. Dehydration is a predisposing factor. The condition typically resolves with rehydration.

Heat exhaustion occurs further along the spectrum of severity of heat illness and primarily results from dehydration and body salt depletion. The illness typically manifests as sweating, weakness, fatigue, headache, nausea, and dizziness. Core body temperature may be only slightly elevated and is usually less than 40°C (104°F). Milder cases of heat exhaustion may respond well to oral salt solutions; however, more severe cases usually require hospitalization, blood chemistry analysis, and intravenous re-hydration.

Heat stroke is a life-threatening form of heat illness that typically occurs in patients with a core temperature greater than 41°C (106°F). Core temperatures of this magnitude result in loss of thermoregulation, tissue damage, and multisystem failure. Neurologic dysfunction is the hallmark of heat stroke and is frequently associated with cerebral edema. Patients typically present extremely dehydrated (often with dry skin) and may exhibit confusion, disorientation, ataxia, psychosis, seizures, unconsciousness, and hemodynamic instability. Treatment of heat stroke typically includes intensive care monitoring, blood chemistry analysis, rehydration and rapid body cooling. The preferred method for rapid cooling is ice water immersion. However, if an immersion tank is not available, evaporative cooling using cold water mists and fans may be effective. Other less effective but potentially useful cooling techniques include ice packs, cooling blankets, peritoneal lavage, and cardiopulmonary bypass.

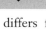

◆ KEY POINTS ◆

1. Fever, as seen with infections, differs from hyperthermia in that it results from a resetting of the temperature set point in the hypothalamus, thereby enabling medications that readjust the set point (e.g., acetaminophen or aspirin) to be effective.

2. Milder forms of heat illness may not present with significantly elevated body temperatures.

3. Heat stroke is a life-threatening form of heat illness that typically occurs in patients with core temperatures greater than 41°C (106°F).

4. Neurologic dysfunction is the hallmark of heat stroke and is frequently associated with cerebral edema.

97

Electrical Injury

In the United States, there are 1,000 deaths annually that result from electrical injury. Electrical exposures may be divided into low voltage (<1000 volts) and high voltage (>1000 volts). Although high voltage has a much greater potential for injury, low-voltage injuries are the most common and account for nearly half of all deaths caused by electrocution. Complications from electrical injury include vascular spasm, burns, bone fractures, gastrointestinal injury, cataracts, tympanic membrane rupture, central and peripheral neurologic injury, myonecrosis, rhabdomyolysis, renal failure, cardiac dysrhythmias, myocardial infarction, cardiac arrest, respiratory arrest, and death. Electrical injury during pregnancy is highly associated with fetal morbidity and mortality.

PATHOPHYSIOLOGY

Tissue damage resulting from electricity is due to the direct effects of the current as well as the thermal energy generated. Injury severity is directly related to the type of current (i.e., alternating or direct), current intensity (i.e., amperage), current path, voltage, the duration of contact, and the resistance of tissues. Ohm's law states that amperage = voltage/resistance. Injury is mostly related to the amount of amperage, and, to a lesser extent, the resistance of the tissues. The following are tissues with different electrical resistances (least resistance to greatest): nerve, blood, muscle, skin, tendon,

and fat. Up to 30% of patients sustaining an electrical shock experience a cardiac dysrhythmia. The most common dysrhythmias are sinus tachycardia and premature ventricular contractions. Ventricular fibrillation most frequently results from lower energy alternating current (AC) exposures, while asystole is more common following exposure to larger energy direct current (DC). Lightning, with its extremely large energy levels, tends to "splash" or "flash over" humans, and rarely causes deep current-related, soft-tissue injury. However, the large pressure gradients and subsequent shock wave that are generated by lightning strikes may cause "blast" injuries similar to explosives.

HISTORY

The diagnosis of electrical injury is usually based on the history. A complete history should be obtained with as much information as possible about the electrical source (e.g., voltage, amperage, type of current [AC versus DC]), body contact point, duration of electrical exposure, losses of consciousness, and postexposure symptoms.

PHYSICAL EXAMINATION

As in other trauma, the physical examination should first focus on evaluation of the more critical cardiovascular and pulmonary systems. A thorough assessment of soft-tissue injuries should also be performed. The overall neurovascular status should be assessed and re-evaluated frequently. All patients should receive an electrocardiogram and be placed on continuous cardiac monitoring. Laboratory blood analysis is typically warranted in more significant exposures and usually includes a complete blood count, electrolytes, BUN, creatine, creatine kinase, cardiac isoenzymes, myoglobin, and coagulation studies. Amylase, lipase, and liver function tests are indicated in the setting of suspected gastrointestinal injury. Imaging with plain films and computed tomography should be individualized and may include a trauma series (i.e., cervical spine, chest, and pelvic x-rays).

TREATMENT

The management of patients with significant electrical injury typically includes the combination of trauma, burn, and cardiac care. All severely injured patients should receive at least one large-bore (e.g., 16- or 14-gauge) intravenous catheter. Since extensive deep-tissue injury may exist under normal skin, fluid calculations proportional to the total surface area burned are not helpful.

Initial treatment should focus on general supportive care including appropriate dysrhythmia management. A urinary catheter is usually required to assure adequate urine output. Victims of lightning strikes who do not suffer cardiac or respiratory arrest tend to recover well with supportive treatment. Rhabdomyolysis resulting from significant muscle injury should typically be treated with alkalinization of the urine to promote myoglobin solubility in the urine, and intravenous fluids to maintain a urine output of 1–1.5 mL/kg/hr. Furosemide or mannitol may also help to prevent renal complications in certain cases of rhabdomyolysis by further increasing diuresis and myoglobin clearance.

Burn treatment typically includes debridement and antibiotic dressings (e.g., Silvadene). Significant burns should be treated in a burn center if possible. Tissue ischemia resulting in confined swelling may require an emergent escharotomy or fasciotomy for decompression. Patients should be admitted to the hospital for at least 24 hours of cardiac observation in the following circumstances: hemodynamic instability, loss of consciousness, abnormal electrocardiogram, dysrhythmia, history of cardiac disease, significant cardiac risk factors, hypoxia, or chest pain.

Pregnant patients beyond the first trimester should usually receive obstetrical consultation. Women within the first trimester may be discharged, but should be counseled about the increased risk of subsequent spontaneous abortion associated with electrocution. Patients with labial burns of the mouth are at increased risk for delayed labial artery hemorrhage and should be followed closely. Asymptomatic victims of low-voltage electrical exposure with a normal electrocardiogram may be safely discharged home after 6 hours of cardiac monitoring.

◆ KEY POINTS ◆

1. Electrical exposures may be divided into low voltage (<1000 volts) and high voltage (>1000 volts), with high voltage having a much greater potential for injury.

2. Injury severity is directly related to the type of current (i.e., alternating or direct), current intensity (i.e., amperage), current path, voltage, the duration of contact, and the resistance of tissues.

3. The following are tissues with different electrical resistances (least resistance to greatest): nerve, blood, muscle, skin, tendon, and fat.

4. Extensive deep-tissue injury may exist under normal skin.

Part XVI
Pediatric
Emergencies

98 Congenital Heart Disease

Congenital heart disease occurs in approximately 8 out of every 1,000 live births. Cyanotic lesions result in marked right-to-left shunting and mixing of desaturated venous blood with arterial blood. Acyanotic defects result in right-to-left shunting with increased pulmonary blood flow (Table 98–1).

CYANOTIC LESIONS

Tetralogy of Fallot

Tetralogy of Fallot (TOF) represents 5–7% of all congenital heart defects diagnosed. It is characterized by a ventricular septal defect (VSD), an aorta that overrides both the right and left ventricles, varying degrees of right ventricular outflow tract obstruction, and hypertrophy of the right ventricle (Fig. 98–1).

Cyanosis in TOF is due to right-to-left shunting across a large VSD and decreased pulmonary blood flow. The degree of shunting is determined by the degree of right ventricular outflow tract obstruction. Thus, a substantial proportion of blood travels from the superior vena cava, to the right ventricle through the right atrium, then across the VSD to the left ventricle into the systemic circulation. In the neonatal period, pulmonary blood flow is maintained by a patent ductus arteriosus, which allows blood to travel back to the right from the systemic circulation. Patients with TOF typically present with cyanosis in the neonatal period. Tet spells are episodes of tachypnea, worsening cyanosis, and hypoxia that occur during periods of increased right-to-left shunting. These spells can last from minutes to hours and may lead to severe respiratory acidosis, syncope, and even death. Physical examination may reveal a palpable right ventricular heave or systolic thrill, which is indicative of turbulent flow over the abnormal right ventricular outflow tract. The pulmonic component of the second heart sound is typically inaudible and a systolic ejection murmur may be heard.

The EKG typically reveals right ventricular hypertrophy (RVH) and right axis deviation (RAD). A boot-shaped heart (the so-called coer en sabot) is the classic finding on chest radiography. Echocardiography provides a means to non-invasively diagnose TOF and can quantify the degree of RVOT. Cardiac catheterization is the diagnostic gold standard and can be used to plan surgical repair.

Surgical repair is accomplished by anastomosis of a systemic artery to a pulmonary artery (PA). Common techniques include the Waterston (ascending aorta to PA), Potts (descending aorta to PA), and Blalock-Taussig (subclavian artery to PA).

Transposition of the Great Arteries

Transposition of the great arteries (TOGA) occurs when the aorta communicates with the right ventricle and the pulmonary artery is connected to the left ventricle (Fig. 98–2). When this occurs, there is complete separation of the right and left circulatory systems and a right to left conduit (either patent foramen ovale, patent ductus

TABLE 98–1

Classification of Pediatric Congenital Heart Disease

1. Left-to-right shunts (acyanotic):
   - Patent ductus arteriosus
   - Ventricular septal defect
   - Atrial septal defect
2. Right-to-left shunts (cyanotic):
   - Transposition of the arteries
   - Tetralogy of Fallot
   - Truncus arteriosus
   - Tricuspid atresia
   - Total anomalous pulmonary venous return

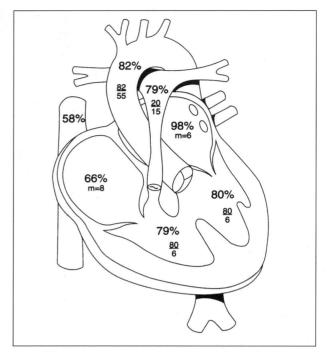

Figure 98–1 Tetralogy of Fallot. Typical anatomic and hemodynamic findings include: (a) an anteriorly displaced infundibular septum, resulting in subpulmonary stenosis, a large ventricular septal defect and overriding of the aorta over the muscular septum; (b) hypoplasia of the pulmonary valve, main and brain pulmonary arteries; (c) equal right and left ventricular pressures; (d) a right-to-left shunt at ventricular level, with a systemic oxygen saturation of 82%.

arteriosus, ventricular septal defect, or atrial septal defect) is required for survival.

TOGA is clinically characterized by varying degrees of cyanosis and tachypnea. A loud, single S2 and harsh, holosystolic ventricular septal murmur are common physical exam findings. RVH and RAD are commonly seen on EKG, and chest radiography reveals increased pulmonary vascularity and an egg-shaped heart. Echocardiography and cardiac catheterization can be used for definitive diagnosis. Prostaglandin E can be used as a temporizing measure to maintain the patency of the ductus arteriosus until surgical repair can be accomplished.

Ebstein's Anomaly

Ebstein's anomaly refers to the congenital defect in which the septal and posterior leaflets of the tricuspid valve are displaced into the right ventricle resulting in an "atrialized" right ventricle (Fig. 98–3). Children typically present with congestive heart failure, cyanosis, or paroxysmal episodes of supraventricular tachycardia. Physical examination reveals widely split first and second heart sounds and a systolic tricuspid regurgitation murmur at the left lower sternal border. Bilateral rales and hepatomegaly indicate congestive heart failure.

Electrocardiographically, Ebstein's anomaly is characterized by tall broad P waves and first-degree atrioventricular block. Chest radiography is typically

non-specific with cardiomegaly being the most common finding. Echocardiography is the mainstay of diagnosis and is used to determine the degree of right atrial dilatation. Surgical repair of Ebstein's anomaly is accomplished by creating an arterial to venous anastomosis in order to increase pulmonary blood flow and the creation of a univentricular heart (the Fontan procedure).

ACYANOTIC LESIONS

Ventricular Septal Defect (VSD)

VSD is the most common congenital heart defect in infants and children. The majority of lesions occurs in the membranous portion of the interventricular septum

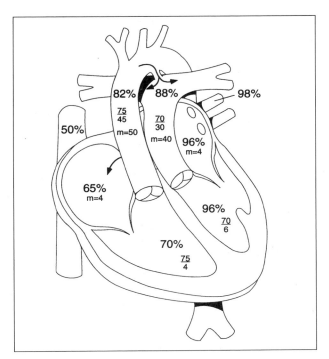

Figure 98–2 Transposition of the great arteries with an intact ventricular septum, a large patent ductus arteriosus (on PGE₁) and atrial septal defect (status post balloon atrial septostomy). Note the following: (a) The aorta arises from the anatomic right ventricle, and the pulmonary artery from the anatomic left ventricle; (b) "transposition physiology," with a higher oxygen saturation in the pulmonary artery than in the aorta; (c) "mixing" between the parallel circulations (see text) at the atrial (after balloon atrial septostomy) and ductal levels; (d) shunting from the left atrium to the right atrium via the atrial septal defect (not shown) with equalization of atrial pressures; (e) shunting from the aorta to the pulmonary artery via the ductus arteriosus; (f) pulmonary hypertension due to a large ductus arteriosus.

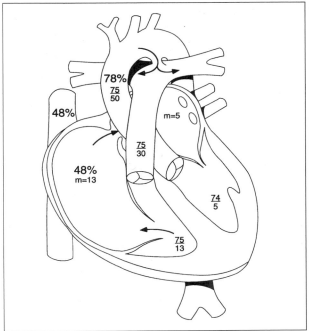

Figure 98–3 Ebstein's anomaly (with large non-restrictive ductus arteriosus). Typical anatomic and hemodynamic findings include: (a) inferior displacement of the tricuspid valve into the right ventricle, which may also cause subpulmonary obstruction; (b) diminutive muscular right ventricle; (c) marked enlargement of the right atrium due to "atrialized" portion of right ventricle as well as tricuspid regurgitation; (d) right-to-left shunting at the atrial level (note arterial oxygen saturation of 78%); (e) a left-to-right shunt and pulmonary hypertension secondary to a large patent ductus arteriosus supplying the pulmonary blood flow; (f) low cardiac output (note low mixed venous oxygen saturation in the superior vena cava).

(70%). The remainder of the defects occurs in the muscular portion of the septum (20%) or between the tricuspid and mitral valves (5%). VSDs are characterized by left-to-right shunting with few clinical consequences unless the shunt is large. The murmur of a VSD is holosystolic and loudest at the left lower sternal border. An apical rumble may be appreciated reflecting increased blood flow through the mitral valve. As the left-to-right shunting begins to cause a degree of pulmonary hypertension, a pulmonary regurgitation murmur (the Graham-Steell's murmur) may be heard. Cyanosis is a late sign and indicates a reversal of the shunt (from left-to-right to right-to-left), which is known as Eisenmenger's syndrome.

Chest radiography and EKG are typically non-specific until pulmonary hypertension develops and then signs of RVH and RAD become evident. Echocar-

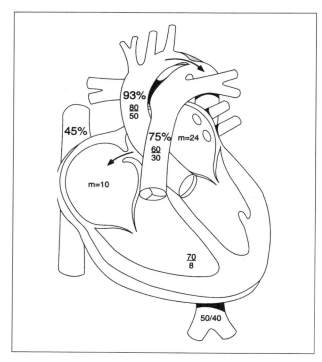

Figure 98–4 Coarctation of the aorta in a critically ill neonate with a nearly closed ductus arteriosus. Typical anatomic and hemodynamic findings include: (a) "juxtaductal" site of the coarctation; (b) a bicommissural aortic valve (seen in 80% of patients with coarctation); (c) narrow pulse pressure in the descending aorta and lower body; (d) a bidirectional shunt at the ductus arteriosus. As in critical aortic stenosis (see Fig. 3–13) there is an elevated left atrial pressure, pulmonary edema, a left-to-right shunt at the atrial level, pulmonary artery hypertension and only a moderate (300 mm Hg) gradient across the arch obstruction. The low measured gradient (despite severe anatomic obstruction) across the aortic arch is due to low cardiac output.

diography and catheterization are used to diagnose and quantify the size of the defect prior to surgical repair.

Coarctation of the Aorta

Coarctation occurs when there is a congenital narrowing of the aortic lumen distal to the left subclavian artery at the site of the ligamentum arteriosum (Fig. 98–4). It is associated with circle of Willis aneurysms, bicuspid aortic valves, Turner's syndrome, and mitral stenosis. Clinically, coarctation is characterized by upper extremity hypertension and relative lower extremity hypotension. The femoral artery pulses are weak and delayed. Notching of the posterior third through eighth ribs due to increased flow through collateral vessels can be seen on chest radiography. Both echocardiography and computed tomography can be used for diagnosis. Early surgical repair is indicated to prevent the long-term complications of uncorrected coarctation (hypertension, aortic dissection, left ventricular failure, and endocarditis).

◆ **KEY POINTS** ◆

1. Cyanotic heart defects are characterized by left-to-right shunting.

2. Ventricular septal defect is the most common congenital heart defect.

3. Tetralogy of Fallot is characterized by RVH, a VSD, right ventricular outflow tract obstruction, and an overriding aorta.

4. Coarctation occurs at the site of attachment of the ligamentum arteriosum.

99 Croup

ETIOLOGY

Croup is a common disease of childhood and a common cause of upper airway obstruction in children. It is a clinical syndrome that is caused by a variety of viral respiratory pathogens, with parainfluenza virus, 1 and 2, respiratory syncytial virus, and adenoviruses being the most common etiologies. So-called "spasmodic croup" is allergic, not infectious, and affects children between the ages of 1 and 5 years. Infectious croup predominantly affects children ages 6 months to 4 years and is most prevalent in the fall to late winter.

PATHOPHYSIOLOGY

Viral infection of the surface epithelium of the respiratory tract, particularly the subglottic regions of the pharynx, leads to a vigorous host response characterized by an increase in vascular endothelial permeability and edema. The characteristic stridor and cough of patients with croup is caused by air being forced through this subglottic "bottleneck."

HISTORY

Patients with croup typically present with a history of a preceding upper respiratory tract infection that has worsened over the preceding 24–72 hours. Fever, rhin-orrhea, and congestion are common presenting symptoms. Patients or family members may report hoarseness, the sudden onset of a bark-like cough, inspiratory stridor, and retractions that worsen at night. Parents may offer that picking their child up and walking outside into the cool night air seems to help alleviate the symptoms.

PHYSICAL EXAMINATION

Patients with croup typically are non-toxic appearing with temperatures less than 39° Celsius. Measurements of oxygen saturation are typically normal until severe obstruction occurs. Retractions, tachypnea, and audible stridor are common.

DIFFERENTIAL DIAGNOSIS

- Inhaled foreign body
- Epiglottitis
- Bacterial tracheitis
- Retropharyngeal abscess
- Peritonsillar abscess

DIAGNOSTIC EVALUATION

The diagnosis of croup is typically made clinically. A soft-tissue neck radiograph (anterior-posterior and

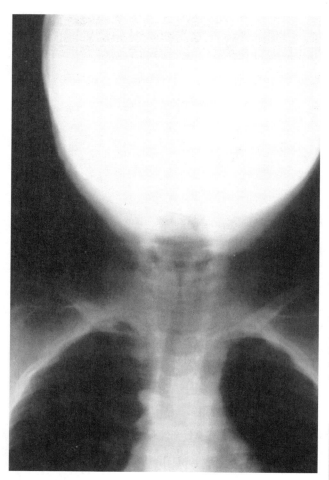

Figure 99–1 Croup in a 3-year-old. Note the "steeple sign" indicative of subglottic narrowing.

lateral views) showing a "steeple sign" may be helpful if the presentation is not classic or can be used to rule out other etiologies for respiratory distress (Fig. 99–1). A mild leukocytosis is typically the only abnormality noted on complete blood count.

TREATMENT

The most important initial step in the emergency department management of a child with croup is to maintain the airway. Children with severe upper airway obstruction with signs of respiratory collapse should be intubated. Post-intubation pulmonary edema, a poorly understood complication of airway management in croup patients, develops in approximately 10% of patients. For those patients who are not in extremis, nebulized cool mist and supplemental oxygen may be all that is required for treatment. Keeping the child calm and in the arms of a care giver will also prevent anxiety-related worsening of the airway obstruction. For those children who fail to respond to these simple measures or who are in severe distress, racemic epinephrine (0.5 cc/2 cc of normal saline) via nebulizer can be used. The vasoconstricting properties of epinephrine are thought to help alleviate the subglottic edema responsible for airway obstruction. If a child exhibits stridor at rest, steroids (typically decadron at a dose of 0.6 mg/kg intramuscularly) are given. Admission is indicated for all children who have stridor at rest or respiratory distress unresponsive to treatment measures.

◆ KEY POINTS ◆

1. Croup is most commonly caused by parainfluenza type 1 and 2.
2. Croup occurs in children aged 6 months to 4 years.
3. Croup is characterized by a seal-like, barking cough and variable degrees of upper airway obstruction.
4. Treatment involves nebulized saline, steroids, and racemic epinephrine, with intubation reserved for severe cases.

100 Bronchiolitis

Bronchiolitis is a lower respiratory tract infection caused by the respiratory syncytial virus (RSV) and affects predominantly infants and young children. RSV bronchiolitis causes almost 100,000 hospitalizations and almost 5,000 deaths per year.

ETIOLOGY

RSV is a single-stranded RNA virus of the Paramyxoviridae family. The virus is found globally and is responsible for outbreaks of upper respiratory tract infection that occur every winter and early spring. Infection most commonly occurs in infants aged 2 to 6 months, with the highest mortality occurring in those children younger than 2 months or those with a history of bronchopulmonary dysplasia. By 3 years of age, virtually 100% of people have been exposed to RSV, though exposure may not confer complete immunity and repeated infections can occur, even in the same year. RSV infection in older children causes upper respiratory type symptoms without the marked respiratory distress that is common among younger patients. Although almost 75% of bronchiolitis cases are caused by RSV, other organisms such as influenza virus, parainfluenza virus, adenovirus, *Mycoplasma pneumoniae*, and *Chlamydia trachomatis* also have been implicated.

PATHOPHYSIOLOGY

RSV is transmitted by the inhalation of aerosolized respiratory secretions or by direct contact with an infected individual. The virus attacks the lining of the bronchioles causing submucosal edema, increased mucous secretion, and sloughing of cellular debris into the airway lumen. The pathologic changes in the small airways lead to decreased gas exchange and a ventilation-perfusion mismatch (V/Q mismatch) with subsequent hypoxia.

HISTORY

Patients with bronchiolitis typically present with signs of upper respiratory tract infection including cough, rhinorrhea, and congestion. Parents may give a history of "fast breathing" and even apnea in younger patients.

PHYSICAL EXAMINATION

Tachypnea (60–80 breaths/minute), fever, and tachycardia are predominant features of bronchiolitis. Hypoxia, nasal flaring, intercostal and subcostal retractions, and cyanosis may be observed. Auscultation of the chest reveals fine rales or audible wheezing and a prolonged expiratory phase of the respiratory cycle secondary to air trapping.

DIFFERENTIAL DIAGNOSIS

- Foreign body
- Asthma

- Pneumonia
- Pneumothorax
- Influenza infection
- Sepsis

DIAGNOSTIC EVALUATION

Chest radiographs in bronchiolitis reveal evidence of air trapping and inflammation with hyperinflation and peribronchial cuffing. Arterial blood gases reveal evidence of hypoxia, while the complete blood count is typically normal. Definitive diagnosis of RSV is accomplished by monoclonal antibody testing of nasopharyngeal swabs.

TREATMENT

Treatment of bronchiolitis is supportive and is based on each individual patient's clinical condition. All but the mildest cases should be given supplemental oxygen and a trial of nebulized beta-agonists such as albuterol. Nebulized racemic epinephrine can be used in patients who do no respond to albuterol. Corticosteroids have been studied extensively in bronchiolitic children and have not been shown to be beneficial. Most children with moderate to severe infections require intravenous

hydration because the increased work of breathing predisposes to dehydration.

Severe cases of bronchiolitis may require mechanical ventilation or even ECMO (extracorporeal membrane oxygenation). Ribavirin, a nucleoside analog with activity against RSV, has been used successfully to treat severe cases of bronchiolitis, especially those with underlying cardiopulmonary diseases that require mechanical ventilation. Admission is indicated for patients who are hypoxic (oxygen saturation <94% after therapy), persistently tachypneic, or who are not feeding secondary to increased work of breathing.

◆ KEY POINTS ◆

1. The majority of cases of bronchiolitis are due to infection with the respiratory syncytial virus.

2. Bronchiolitis involves the lower airways and results in air trapping and ventilation-perfusion mismatch.

3. Tachypnea, tachycardia, fever, and hypoxia are the clinical hallmarks of RSV infection.

4. Treatment of bronchiolitis involves oxygen, nebulized beta-agonists, and nebulized epinephrine.

101

Kawasaki's Disease

Kawasaki's disease, also known as mucocutaneous lymph node syndrome, refers to a condition characterized by fever and a diffuse vasculitis that affects children, predominantly before the age of 5 years. Although most cases resolve spontaneously, up to 25% of affected children will go on to suffer serious consequences such as coronary artery aneurysms.

EPIDEMIOLOGY

The incidence of Kawasaki's disease in the United States is approximately 60/100,000 per year, with many atypical cases going unrecognized and unreported. The disease typically occurs in children between the ages of 2 and 5, with only rare cases occurring in late childhood or adulthood. Male children are affected more commonly than females and clustering of cases can occur. Risks for the development of Kawasaki's disease include such seemingly unrelated factors as a recent (within 30 days) respiratory illness and shampooing or cleaning carpet in the last 30 days (supporting a dust mite vector for the disease).

PATHOPHYSIOLOGY

The exact cause of Kawasaki's disease remains unknown, though the clinical presentation, seasonal variation, and clustering of cases suggests an infectious agent. Regardless of the cause, there appears to be an exaggerated host immune response against the unknown stimulus, which results in damage to the endothelial layer of blood vessels. The immune hyperresponse leads to a diffuse antibody-mediated vasculitis resulting in the long-term clinical sequelae of the disease.

CLINICAL MANIFESTATIONS

For a diagnosis of Kawasaki's disease, a patient must have fever for at least 5 straight days and at least four of the following five clinical manifestations:

- Cervical lymphadenopathy
- Bilateral conjunctivitis
- Mucositis characterized by strawberry tongue, an injected pharynx, or cracked lips
- Rash
- Erythema of the palms or soles combined with edema of the hands or feet that progresses to periungual desquamation.

These clinical criteria are neither 100% sensitive nor 100% specific for the diagnosis of Kawasaki's disease. Laboratory evaluation typically reveals signs of systemic inflammation with elevated erythrocyte sedimentation rate and C-reactive protein. Urinalysis may show pyuria that is of urethral origin. The hepatic transaminases may be mildly elevated and a normocytic, normochromic anemia may be evident on complete blood count.

DIFFERENTIAL DIAGNOSIS

- Measles
- Toxic shock syndrome
- Erysipelas
- Stevens-Johnson syndrome
- Toxic epidermal necrolysis

COMPLICATIONS

Up to 25% of untreated cases of Kawasaki's disease will go on to have serious vascular complications including coronary artery aneurysms and acute peripheral arterial occlusion. With treatment, the incidence of vascular complications drops to 4%.

TREATMENT

IVIG (intravenous immune globulin) and aspirin are the mainstays of therapy for Kawasaki's disease. IVIG has been shown to reduce the incidence of coronary artery aneurysms when given within the first 10 days of illness. It is usually administered intravenously in a single dose of 2 grams/kilograms.

High-dose aspirin (100 mg/kg/day) is typically given during the acute phase of illness and then at more standard doses (3–5 mg/kg/day) after the fever of Kawasaki's disease has resolved. All patients with Kawasaki's disease should be followed indefinitely with periodic echocardiograms to ensure normal cardiac contractility and the absence of coronary artery aneurysms.

◆ KEY POINTS ◆

1. Kawasaki's disease causes a vasculitis that affects the coronary arteries.
2. The exact cause of Kawasaki's disease is unknown.
3. Kawasaki's disease is characterized by fever, rash, lymphadenopathy, conjunctivitis, strawberry tongue, and peripheral extremity swelling.
4. Aspirin and IVIG are the mainstays of therapy for patients with Kawasaki's disease.

102

Sudden Infant Death Syndrome

Sudden infant death syndrome (SIDS) is defined as sudden death in an infant that remains unexplained after a thorough investigation of the death scene, medical records, and autopsy data. A plausible cause of death, whether it is abuse; undiagnosed cardiac, neurologic, or infectious illness; or inborn errors of metabolism, can be found in up to 15–20% of "unexplained" deaths that occur in the infant age group.

EPIDEMIOLOGY

SIDS typically occurs between 2 and 4 months of age and greater than 90% of cases occur before 6 months of age. This is a time of tremendous cardiac, neurologic, and pulmonary development in an infant, and aberrations of this normal maturation process are hypothesized to be factors in SIDS. Several factors have been identified that place infants at increased risk of sudden death, although none appears to be sensitive or specific. Infants of young mothers (less than 20) and mothers who smoke are 2 to 4 times more likely to succumb to SIDS. Maternal drug use, low socioeconomic class, and low birth weight also appear to be risk factors. Siblings of SIDS victims have an increased (approximately five-fold) risk of subsequent SIDS deaths. Perhaps the most well-publicized risk factor for SIDS is allowing an infant to sleep prone.

PATHOPHYSIOLOGY

Despite intense research, the exact cause of SIDS remains unknown. Several pathologic changes have been found at autopsy that appear to be linked to an increased risk of SIDS, including brainstem gliosis, persistent periadrenal brown fat, and persistent hepatic hematopoiesis. The evaluation of alarm monitors from children who later died from SIDS reveals that bradycardia and apnea appear to be the predominant prearrest abnormalities. Prone sleeping, especially on mattresses filled with polystyrene, increases the degree of "rebreathing" and may lead to suffocation in an infant who does not have the strength and coordination to move its head in order to obtain fresh air. Though the exact number is unknown, it is estimated that between 2 and 10% of all cases of SIDS are actually due to undiagnosed child abuse.

MANAGEMENT

Unfortunately, the vast majority of infants with SIDS cannot be resuscitated despite heroic efforts in the emergency department. Parents should be comforted and allowed to see their child after a pronouncement of death has been made. Most states require a postmortem examination in all cases of infant death and the parents should be informed of this at an appropriate time.

Prevention remains the key to decreasing the incidence of SIDS. Good prenatal care, smoking abstinence, and refraining from illicit drug use are three steps that have been shown to be protective. The role of home apnea monitors is controversial. Apnea monitors became popular in the late 1970s though no study has shown that they reduce the incidence of SIDS deaths.

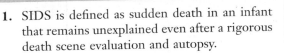

◆ KEY POINTS ◆

1. SIDS is defined as sudden death in an infant that remains unexplained even after a rigorous death scene evaluation and autopsy.

2. Smoking, young maternal age, and drug use are risk factors for SIDS.

3. Siblings of SIDS victims are at increased risk of sudden death.

4. Sleeping supine rather than prone seems to protect infants from SIDS.

103 Pyloric Stenosis

Pyloric stenosis is characterized by a concentric hypertrophy of the pylorus leading to profound gastric outlet obstruction. It is an important cause of vomiting in children, especially during the first few months of life.

EPIDEMIOLOGY

The incidence of pyloric stenosis is approximately 3 per 1000 live births. The condition typically presents within the first 2 months of life and males are affected 4 times more than females. For unclear reasons, first-born males are particularly at risk. The cause of pyloric stenosis is undoubtedly multifactorial with environmental and genetic factors playing a role. There is an association between pyloric stenosis and infants treated with erythromycin for pertussis.

CLINICAL MANIFESTATIONS

Pyloric stenosis classically presents as projectile vomiting in an otherwise healthy infant. Despite repeated bouts of vomiting, affected children typically appear well and will readily feed, even immediately after emesis. Weight loss and varying degrees of dehydration are common. Careful observation of the abdomen may reveal a peristaltic wave traveling left to right across the upper abdomen. Palpation of the abdomen is significant for an "olive-shaped" mass representing the hypertrophic pylorus. Although the olive is present in as many as 85% of patients with pyloric stenosis, a tense, distended abdomen often makes palpation difficult.

DIAGNOSTIC EVALUATION

Laboratory evaluation reveals a hypochloremic metabolic alkalosis from repeated vomiting of gastric acid. Ultrasonography is the first recommended imaging study if the diagnosis cannot be made on clinical grounds alone. Ultrasonography is very specific, but sensitivity suffers in patients with large amounts of bowel gas or a large body habitus. An upper GI (gastrointestinal) contrast study can also be used to establish the diagnosis of pyloric stenosis. Positive studies demonstrate the "string sign," a thin stream of contrast flowing through a narrowed pylorus.

TREATMENT

The definitive treatment of pyloric stenosis is surgery. Laparoscopic pyloromyotomy has replaced the traditional open Ramstedt pyloromyotomy. Prior to surgical pyloromyotomy, aggressive fluid resuscitation with intravenous crystalloid is indicated.

◆ KEY POINTS ◆

1. Pyloric stenosis is common in first-born males.
2. Projectile vomiting is a common presenting complaint.
3. The "olive" is the classic physical exam finding.
4. Surgical pyloromyotomy is curative.

104 Intussusception

Intussusception occurs in late infancy and early childhood (between 2 months and 6 years), with the peak incidence occurring in the 6–9 month age group. It typically occurs in the late fall and early winter and has been associated with viral upper respiratory and gastrointestinal infection (rotavirus and adenovirus in particular). The overall mortality (1%) of this condition has declined over the years with modern treatment modalities.

PATHOPHYSIOLOGY

Intussusception occurs when a proximal piece of bowel telescopes into the lumen of a piece of distal bowel (Fig. 104–1). The most common site of occurrence is at the ileocecal valve with a piece of ileum telescoping into the ascending large colon. A "lead point" is found in a small minority of patients (5%), with benign polyps, hypertrophied lymph nodes (Peyer's patches), lymphoma, or a Meckel's diverticulum being most common.

As the proximal piece of bowel invaginates into the distal lumen, edema develops and the blood supply is strangulated. Strangulation initially presents as bloody, mucus-filled stools (so-called currant jelly stools) that progresses to bowel infarction, necrosis, and perforation.

CLINICAL MANIFESTATIONS

Patients with intussusception present with abdominal pain and vomiting. Pain in the preverbal child often manifests as "colic," inconsolable crying, or "drawing up of the legs." Bilious vomiting is uncommon, though blood-stained vomitus does occasionally occur. As the disease progresses and the mucosa begins to slough, the patient begins to pass stool composed predominantly of blood and mucous. Untreated, these early signs progress over 24 to 48 hours to lethargy, dehydration, and shock.

Physical examination may reveal signs of shock and bowel perforation including tachycardia, tachypnea, fever, and hypotension. Earlier in the presentation, the exam may be remarkable only for a palpable sausage-like mass in the abdomen. Abdominal pain is almost universal, though the examination of infants is difficult. Rectal exam typically reveals heme-positive stool.

DIAGNOSIS AND TREATMENT

Patients suspected of having intussusception should be placed on a cardiac monitor, have an intravenous line established, and blood sent for chemistries, complete blood count, coagulation studies, and type and cross. Intravenous fluid bolus should be initiated (20 cc/kg of normal saline). If the patient shows signs of perforation or shock, immediate surgical intervention is indicated. If the patient is early in the disease course, further radiographic study is warranted. Plain abdominal radiographs are often the first study obtained on patients suspected of having intussusception. Characteristic find-

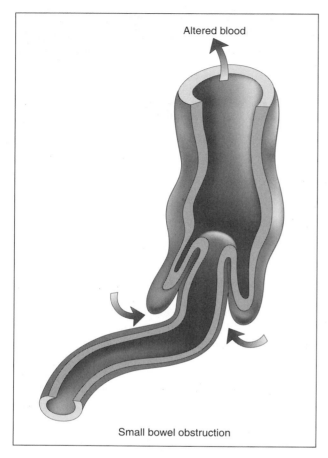

Altered blood

Small bowel obstruction

Figure 104–1

ings include evidence of bowel obstruction with dilated loops of small bowel and air-fluid levels, or signs of a mass in the area of the lesion. Ultrasound is a useful, non-invasive tool for the diagnosis of intussusception with a high degree of sensitivity and specificity in the hands of an experienced operator.

Barium or air-contrast enemas can be used as both a diagnostic and therapeutic maneuver. Air-contrast enemas have become the procedure of choice in the treatment of intussusception, with a success rate approaching 75% in several large studies. Once the intussusception is reduced, the patient should be observed in the hospital for 24 to 48 hours in case of recurrence, which occurs in approximately 10% of cases. Surgical intervention may be necessary in cases of recurrent disease.

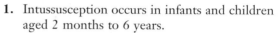

◆ **KEY POINTS** ◆

1. Intussusception occurs in infants and children aged 2 months to 6 years.
2. A lead point is found in a minority of patients and includes such conditions as Meckel's diverticulum, lymphoma, or hypertrophied lymph nodes.
3. Currant jelly stools composed of blood and mucus are characteristic of intussusception.
4. Air enemas are both diagnostic and therapeutic.

105

Meckel's Diverticulum

Meckel's diverticulum is a remnant of the embryonic yolk sac. It is formed when the omphalomesenteric duct that connects the yolk sac with the developing fetal gut fails to involute.

EPIDEMIOLOGY

Meckel's diverticulum occurs in approximately 2% of the population with fewer than 10% of these patients ever becoming symptomatic. It is the most common congenital small bowel abnormality and is a common cause of painless rectal bleeding in children. Symptomatic patients are typically boys less than 5 years of age.

PATHOPHYSIOLOGY

A Meckel's diverticulum is typically a small sausage-like projection of the ileum approximately 2 feet from the cecum receiving its blood supply from the terminal branch of the superior mesenteric artery. The outpouching consists of all layers of the bowel wall and occurs on the anti-mesenteric side of the intestine. Often, gastric mucosa can be found in the pit of the diverticulum, predisposing to ulcer formation and bleeding.

CLINICAL MANIFESTATIONS

Patients with Meckel's diverticuli are typically young children who present with painless rectal bleeding.

Although the bleeding is rarely life threatening, it is often hemodynamically significant. Bleeding is more common in cases where heterotopic gastric mucosa is found in the diverticulum. Due to the cathartic effect of blood in the gastrointestinal tract, stools are often dark, brick red in color due to increased transit time.

Some Meckel's diverticuli become symptomatic in older children or adults. In this age group, the presentation is commonly one of small bowel obstruction or intussusception (where the diverticulum acts as the lead point).

DIFFERENTIAL DIAGNOSIS

- Appendicitis
- Intussusception
- Small bowel obstruction
- Hernia
- Arteriovenous malformation
- Volvulus
- Inflammatory bowel disease

DIAGNOSTIC EVALUATION

The diagnosis of Meckel's diverticulum can be made by technetium scanning. This test is highly sensitive (90%) in cases where heterotopic gastric mucosa is present.

The sensitivity can be increased by pre-scan administration of pentagastrin or an H_2-receptor antagonist (ranitidine or cimetidine). Other imaging modalities such as angiography can make the diagnosis but are invasive and less sensitive.

TREATMENT

All patients with a suspected symptomatic Meckel's diverticulum should be placed on a monitor and have an intravenous line established. Blood should be sent for complete blood count, coagulation studies, and type and screen. Any hemodynamically unstable patient should be aggressively resuscitated with crystalloid (normal saline or lactated Ringer's) and have blood products

available. Surgical resection is the treatment of choice for cases of symptomatic Meckel's diverticulum.

◆ KEY POINTS ◆

1. Meckel's diverticuli occur in 2% of the population.
2. They commonly occur in patients 2 years of age.
3. They occur in the small intestine, approximately 2 feet from the ileocecal valve.
4. Surgical resection is the treatment of choice.

Part XVII
Questions and
Answers

Questions

1. A 65-year-old male with a history of hypertension and high cholesterol presents after a syncopal episode. His wife states that he has been complaining of abdominal pain for several days but denied nausea, vomiting, or fever. His vital signs at presentation include a heart rate of 110, blood pressure of 90/60, respiratory rate of 12, and oxygen saturation of 99% on 2 L. On exam, he is diaphoretic with diminished peripheral pulses and a pulsatile abdominal mass. What is the most likely diagnosis?

   a. Diverticulitis

   b. GI hemorrhage

   c. Ruptured abdominal aortic aneurysm

   d. Myocardial infarction

2. After initial stabilization and a normal ECG, what is the most appropriate first test for this patient?

   a. KUB and upright

   b. Bedside abdominal ultrasound

   c. Abdominal CT

   d. Abdominal MRI

3. A 35-year-old male presents with sudden onset of ripping chest pain that radiates to his back between his scapula. He denies smoking or history of cocaine use. On physical exam, he is a tall thin male with unusually long fingers. His blood pressure is 170/80 in the left arm and 140/60 in the right arm, heart rate is 80, and respiratory rate is 20 with an oxygen saturation of 99% on 2 L nasal canula. There is a soft diastolic murmur over the left upper sternal border, and clear lungs. An ECG shows a sinus rhythm with nonspecific changes. The most likely cause of his chest pain would be:

   a. Dissecting aortic aneurysm

   b. Acute myocardial infarction

   c. Pulmonary embolism

   d. Acute pericarditis

4. A 55-year-old female with hypertension and diabetes presents with substernal chest pain radiating to her left arm, associated with diaphoresis and mild shortness of breath. On presentation her heart rate is 90, blood pressure is 140/80, respiratory rate is 18, and oxygen saturation is 99% on 2 L NC. The nurse yells from the bay that the patient just passed out. You find the patient to be pulseless with the following rhythm strip (Fig. Q–4). What should be your first intervention?

   a. Intubation

   b. Defibrillate at 200J

   c. IV adenosine

   d. IV thrombolytics

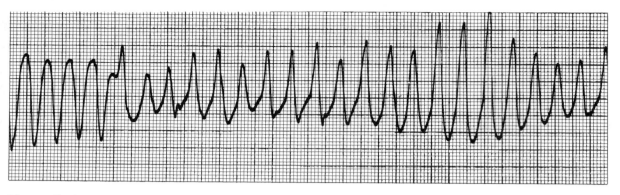

Figure Q–4

5. A 67-year-old male with a history of high cholesterol and smoking presents 2 hours after eating a large meal with burping and chest discomfort. He attempted antacids at home with only mild relief but his symptoms worsened and he arrives in the emergency department. The most useful initial test to help with the diagnosis is:

   a. A right upper quadrant US

   b. An ECG

   c. A CXR

   d. KUB and upright

6. A 60-year-old female presents with pleuritic chest pain that woke her up from sleep. She also complains of shortness of breath and palpitations. On further history, it is discovered that the patient recently returned from a trip to Japan and wondered if she may have been exposed to something during her travels. Her past medical history is significant for arthritis. Her medications include estrogen and Tylenol. On physical exam she is tachypneic with a temperature of 100.2°F, a heart rate of 110, blood pressure of 130/80, respiratory rate of 24, and oxygen saturation of 93% on RA. Her ECG shows sinus tachycardia with nonspecific ST-T wave changes. Her chest x-ray is clear. A ventilation-perfusion scan shows a large defect in the right lower lobe. Treatment in the emergency department should begin with:

   a. IV antibiotics

   b. Indomethacin

   c. IV thrombolytics

   d. IV heparin

   e. Greenfield filter

7. A 62-year-old male with a smoking history, hypertension, and angina presents with substernal chest pain at rest. The patient states that he typically gets chest pain with exertion but today he developed chest pain while sitting eating dinner. He denies shortness of breath, nausea, vomiting, or diaphoresis. The patient states his chest pain was not relieved until he took 2 SL nitroglycerine. He arrives in the emergency department with recurrent chest pain that is again relieved after 2 SL nitroglycerine. His ECG shows nonspecific ST-T wave changes in V4-V6. His chest x-ray is clear. His cardiac enzymes are normal. What is the best treatment option?

   a. Discharge patient with nitrates and have him follow up with his cardiologist next week

   b. Admit him to a monitored bed with IV heparin and beta-blockers

   c. Administer thrombolytics

   d. Administer Maalox and discharge patient home on an H_2 blocker

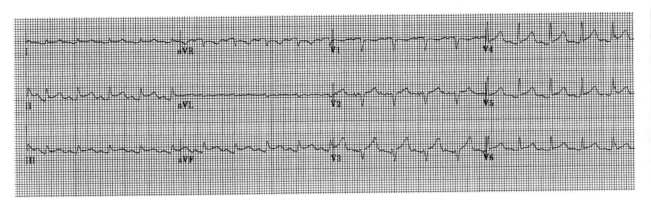

Figure Q–8

8. A 25-year-old male presents with pleuritic CP. The patient states that last week he had an upper respiratory infection associated with dry cough and sore throat. He denies fever, chills, nausea, vomiting, or abdominal pain. The patient states his chest pain is better when he sits up and leans forward. His ECG is shown below (Fig. Q–8). What is the best treatment option?

   a. Azithromycin

   b. Nitroglycerine

   c. Lopressor

   d. Indomethacin

9. A 30-year-old male presents with sudden onset of left flank pain radiating to his groin. The patient complains of nausea and 1 episode of vomiting but denies fever, chills, or abdominal pain. He denies any past medical history and does not take any medications. He is writhing on the stretcher in pain. His heart rate is 110, blood pressure is 120/70, respiratory rate is 15, temperature is 98.7°F, and oxygen saturation is 100% on RA. His physical exam is remarkable for mild CVA tenderness on the left. His urinalysis shows no bacteria, 0–2 WBC, and 50–100 RBC. What is the most likely diagnosis?

   a. Acute pyelonephritis

   b. Kidney stone

   c. Musculoskeletal back spasm

   d. Testicular torsion

10. A 25-year-old female presents with left lower quadrant pain and vaginal spotting. The patient denies nausea, vomiting, or fever. She states that she has always had very irregular periods. On physical exam, her heart rate is 90, blood pressure is 120/70, respiratory rate is 12, oxygen saturation is 99% on RA, and temperature is 98.7°F. Her pelvic exam is remarkable for blood at cervical OS with mild left adnexal fullness and tenderness. What is the most important initial test?

    a. Urinalysis

    b. Beta-hCG

    c. CBC

    d. Type and screen

11. A 45-year-old female with end-stage renal disease on hemodialysis presents to the emergency department with shortness of breath. Pt states she missed her past two dialysis appointments because her car broke down. On physical exam she is in moderate respiratory distress, heart rate is 110, blood pressure is 160/95, respiratory rate is 24, and oxygen saturation is 90% on RA. She has an elevated JVD, her heart is tachycardic without murmurs, her lungs have bilateral crackles halfway up, and she has 2+ pitting edema in her lower extremities. The following ECG is obtained (Fig. Q–11). Of the following treatment options, which should be given first?

    a. PO or rectal Kayexalate

    b. IV insulin and glucose

    c. IV calcium gluconate or calcium chloride

    d. IV sodium bicarbonate

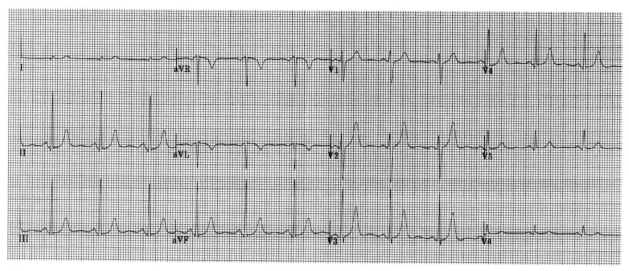

Figure Q–11

12. A 70-year-old female with history of HTN presents with mental status changes. The patient's daughter states her mother had been complaining of increased thirst and urination over the past few weeks and today had a near syncopal episode at home. Her medications include hydrochlorothiazide. The patient is somnolent but responds to voice. Her vital signs include a heart rate of 120, blood pressure of 90/70, respiratory rate of 20, oxygen saturation of 96% on RA, and temperature of 98.7°F. On exam, she has dry mucous membranes, a supple neck, and she moves all of her extremities equally. Her FS glucose is greater than 600. Her initial labs show:
Na = 124 mmol/L (135–145 mmol/L)
K = 5.0 mmol/L (3.4–4.8 mmol/L)
Bun = 45 mg/dL (8–25 mg/dL)
Cr = 1.8 mg/dL (0.6–1.5 mg/dL)
Glucose = 875 mg/dL (70–110 mg/dL)
Osmolarity = 360 mOsm/kg (280–296 mOsm/kg)
Her urinalysis is positive for glucose but negative for ketones. What is the most likely diagnosis?

a. Stroke

b. Hyperosmolar hyperglycemic nonketonic coma

c. Diabetic ketoacidosis

d. Hyponatremia

13. What is the best initial treatment for the above diagnosis?

a. IV insulin

b. IV normal saline

c. IV naloxone

d. IV thrombolytics

14. A 16-year-old female is found unconscious in her bedroom at home. Her mother finds a suicide note and 2 empty pill bottles beside her. When EMS arrived, the patient responded to sternal rub with shallow respirations and a finger stick glucose of 80. On arrival to the emergency department, her vital signs are a heart rate of 80, blood pressure is 110/60, respiratory rate is 10, temperature is 98.7°F, oxygen saturation is 100% on 2 L NC. Her physical exam is unremarkable except for somnolence. Her pupils are 3 mm and reactive bilaterally. Her toxicologic screen is positive for benzodiazepines and Tylenol. What it the treatment for Tylenol overdoses?

a. Naloxone

b. Sodium bicarbonate

c. N-acetylcysteine (NAC)

d. Flumazenil

15. A 25-year-old female presents with shortness of breath after eating fried rice. She has a history of allergic reaction to shellfish and is not sure if there may have been some in the fried rice. She states it feels like there is a lump in her throat. On initial presentation she is in mild respiratory distress. Her vital signs show a heart rate of 100, blood pressure of 130/70, respiratory rate of 20, and oxygen saturation of 99% on RA. Her physical exam is remarkable for a swollen uvula and stridor. Which is the most appropriate medication at this time?

    a. SC epinephrine

    b. Benadryl

    c. Albuterol nebulizer

    d. Prednisone

16. A 22-year-old female presents with fever, flank pain, and dysuria. The patient states she developed dysuria and increased urinary frequency 2 days ago. This morning she woke up with a fever of 102°F, nausea, and left flank pain. Her vital signs include a heart rate of 100, blood pressure of 120/70, respiratory rate of 12, oxygen saturation of 100% on RA, and a temperature of 102.5°F. Her exam is remarkable for left flank tenderness. The most likely organism that caused this infection is:

    a. *Chlamydia trachomatis*

    b. *Escherichia coli*

    c. *Clostridium perfringens*

    d. *Streptococcus pyogenes*

17. A 35-year-old female GIPI presents with nausea, vomiting, and right upper quadrant pain radiating to her back. Her pain began this evening approximately I hour after eating dinner. She recalls having similar episodes during her pregnancy last year and usually they would resolve after I to 2 hours but tonight the pain did not subside after 10 hours. She is an obese female in moderate distress. Her vital signs are a heart rate of 110, blood pressure of 120/70, respiratory rate of 20, oxygen saturation of 100%, and temperature of 100.9°F. Her exam is remarkable for right upper quadrant tenderness with a positive Murphy's sign. Her labs are remarkable for:

WBC = 15.0×10^3/mL ($4.5–11.0 \times 10^3$/mL)
AST = 65 U/L (15–40 U/L)
ALT = 70 U/L (10–40 U/L)
Total Bilirubin = 1.9 mg/dL (0.1–1.0 mg/dL)
Direct Bilirubin = 0.7 mg/dL (0.0–0.3 mg/dL)
Amylase = 75 U/L (25–125 U/L)
Lipase- = 4 U/L (3–19 U/L)

A right upper quadrant ultrasound is obtained and shows gallbladder wall thickening with some pericholecystic fluid. What is the most likely diagnosis?

    a. Biliary colic

    b. Acute cholecystitis

    c. Acute pancreatitis

    d. Ascending cholangitis

18. What is the next best intervention?

    a. Discharge the patient home with close follow-up by her primary care physician in several days if her pain does not resolve

    b. IV antibiotics and prompt surgical consultation

    c. Nasogastric tube placement, IV fluids, NPO, and observation

    d. Abdominal CT

19. A 27-year-old female G3P2 at 29 weeks' gestation presents with vaginal bleeding. The patient woke up this morning and noted bright red vaginal bleeding. She states the bleeding stopped but was concerned and thought it should be evaluated. The patient denies abdominal pain or cramping, clear watery discharge, or trauma. She has noted good fetal movement all day. Her vital signs include a heart rate of 80, blood pressure of 125/70, respiratory rate of 12, oxygen saturation of 100%, temperature of 98.7°F, and a fetal heart rate of 130. Her labs show a hematocrit of 32 (36–46) and she is Rh positive. The patient is attached to a monitor, supplemental oxygen, and 2 large-bore IVs placed. What is the most appropriate next step in this patient's management?

    a. Vaginal examination

    b. Ultrasound

    c. Emergent transfusion

    d. Stat cesarean section

20. An 18-year-old female presents with 24 hours of right lower quadrant pain accompanied by low-grade fever, malaise, 2 episodes of vomiting, and loose stools. Upon presentation to the emergency department, the patient was febrile with a temperature of 101.2°F and had tenderness in the right lower quadrant without evidence of rebound or involuntary guarding. In this case, which of the following should be considered in the differential diagnosis?

    a. Appendicitis

    b. Ectopic pregnancy

    c. Tubo-ovarian abscess

    d. Pelvic inflammatory disease

    e. Gastroenteritis

    f. All of the above

21. Which of the following agents should be considered as the **initial** treatment of patients with an asthma flare?

    a. Oral steroids

    b. Intravenous steroids

    c. Inhaled beta-agonists

    d. None of the above

22. A 6-month-old male infant presents to the emergency department in respiratory distress. His parents report that he has been congested and coughing for the past day, but now he seems to be having problems breathing. His triage vital signs include fever of 101°F and a respiratory rate of 60 with a room air saturation of 90%. His physical exam is significant for supraclavicular and subcostal retractions and fine wheezes throughout the lung fields. The most likely diagnosis in this case is:

    a. Croup

    b. Pneumonia

    c. Bronchiolitis

    d. Congestive heart failure

23. The most likely organism responsible for this presentation is:

    a. *Streptococcus pneumoniae*

    b. *Chlamydia*

    c. Parainfluenza virus

    d. Respiratory syncytial virus

24. Steroids have been shown to be beneficial in the treatment of this condition: True or False.

25. Which of the following is not a characteristic of fulminant hepatic failure?

    a. Hepatic encephalopathy

    b. Elevated bilirubin

    c. Coagulopathy

    d. Cerebral edema

26. Upper gastrointestinal bleeding refers to bleeding that occurs proximal to the:

    a. Hepatic flexure

    b. Splenic flexure

    c. Ligament of Treitz

    d. Ileocecal valve

27. A 42-year-old male with a history of substance abuse presents to the emergency department unresponsive. Initial vital signs include a heart rate of 110, blood pressure of 142/75, respiratory rate of 26, and temperature of 97.8°F. Initial blood glucose is 99. Which of the following conditions is **least** likely the cause of this presentation?

    a. Methanol intoxication

    b. Diabetic ketoacidosis

    c. Ethanol intoxication

    d. Ethylene glycol intoxication

28. Initial laboratory evaluation reveals an anion gap metabolic acidosis. Which of the following would help to distinguish between ingestions of methanol and ethylene glycol?

    a. An osmolal gap

    b. An elevated creatinine

    c. Urinary fluorescence under Wood's lamp

    d. None of the above

29. Treatment of methanol and ethylene glycol poisoning involves antagonism of alcohol dehydrogenase with which substance?

a. Fomepizole

b. Ethanol

c. Both

d. Neither

30. An 85-year-old female presents to the emergency department complaining of the acute onset of severe abdominal pain. She has a past medical history notable for atrial fibrillation and was taking warfarin up until 4 days ago when she stopped it in preparation for cataract surgery. She is also taking digoxin to control her heart rate. On exam, she is afebrile, mildly tachycardic, and in obvious distress. Her abdomen is soft and diffusely tender without evidence of generalized peritonitis. The most likely diagnosis is:

a. Mesenteric ischemia

b. Appendicitis

c. Diverticulitis

d. None of the above

31. An 18-year-old male presents to the emergency department obtunded with a fever of 103°F. He is a college freshman and was found by his roommates with a markedly elevated level of consciousness. For the three days prior to presentation, he had been complaining of upper respiratory symptoms of cough, congestion, and mild headache. Which would be the most likely diagnosis in this case?

a. Bacterial meningitis

b. Subarachnoid hemorrhage

c. Stroke

d. Heroin overdose

32. Of the following etiologic agents, which should be considered as the most likely cause in this case?

a. *Neisseria meningitidis*

b. *Cryptococcus neoformans*

c. *Listeria monocytogenes*

d. *Haemophilus influenzae*

33. Viral and bacterial meningitis can be distinguished by history and physical alone: True or False.

34. The recommended empiric antibiotic coverage in this case would be:

a. Vancomycin

b. Ampicillin

c. Vancomycin and ceftriaxone

d. Penicillin G

35. Toxic shock syndrome is caused by a toxin produced by which organism?

a. *E. coli*

b. *Pseudomonas aeruginosa*

c. *Streptococcus pyogenes*

d. *Staphylococcus aureus*

36. Which of the following conditions is not transmitted by a tick?

a. Rocky Mountain spotted fever

b. Tularemia

c. Lyme disease

d. Malaria

37. Risk factors for the development of tuberculosis include which of the following:

a. Age (higher risk in infants and the elderly)

b. Close contact with a person known to have TB

c. HIV infection

d. Residing in a nursing home

e. All of the above

38. A tall, thin 25-year-old male presents to the emergency department complaining of severe, pleuritic chest pain, shortness of breath, and lightheadedness. His triage blood pressure is 75/45 with a pulse of 135. The most likely diagnosis in this case is:

a. Pneumothorax

b. Tension pneumothorax

c. Myocardial infarction

d. Pulmonary embolism

39. The first step in management is:

a. Obtain a chest radiograph to document a pneumothorax

b. Immediate needle decompression of the affected hemithorax

c. Tube thoracostomy

d. Administer thrombolytics

40. Which of the following are risk factors for the development of spontaneous pneumothoraces?

a. Smoking

b. History of prior pneumothoraces

c. Tuberculosis

d. All of the above

41. A 65-year-old man presents to you with spontaneous epistaxis of 30 minutes' duration. What is the most likely source of the hemorrhage?

a. Arterial from the anterior nasopharynx

b. Venous from the anterior nasopharynx

c. Arterial from the posterior nasopharynx

d. Venous from the posterior nasopharynx

42. A 55-year-old woman presents to the emergency department complaining of blurry vision in her left eye and a headache. Upon examination of her eyes, you notice that her right eye is normal, but her left eye is tearing, has a midway dilated pupil, an injected conjunctiva, and a "steamy"-appearing cornea. This constellation of symptoms is most consistent with which diagnosis?

a. Conjunctivitis

b. Migraine

c. Orbital hemorrhage

d. Acute angle closure glaucoma

43. A 60-year-old man with atrial fibrillation presents with acute, painless vision loss in his right eye. On funduscopic exam, you notice a "cherry red spot" on his retina. Initial therapy should consist of which of the following?

a. Massage of the eye globe

b. Intravenous thrombolytic therapy

c. Prednisolone eyedrops

d. Intravenous saline

44. A 40-year-old man with recurrent sinusitis presents with 4 days of progressively worsening red, swollen, warm skin overlying his left lower eyelid and cheek. His left conjunctiva is slightly injected, but he states that he has been rubbing his left eye. He has no pain with eye movement. His intraocular pressure is 11 mmHg. His presentation is most consistent with which diagnosis?

a. Orbital cellulitis

b. Periorbital cellulitis

c. Glaucoma

d. Sinusitis

45. A 75-year-old man with atrial fibrillation presents via ambulance with a left facial droop, left-sided weakness (greatest in his left arm), and left-sided sensory deficits. Which branch of his cerebral circulation is most likely affected?

a. Right anterior cerebral artery

b. Right middle cerebral artery

c. Left anterior cerebral artery

d. Left middle cerebral artery

46. If intravenous thrombolytics are to be considered, his symptoms should have definitively been present no longer than:

a. 30 minutes

b. 3 hours

c. 12 hours

d. 24 hours

47. Which of the following diseases most often present with a headache?

a. Ménière's disease

b. Benign positional vertigo

c. Ischemic stroke

d. Temporal arteritis

48. A 30-year-old epileptic woman presents to the emergency department via ambulance with continuous generalized seizure activity that has lasted for 15 minutes. Which of the following is a complication of prolonged seizure activity?

    a. Myocardial infarction
    b. Malignant hyperthermia
    c. Rhabdomyolysis
    d. Hypoglycemia

49. After how many minutes of continued, generalized seizure activity may irreversible neurologic damage occur?

    a. 15–30 minutes
    b. 30–60 minutes
    c. 2–3 hours
    d. 3–5 hours

50. Which medication acts the fastest to terminate seizure activity in the brain?

    a. Dilantin
    b. Lorazepam
    c. Valproic acid
    d. Succinylcholine

51. A 74-year-old man presents to the emergency department with a headache and vertigo that has slowly worsened over the last 4 hours and is not improved by remaining still. On physical examination, you notice that his nystagmus has an upward fast beat component. Which diagnosis is most consistent with his presentation?

    a. Benign positional vertigo
    b. Brainstem hemorrhage
    c. Posterior cerebral artery ischemic stroke
    d. Viral labyrinthitis

52. A 55-year-old woman presents with vertigo that began suddenly, is worse with movement, and completely resolves when she remains still for 30 seconds. What is most likely the cause of her vertigo?

    a. Transient ischemic attack
    b. Viral infection of the semicircular canals
    c. Infarction within the semicircular canals
    d. A free-floating otolith within the semicircular canals

53. A 40-year-old man is brought to the emergency department by ambulance with 3 days of progressively worsening, ascending weakness in both of his legs and difficulty "getting a full breath of air." His past medical history is remarkable for intravenous heroin abuse that he reportedly quit 5 years ago. On physical examination, his lower extremity reflexes are absent. What is the most likely cause of his weakness?

    a. Epidural abscess
    b. Myasthenia gravis
    c. Guillain-Barré syndrome
    d. Multiple sclerosis

54. A 45-year-old electrician was witnessed to fall to the ground in cardiac arrest after he was exposed to a 300 volt AC electrical current. Which of the following cardiac rhythms are the paramedics most likely to find when they quickly arrive at the scene?

    a. Ventricular fibrillation
    b. Ventricular tachycardia
    c. Asystole
    d. Third-degree heart block

55. Which of the following choices lists the different tissue types from most resistant to electrical current to the least resistant?

    a. Fat, tendon, skin, muscle, blood, nerve
    b. Nerve, fat, muscle, tendon, skin, blood
    c. Blood, muscle, skin, tendon, fat, nerve
    d. Nerve, blood, muscle, tendon, blood, fat

56. A 19-year-old football player is brought to your emergency department by paramedics after he collapsed on the field at the end of a 4-hour practice on a hot summer day. On examination, you find a large, obtunded male with a body temperature of 106°F, heart rate of 126, blood pressure of 130/70,

respiratory rate of 18, oxygen saturation of 100% on room air, and flushed, dry skin. Which of the following is the initial therapy of choice?

a.   Acetaminophen suppository

b.   Aggressive intravenous saline rehydration

c.   Cold packs placed in the armpits and groin

d.   Body immersion in a tank of cold water

57.   A 19-year-old male is brought to your emergency department by paramedics after being struck on his left side by a car traveling 30 mph as he was walking across the street. His vital signs reveal a heart rate of 130 bpm, blood pressure of 90/65, respiratory rate of 40, and a blood oxygen saturation of 93%. On examination, he is alert and oriented, with chest wall tenderness and decreased breath sounds on the left. What should happen next?

a.   Endotracheal intubation

b.   Left tube thoracostomy

c.   Diagnostic peritoneal lavage

d.   CT scan of the chest and abdomen

58.   A 24-year-old male presents to the emergency department 30 minutes after being stabbed with a knife in his middle abdomen. He is alert and oriented with normal vital signs. Further examination is remarkable for the protrusion of 10 cm of small intestine from a 3 cm laceration located just above his umbilicus. Which of the following should happen next?

a.   Focused abdominal ultrasound

b.   CT scan of the abdomen

c.   Diagnostic peritoneal lavage

d.   Transport to the operating room

59.   A 20-year-old woman presents to your emergency department 10 minutes after being shot with a handgun in her left upper chest just below her clavicle. She is alert and oriented with a heart rate of 110 bpm, respiratory rate of 30, and blood oxygen saturation of 94%. Further examination reveals an expanding hematoma over the left clavicle and neck, and decreased breath sounds over the left chest. Which of the following should happen next?

a.   Left tube thoracostomy

b.   Immediate portable chest x-ray

c.   Endotracheal intubation

d.   Emergent thoracotomy

60.   A 40-year-old man is accidentally struck in the head with a baseball bat as he walks by a baseball player practicing his swing. After initially losing consciousness for 2 minutes, he wakes up, states that he is fine, walks over to his car, sits in the driver's seat, and loses consciousness again. Ten minutes later, he is still unresponsive. Which diagnosis is most consistent with his presentation?

a.   Subarachnoid hemorrhage

b.   Subdural hematoma

c.   Epidural hematoma

d.   Diffuse axonal injury

61.   An 8-year-old boy is carried into your emergency department by his father after "badly spraining his ankle" while running around the house. His physical examination is remarkable for moderate to severe swelling and tenderness over the anterior and lateral aspects of his right ankle. Plain film imaging of his right ankle is normal. What is the next best step?

a.   Discharge the patient with a "sprained ankle" instruction sheet

b.   Admit the patient to the hospital for observation

c.   Immobilize the right ankle in a splint, instruct the patient to be non-weight bearing on his right foot, and arrange outpatient orthopedic follow-up for the concern of a growth plate injury

d.   Obtain "stress views" of the ankle mortise on x-ray to rule out an unstable ligamentous injury

62.   A 64-year-old woman on digoxin for congestive heart failure and atrial fibrillation presents to the emergency department complaining of weakness, nausea, new palpitations, and a yellowing of her vision. Her vital signs are normal. An ECG

reveals atrial fibrillation at 60 beats per minute with frequent premature ventricular contractions. Which of the following is an indication for digoxin-specific antibodies in the setting of digoxin toxicity?

a. Atrial fibrillation

b. A digoxin level 2 ng/L

c. A potassium level greater than 5 meq/L

d. Premature ventricular contractions

63. The woman's cardiac rhythm changes from atrial fibrillation to ventricular tachycardia in front of your eyes on the monitor. Her symptoms and physical examination otherwise remain unchanged. Which medication is a reasonable choice to treat her stable ventricular tachycardia?

a. Procainamide

b. Quinidine

a. Phenytoin

d. Calcium chloride

Answers

1. c (chapter 23)

A pulsatile abdominal mass is the classic finding on physical exam of a ruptured AAA. Patients may present with hypotension but they also can be hemodynamically stable initially. Patients with diverticulitis typically present with left lower quadrant pain, nausea, and low-grade fever and are often hemodynamically stable. Patients with GI hemorrhage typically present with bloody or melanotic stool that is usually painless. Patients having an acute myocardial infarction can present with abdominal pain and hypotension. Thus, an ECG should be obtained to rule out cardiac causes.

2. b (chapter 23)

An ultrasound is the ideal test, especially in unstable patients, as it is extremely accurate for making the diagnosis of an AAA and measuring its diameter. However, it is not as sensitive in determining whether an AAA has ruptured. Prompt surgical consultation should be obtained. For stable patients, an abdominal CT will demonstrate both aneurysmal size and site of rupture, either intraperitoneal or retroperitoneal. A plain abdominal radiograph may show an arch of calcification of the aortic wall or paravertebral soft tissue mass but is least helpful. An MRI is not an ideal test as it can take several hours to obtain and is often not emergently available.

3. a (chapter 22)

Most cases of aortic dissection occur between the ages of 50 and 70. However, they can present in younger age groups with certain predisposing conditions, for example, Marfan's syndrome. A classic physical exam finding includes unequal blood pressures. A diastolic murmur of aortic insufficiency can occur when the dissection involves the aortic valve. Young patients, especially with a history of cocaine use or strong family history of early death, can present with acute MI. Thus, an ECG should be immediately obtained in all patients who present with chest pain. However, it is not typically associated with blood pressure differential. Pulmonary embolism typically presents with sudden onset of pleuritic CP and patients are often hypoxic and tachycardic with equal blood pressure. Acute pericarditis patients typically have pleuritic CP that is relieved by sitting forward and associated with a recent viral upper respiratory infection.

4. b (part III)

The rhythm strip shows ventricular fibrillation (VF). The first intervention is to defibrillate with 200 J. If the patient is still in VF arrest, then defibrillate at 300 J, 360 J, and follow the ACLS protocol for VF arrest. Intubation, IV access, or drug treatment should not delay the life-saving potential of early defibrillation. Adenosine is not part of the ACLS protocol for VF arrest. Thrombolytics are not the first-line intervention for VF arrest.

5. b (chapter 17)

An ECG should be the first test obtained in patients with risk factors for coronary artery disease. An acute MI can mimic GI symptoms. A right upper quadrant ultrasound is helpful when cholecystitis or gallbladder disease is suspected. A CXR will be helpful to rule out other causes of chest discomfort but should not be the first test ordered. A KUB and upright would not be beneficial in this case.

6. d (chapter 26)

Treatment of pulmonary embolus (PE) should be initiated once the diagnosis is confirmed. Begin treatment with either IV unfractionated heparin or low molecular weight heparin (LMWH). IV antibiotics are used to treat pneumonia not PE. Indomethacin would be used to treat pericarditis. Unstable patients with PE who are in shock or significant respiratory distress should be assessed for thrombolytic therapy with urokinase, streptokinase, or recombinant tissue plasminogen activator. Greenfield filters should be used for patients who have contraindications for anticoagulation or with recurrent PE despite therapeutic anticoagulation.

7. b (part III)

Patients who have unstable angina or new-onset angina need to be admitted to a CCU or monitored bed and ruled out for myocardial infarction by serial enzymes. These patients should also receive IV heparin and beta-blockers. A nitroglycerin IV drip may be needed to control their pain. Patients with unstable angina need to be admitted to the hospital as unstable angina has a higher chance of progressing to an acute myocardial infarct. Thrombolytics are not indicated in this patient. Maalox and H_2 blockers are used to treat reflux disease, not unstable angina.

8. d (chapter 24)

Patients with idiopathic, viral, rheumatologic, and post-traumatic pericarditis are usually treated with non-steroidal anti-inflammatory drugs (i.e., aspirin, ibuprofen, or indomethacin).

9. b (part VI)

This is a classic presentation of kidney stones. Patients with acute pyelonephritis are febrile with bacteria and WBC in the urinalysis. Patients with musculoskeletal back spasm typically present with a history of trauma or back strain while lifting a heavy object prior to onset of pain. They also have a normal urinalysis. Testicular torsion involves acute onset of severe testicular pain, radiating to groin or abdomen, associated with nausea or vomiting. On physical exam there is a high riding, horizontally lying testis.

10. b (chapter 43)

An ectopic pregnancy should be considered in all women of childbearing age. Thus, a beta-hCG should be the first test ordered. Urinalysis, CBC, type, and screen are part of the workup for vaginal bleeding, but the most important thing is to determine if the patient is pregnant.

11. c (chapter 77)

This patient has hyperkalemia and needs emergent hemodialysis. Treatment in the emergency department should begin with calcium gluconate or calcium chloride for cardiac membrane stabilization. Answers a, b, and d are all part of the treatment for symptomatic hyperkalemia and should be given in the following order. Give insulin and glucose to shift potassium into cells. In addition, albuterol nebulizer and sodium bicarbonate can also be used to shift potassium into cells. Then consider furosemide and Kayexalate to remove potassium from the body.

12. b (chapter 76)

Hyperosmolar hyperglycemic nonketonic coma (HHNC) is defined as a plasma glucose greater than 600 mg/dL and a plasma osmolarity greater than 350 mOsm/kg in the absence of ketoacidosis in patients with a decreased level of consciousness. Certain medications, including beta-blockers, dilantin, corticosteroids, and thiazide diuretics, have been implicated in the development of HHNC. A stroke needs to be considered in the differential diagnosis. However, with an abnormally high glucose to explain the mental status changes, stroke is lower on the differential. Diabetic ketoacidosis again is part of the differential but it typically occurs in patients with a history of type I diabetics and the presence of ketosis. The hyponatremia can be explained by the high glucose. For each 100 mg/dL increase in plasma glucose concentration (above 100 mg/dL), plasma sodium concentration will decrease by 1.6 mEq/L.

13. b (chapter 76)

The average fluid deficit for patients with HHNC is between 9 and 12 L. Begin fluid resuscitation with normal saline. Replete electrolyte abnormalities as needed. Insulin is typically reserved for patients who are acidotic, hyperkalemic, or in renal failure since usually fluid alone resolves the hyperglycemia. Naloxone is typically given to patients who present with mental status changes due to opiate overdose. On exam they usually have pinpoint pupils and respiratory depression. Thrombolytics are used for patients who present with large acute strokes. These patients often present with hemiparesis or other focal neurologic signs.

14. c (chapter 86)

The mainstay of treatment for acetaminophen poisoning is the administration of the antidote N-acetylcysteine (NAC). NAC, a glutathione precursor, works by replenishing glutathione stores and inhibiting the binding of toxic metabolites to hepatic proteins. Naloxone is used for opiate overdose. Sodium bicarbonate is used for tricyclic overdoses. Flumazenil may be used with caution for pure acute benzodiazepine overdose, but should not be used if chronic benzodiazepine use is a possibility, as acute benzodiazepine withdrawal, including seizures, may be precipitated.

15. a (chapter 83)

Patients with systemic signs of anaphylaxis, including those with airway involvement, should receive epinephrine. All patients with significant allergic reactions should receive corticosteroids to prevent late-phase reactions.

Patients should also receive antihistamines—both H_1 and H_2 blockers—including diphenhydramine (Benadryl) and ranitidine (Zantac). Patients with persistent bronchospasm can be treated with beta-agonists (e.g., albuterol).

16. b (chapter 38)

Escherichia coli accounts for approximately 80 to 90% of all urinary tract infections. *Clostridium perfringens* causes cellulites. *Streptococcus pyogenes* causes skin infections and abscesses. *Chlamydia trachomatis* causes conjunctivitis, urethritis, cervicitis, and pelvic inflammatory disease.

17. b (chapter 37)

Acute cholecystitis presents similar to biliary colic but the pain is usually more severe and lasts longer than 6 hours. Patients with acute cholecystitis typically have elevated white counts, liver functions, and bilirubin. Patients with biliary colic usually have normal laboratory studies and their pain typically resolves in less than 6 hours. They can have RUQ tenderness during the acute episode. Patients with acute pancreatitis can present with RUQ pain radiating to the back but will have elevated amylase and lipase. Patients with ascending cholangitis present with fever or chills, jaundice, and RUQ pain (i.e., Charcot triad).

18. b (chapter 37)

Patients with acute cholecystitis require prompt surgical consultation. These patients should receive broad-spectrum antibiotics. Definitive treatment of acute cholecystitis is an urgent cholecystectomy usually within 24 to 72 hours. Patients with biliary colic can be discharged home, with close follow-up, if their pain has completely resolved and they can maintain oral hydration. However, this patient has acute cholecystitis. Patients with acute cholecystitis need broad-spectrum antibiotics. NG tube placement, IV fluids, NPO, and observation would be the treatment for acute pancreatitis. A right upper quadrant ultrasound is the diagnostic study of choice. Thus, no further imaging study is necessary to make the diagnosis.

19. b (part VII)

The diagnosis of placenta previa can be made by ultrasound with 95% accuracy. A vaginal exam should not be performed in the emergency department until an ultrasound can be obtained to rule out placenta previa as a digital exam could trigger a hemorrhage. This patient is hemodynamically stable and there is no indication at this time for emergent transfusion. Recall that during pregnancy the plasma volume increases by 50% and the red blood cell volume increases by only 20–30% causing a decrease in hematocrit. Unstoppable labor, fetal distress, and life-threatening hemorrhage are indications for immediate cesarean delivery. However, there is no indication at this time.

20. f (parts V and VII)

In females of reproductive age, appendicitis, ectopic pregnancy, tubo-ovarian abscess, pelvic inflammatory disease, and gastroenteritis should all be considered in the differential of right lower quadrant abdominal pain. Patients in this age group should be considered to be pregnant until proven otherwise, and a complete physical examination including pelvic and rectal examination should be performed as part of the evaluation. In the non-pregnant patient, CT scanning provides important information in cases that are diagnostically ambiguous.

21. c (chapter 29)

Inhaled beta-agonists are the cornerstone of therapy of an acute exacerbation of asthma. Substances such as albuterol should be used liberally and act in minutes to dilate the airways. Steroids are essential to the long-term management of an asthma flare as well, but their effect is delayed 6–8 hours. Steroids, whether oral or parenteral, treat the underlying inflammatory process responsible for the exacerbation.

22. c (chapter 100)

23. d (chapter 100)

24. False (chapter 100)

Bronchiolitis is a disease of the lower respiratory tract caused predominantly by the respiratory syncytial virus that classically affects infants in the first year of life. Treatment is supportive and involves liberal use of inhaled beta-agonists and racemic epinephrine. Steroids have not been shown to be effective in the treatment of bronchiolitis. Croup is an upper respiratory tract disease characterized by stridor and upper airway obstruction and a characteristic bark-like cough. It affects a slightly older age group (6 months to 4 years). Racemic epinephrine and steroids are used in the treatment of croup.

25. b (chapter 34)

Fulminant hepatic failure (FHF) is a clinical syndrome characterized by cerebral edema, hepatic encephalopathy, coagulopathy, infection, and acute renal failure. Although an elevated bilirubin is typically found in cases of FHF, it is neither required nor specific to the condition. FHF is typically caused by infection with the hepatitis B or C viruses. It is one of the leading causes of liver failure leading to transplantation.

26. c (chapter 31)

Common causes of upper gastrointestinal bleeding include esophageal varices, peptic ulcers, and duodenal ulcers. Lower gastrointestinal bleeding is most commonly caused by diverticulosis, arteriovenous malformations, hemorrhoids, or colon cancer.

27. b (chapter 75)

28. c (chapter 75)

29. c (chapter 75)

The patient in question presented with markedly altered level of consciousness, tachypnea, and tachycardia. Although methanol, diabetic ketoacidosis (DKA), ethanol, and ethylene glycol intoxication are all on the differential in patients presenting obtunded to the emergency department, a normal blood glucose level all but eliminates DKA as a possibility. Methanol intoxication is characterized by an elevated anion gap metabolic acidosis and osmolal gap. Formic acid is the toxic metabolite and typically affects the kidneys and eyes (snowstorm vision). Ethylene glycol also causes a gap acidosis and renal failure. The toxic metabolite responsible for the kidney dysfunction in ethylene glycol poisoning is calcium oxalate. A Wood's lamp can be used to detect fluorescein (a common additive to ethylene glycol) in the urine. Both methanol and ethylene glycol act by competitively inhibiting alcohol dehydrogenase. Ethanol and fomepizole both can be used as antidotes.

30. a (chapter 36)

One of the major risk factors for the development of mesenteric ischemia is intracardiac thrombus formation in the setting of atrial fibrillation. Preexisting atherosclerotic vascular disease and the use of digoxin are also risk factors. Clinically, mesenteric ischemia is characterized by lactic acidosis and "pain out of proportion to the physical exam."

31. a (chapter 68)

32. a (chapter 68)

33. False (chapter 68)

34. c (chapter 68)

Meningitis is inflammation of the meninges of the brain. It can be caused by a host of agents including various bacteria, viruses, and fungi. It is characterized clinically by fever, headache, altered level of consciousness, and meningismus. Common etiologies include *Streptococcus pneumoniae*, *Neisseria meningitidis* (especially in college dormitories, army barracks, etc.), and *Listeria monocytogenes* (immunocompromise). The rate of *Haemophilus influenzae* meningitis has decreased markedly since the institution of routine vaccination of young children. Empiric treatment typically involves parenteral administration of vancomycin and ceftriaxone, with ampicillin added if *Listeria* is suspected.

35. d (chapter 65)

The cascade leading to sepsis is initiated by exotoxins that are made and released by an organism. Examples include the toxic shock syndrome toxin (TSST-1) produced by *Staphylococcus aureus* and toxin A by *Pseudomonas aeruginosa*. Organisms such as staphylococci (techoic acid) and *Streptococcus pneumoniae* (polysaccha-

ride capsule) each have an antigenic surface component that initiates the sepsis cascade. Gram-negative organisms, such as *Escherichia coli,* have a distinct endotoxin called lipopolysaccharide (LPS) that is a component of their cell membranes and is associated with the sepsis syndrome.

36. d (chapter 69)

Rocky Mountain spotted fever (RMSF), tularemia, and Lyme disease are all carried by ticks. RMSF is a rickettsial illness carried by the tick *Dermacentor andersoni* or *Dermacentor variabilis*. Tularemia is caused by a protozoan and carried by *Ixodes scapularis*. Lyme disease is caused by a spirochete and carried by *Ixodes scapularis*. Malaria is caused by a protozoan and is carried by the mosquito.

37. e (chapter 66)

Tuberculosis caused by infection with *Mycobacterium tuberculosis* is the leading infectious cause of death in the world. Risk factors for infection include extremes of age, close contact with a person known to have TB, HIV infection, residing in a nursing home, low socioeconomic status, and travel to endemic areas.

38. b (chapter 28)

39. b (chapter 28)

40. d (chapter 28)

Spontaneous pneumothoraces occur classically in tall, thin males and are characterized by pleuritic chest pain and shortness of breath. Hemodynamic instability (tachycardia, hypotension, elevated jugular venous distention) herald a tension pneumothorax, which is a potentially life-threatening condition that must be promptly treated with needle decompression followed by tube thoracostomy.

41. a (chapter 7)

Nearly all cases of epistaxis are arterial in origin and originate in the anterior nasopharynx in a region known as "Keisselbach's plexus."

42. d (chapter 14)

Acute angle closure glaucoma results from an outflow obstruction of aqueous humor from the anterior chamber of the eye. By definition, the measured intra-ocular pressure is above 20 mmHg. The physical examination of patients with acute angle closure glaucoma may reveal visual acuity deficits, conjunctival injection, a cloudy or steamy-appearing cornea, and a midway positioned or dilated pupil that is fixed or sluggish to react to light.

43. a (chapter 13)

The patient's symptoms are most consistent with non-compressive, central retinal artery occlusion likely resulting from an embolized clot of cardiac origin. Patients with noncompressive CRAO should initially be treated with global (i.e., eyeball) massage that attempts to dislodge the clot by applying digital pressure over the closed eye for 5-second intervals. Intra-arterial thrombolytic therapy may be warranted in certain cases, but global massage should be performed first in the hope of providing some retinal perfusion to severely ischemic retinal tissue.

44. b (chapter 10)

The patient's symptoms are most consistent with perior-bital cellulitis, which usually results from sinus infections and local skin trauma. Periorbital (preseptal) cellulitis does not enter the orbit (eye socket) and therefore is not typically associated with painful eye movement.

45. b (chapter 47)

The regions of the brain most responsible for the above symptoms are located in the more lateral aspects of the frontal and parietal lobes. These areas receive most of their blood supply via the right middle cerebral artery.

46. b (chapter 47)

To date, all studies evaluating the role of intravenous thrombolytics in acute stroke have shown a worse outcome if administered after 3 hours from symptom onset.

47. d (chapter 46)

Vascular inflammation is one cause of headache. Cerebral arteries significantly distal to the circle of Willis are not well innervated with pain receptors and therefore explain the absence of headache in most ischemic strokes. Headache is not typically associated with peripheral vertigo.

48. c (chapter 48)

As with intense exercise, muscle breakdown often accompanies convulsive seizure activity. Prolonged convulsive seizures may result in significant muscle breakdown and rhabdomyolysis.

49. b (chapter 48)

After 30 to 60 minutes of continuous seizure activity, irreversible neurologic injury may result from the rapid depletion of metabolic substrates and worsened by hypotension associated with autonomic instability.

50. b (chapter 48)

Lorazepam (Ativan) exerts its effects within approximately 1 minute. Phenytoin (Dilantin) takes approximately 20 minutes to reach therapeutic levels due to the long infusion time required and since phosphenytoin requires hepatic metabolism for activation. Valproic acid must be administered orally and requires time for intestinal absorption. Succinylcholine paralyzes muscles, thus suppressing the visual convulsions. However, it does not suppress seizure activity within the brain.

51. b (part VIII)

Headache is not typically associated with peripheral vertigo or ischemic stroke. Brainstem hemorrhage may result in headache and is one of the few possible causes of vertical nystagmus.

52. d (chapter 51)

The patient's symptoms are most consistent with benign positional vertigo, which results from a free-floating otolith that has broken free from its usual attachment within the semicircular canals. Although the other diagnoses may be associated with vertigo that is worsened with movement, resolution of symptoms by remaining still is not typical.

53. c (chapter 50)

Guillain-Barré syndrome is a demyelinating neurologic disease that usually manifests as absent lower extremity reflexes and ascending paralysis that may involve the diaphragm. A distant history of intravenous drug abuse does not increase the likelihood of newly developing an epidural abscess, which is typically associated with back pain.

54. a (chapter 97)

Ventricular fibrillation most frequently results from lower energy alternating current (AC) exposures, while asystole is more common following exposure to higher energy and direct current (DC).

55. a (chapter 97)

Injury severity is directly related to the type of current (i.e., alternating or direct), current intensity (i.e., amperage), current path, voltage, the duration of contact, and the resistance of tissues.

56. d (chapter 96)

Body immersion in cold water is the most effective means of rapidly lowering body temperature. Acetaminophen is only helpful as an antipyretic in cases such as infectious illness where the body's temperature set point in the hypothalamus has been reset.

57. b (chapter 60)

In evaluating a trauma patient, the most important systems are evaluated and treated first. In this scenario, the most likely diagnosis is a tension pneumothorax resulting from rib fractures. Tension pneumothorax is a clinical diagnosis that should be treated prior to obtaining radiologic confirmation. Since the patient is speaking normally

(airway), his tension pneumothorax should be treated next with needle or tube thoracostomy (breathing).

58. d (chapter 61)

Abdominal evisceration is an indication for laparotomy. Further abdominal investigation, if necessary, should occur in the operating room.

59. c (chapter 60)

In evaluating a trauma patient, the most important systems are evaluated and treated first. An expanding hematoma of the neck may rapidly obstruct the airway due to the significant swelling and soft tissue distortion. Delaying endotracheal intubation and airway protection may make future attempts impossible. The patient's likely left-sided pneumothorax (breathing) should be decompressed after endotracheal intubation.

60. c (chapter 57)

Epidural hematomas are associated with a lucid interval between periods of loss of consciousness following head trauma. The other diagnoses are not typically associated with a regaining of consciousness once loss of consciousness occurs.

61. c (chapter 63)

In children, the epiphyseal growth plate is generally weaker than the supporting ligaments and tendons, thereby placing children at greater risk for growth plate injuries.

62. c (chapter 94)

Hyperkalemia above 5 meq/L is associated with worse outcomes and is therefore one of the indications for digoxin-specific antibody (Digibind) therapy.

63. c (chapter 94)

Phenytoin and lidocaine are the antiarrhythmics of choice for treating ventricular dysrhythmias associated with digoxin toxicity.

Index

Urogenital emergencies, 113–122
Urticaria, 264
Uterine bleeding, 123–128. *See also*
    Vaginal bleeding
UTIs. *See* Urinary tract infections
Uveitis, 19

Vaginal bleeding, 123–129, 135–136
    causes of, 123–124, 126
        first-trimester, 127–129
        third-trimester, 135–136
    treatment of, 125, 128–129, 136
Vaginal discharge, 232–233
Valgus deformity, 195, 197
Vancomycin, 228
Varicella-zoster virus, 33, 215
Varus deformity, 195, 197
Vasculitis, 141–142, 313–314
Ventricular fibrillation, 42, 44
    treatment of, 44–46

Ventricular septal defect, 305–308
Ventricular tachycardia, 42, 44
    treatment of, 44–46
Vertigo, 153–155
    causes of, 137
    physical examination for, 153–
        154
    treatment of, 154–155
Vibrio, 225–226, 228
Virchow's triad, 60
Visual acuity, 19, 22. *See also* Eye
Vitamin A toxicity, 253
Vitamin B12 deficiency, 138
Vitamin D, deficiency of, 252
    toxicity of, 253–254
Vitreous humor, 32
    inflammation of, 19
Volvulus, 99–100
VSD. *See* Ventricular septal defect
VZV. *See* Varicella-zoster virus

Waterhouse-Friderichsen syndrome, 260
Waterson technique, 305
Wedge fracture, 180–181
Westermark's sign, 77
Willis, circle of, 144, 308
Wolff-Parkinson-White syndrome,
    42–43
    treatment of, 45
Woodruff's plexus, 15
Wound care, 192–194
WPW. *See* Wolff-Parkinson-White
    syndrome

Yaws, 233
Yersinia enterocolitica, 224–226, 228
Yolk sac remnant, 321

Ziehl-Neelson technique, 211
Zollinger-Ellison syndrome, 253
Zygoma fracture, 178

RE

RI   )06